RECONCEIVING MIDWIFERY

Reconceiving Midwifery

Edited by
Ivy Lynn Bourgeault
Cecilia Benoit
and
Robbie Davis-Floyd

McGill–Queen's University Press
Montreal & Kingston · London · Ithaca

© McGill-Queen's University Press 2004
ISBN 0-7735-2689-7 (cloth)
ISBN 0-7735-2690-0 (paper)

Legal deposit second quarter 2004
Bibliothèque nationale du Québec

Printed in Canada on acid-free paper that is 100% ancient forest free
(100% post-consumer recycled), processed chlorine free.

This book has been published with the help of a grant from the
Canadian Federation for the Humanities and Social Sciences, through
the Aid to Scholarly Publications Programme, using funds provided
by the Social Sciences and Humanities Research Council of Canada.

McGill-Queen's University Press acknowledges the support of the Canada
Council for the Arts for our publishing program. We also acknowledge the
financial support of the Government of Canada through the Book Publishing
Industry Development Program (BPIDP) for our publishing activities.

National Library of Canada Cataloguing in Publication

Reconceiving midwifery /
    edited by Ivy Lynn Bourgeault, Cecilia Benoit and Robbie Davis-Floyd.

Includes bibliographical references and index.
ISBN 0-7735-2689-7 (bnd)
ISBN 0-7735-2690-0 (pbk)

    1. Midwifery – Canada. 2. Midwifery – Canada – History.
I. Bourgeault, Ivy Lynn, 1967– II. Benoit, Cecilia, 1954– III. Davis-Floyd, Robbie

RG950.R42 2004   362.1'982'00971   C2003-906107-8

This book was typeset by Dynagram Inc. in 10/12 Sabon.

Contents

Acknowledgments

This collected work – albeit directed by the three of us as editors – is the result of the effort and energy of several individuals and agencies, some of whom we feel deserve special mention here.

First, we would like to acknowledge the financial support for this lengthy project from the Social Sciences and Humanities Federation of Canada through its Aid to Scholarly Publications Program and from the Social Sciences and Humanities Research Council of Canada through their Aid to Occasional Research Conferences fund. Additional funds for the completion of the project were also generously provided by the Department of Sociology and Faculty of Health Sciences at the University of Western Ontario, and by the Department of Sociology and Health Studies Programme at McMaster University through an arrangement of discretionary funds to Ivy Bourgeault as a result of her being awarded a Canadian Institutes for Health Research New Investigator Award.

We would also like to acknowledge all of the support we received from our contributors. This made our work as editors that much easier and more successful. We would particularly like to thank Margaret MacDonald for her added assistance in helping co-organize the 1999 conference in Toronto that enabled us to come together and present, discuss, and more fully integrate our separate pieces into this collaborative volume.

We would like to thank the anonymous reviewers for their helpful comments and advice on suggested revisions to improve the clarity and impact of our volume. We particularly appreciated their supportive comments on the collection we have put together.

Terri Tomchick also deserves a special mention for her patient and meticulous copy editing of the multi-formatted chapters she initially received into a uniformly formatted and organized manuscript. Without her, this book would still exist in pieces at the back of our filing cabinets.

We would like to thank Aurèle Parisien and the rest of the staff at McGill-Queen's University Press for all of their support and advice in helping us bring this project to completion. Our thanks also goes to Ruth Pincoe, who assisted in the indexing of this volume.

Finally, we would like to offer our sincerest gratitude to all the midwives, birthing women, and their supporters across our fine country who in many ways made this an extraordinary topic to research, write about, and publish.

Thanks to you all.

Foreword

This book tells the story of the midwifery renaissance that began in Canada during the 1970s and continues today: its chapters describe and analyse how Canadians came to "reconceive" midwives and midwifery and generate a new model of midwifery care, funding, and education – one that is unique in the Americas and rare in the world – and how that new model has integrated into the various provincial health care systems known collectively as medicare. To their credit, many of the book's contributors have been there from the beginning, documenting, describing, recording, analysing, and supporting the remarkable developments to date, and fully committed to promoting the benefits of the new Canadian midwifery into the future.

Back in 1997, when I was still unaware of the rich literature that already existed on Canadian developments in midwifery and maternity care, I had intended to carry out an independent study of "The Development of Direct-Entry Midwifery in North America," a rather grandiose title indicating my original intention to investigate midwifery in Canada, the U.S., and Mexico. When my first proposal was funded by the Wenner-Gren Foundation for Anthropological Research, I must admit that I panicked a bit about the scale of the proposed project. But this panic was quickly alleviated when I turned my attention toward Canada and discovered the many social scientists who had for some time been engaged in studying midwifery and the organization of maternity care in the Canadian context. It became obvious that my job was not to reinvent the wheel but rather to simply bring these Canadian researchers together on an academic panel in hopes of generating an edited book. In this endeavour I asked for help from my long-time colleague Patricia Kaufert to co-organize a panel called "The Development of Direct-Entry Midwifery in North America: Politics, Professionalization, and Change." The panel presented at the joint meetings held by the Society for Medical Anthropology (SMA) and the Society for Applied Anthropology (SfAA) in Seattle in 1997. Twelve out of the fourteen papers on that panel were given by Canadian social scientists on various aspects of what Ivy Bourgeault had been calling "the new Canadian midwifery" (the two exceptions were my own paper on American direct-entry midwifery and a paper by Raymond DeVries on midwifery in the Netherlands).

After the panel we held a group discussion on creating a co-edited collection. I said that I would prefer to have two Canadian social scientists as first editors, because of their greater familiarity with midwives and midwifery research in Canada and because it did not seem appropriate for an American to be first editor of a book about Canada. Pat Kaufert was unable to participate as an editor, and it quickly became apparent that the two most outstanding scholars on Canadian midwifery were Ivy Bourgeault, whose dissertation addressed the development of this "new midwifery" in Ontario, and Cecilia Benoit, who had published widely on midwifery in Newfoundland and had also carried out research comparing developments in Canadian midwifery with those of a number of other countries, including the U.S., Sweden, and Finland. With the consent of the other panel participants, the three of us proceeded as co-editors of this collection. In its design, selection of its contributors, as well as many of its underlying understandings, we are greatly indebted to midwife and social scientist Betty Anne Daviss, who generously shared with us her experience and expertise.

As word of the book's inception spread to the Canadian midwifery community, we editors began to receive expressions of concern from a number of midwives about how they would be represented by the social scientists writing for the collection and whether they would have a voice in those representations. In response, Ivy and Cecilia obtained funding from the Social Science and Humanities Research Council of Canada (SSHRC) to put on a conference in Toronto in July 1999 in preparation for the book. The conference was attended by approximately fifty people drawn from across the country, a felicitous mix of social scientists and midwives. Chapter authors presented what they intended to say, and attendees had plenty of opportunity to discuss each chapter and offer words of praise and, when deemed appropriate, suggestions for improvement. In other words, finding ourselves involved in the politics of representation, we created a model for collaboration between practitioners and the social scientists who study them. All of us sharcd a commitment to fostering midwifery in Canada and to producing the best possible book about it that we could. Everyone attended carefully to every presentation; the discussions were extremely productive; and the collaborative spirit has continued to characterize the development of this book.

At least in the case of the social science of midwifery, like attracts like: midwives are deeply committed to the care and well-being of mothers and babies, and so are the social scientists who study midwifery and birth. The authors in this volume make no pretense toward disengagement from their subjects; rather, they care about them passionately and try to make their research of practical value as well as of theoretical importance. The chapters in this book reflect that shared dedication. We are pleased with the results and hope that our readers are in agreement.

And here I must add a personal note. On 12 September 2000, my daughter, Peyton Floyd, was killed in an auto accident, four days before her twenty-first birthday. Up until that point, while Ivy and Cecilia had certainly led the editorial process, we had engaged in a good deal of collaboration with each other, meeting when we could and co-editing various chapters together. But after my daughter's death, I had to withdraw from work on this book and leave its final production to Ivy and Cecilia. They rose gallantly to the task, turning in an outstanding manuscript. But they did not stop with the professional. Wanting to do something to ease my pain, they turned their passionate commitment to the welfare of mothers toward me, a mother who had lost a child. On a day full of grief and pain, a large brown envelope with Ivy's return address on it arrived in the mail. Thinking it probably contained some chapters for the book, I was surprised to find that it felt squishy when I picked it up. I opened it carefully and found a gorgeous handmade quilt spread out in my hands. Its primary colours, chosen by Ivy (who conceived the quilt and created its overall design) are primarily ivory and burgundy, but many other colours are present, for each square was designed and decorated by an individual contributor to the book in honour of Peyton. And in the centre of the quilt, two ribbons tie together two sides of a burgundy heart. You open the heart, and discover inside a graphic of a dancer who looks much like Peyton did during the years she danced *en pointe*. It is the most incredible gift I have ever received. And it is a gift to you, the reader, as well, for the love, commitment, and understanding it encapsulates are also to be found in these pages.

Robbie Davis-Floyd
Austin, Texas, January 2002

RECONCEIVING MIDWIFERY

Reconceiving Midwifery in Canada

Ivy Lynn Bourgeault, Cecilia Benoit, and Robbie Davis-Floyd

Midwifery today is in a state of ferment and change. The phenomenon referred to as the *new midwifery* – which denotes a critical shift in thinking and action by midwives, birthing women, and sympathetic supporters in regard to the significance of midwifery for the health and well-being of mothers and infants – is emerging increasingly around the world (Burtch 1994; Bourgeault 1996, 2000; Bourgeault and Fynes 1996/97, 1997; Shroff 1997; Page and Percival 2000). Perhaps in no other country is this change in maternity care organization more apparent than in Canada.

Until the 1990s, Canada held the dubious distinction of being the only industrialized nation without formal provisions for midwifery practice. Then, between the mid to later years of that decade, midwifery was legalized and integrated into nearly half of its provincial jurisdictions: first in Ontario and subsequently in Quebec, British Columbia, Alberta, Manitoba, and Saskatchewan. In most other provinces and the territories, discussion is currently underway about whether midwifery should be integrated into existing maternity care services and, if so, in what manner. It is anticipated that most if not all of these other areas of the country will soon follow suit to legalize midwifery and integrate it into their respective health care systems. In doing so, midwives and their advocates in Canada are creating unique styles of midwifery practice inspired by both international models and local initiatives, some national in nature and others peculiar to provincial/territorial circumstances. Canadian midwives and their supporters are being watched with great interest. Both at home and abroad, midwives, social scientists, health policy analysts, health care advocates, childbearing women, and their partners are asking how this new conception of the midwifery profession has evolved, how it has become integrated into provincial health care systems that have until recently excluded midwifery care, and what integrating midwifery practice will do to help improve maternity care more broadly.

As with all service occupations, the new midwifery in Canada did not appear overnight nor in a national vacuum. Its development is a compilation of indigenous, provincial, national, and international influences at various levels – government, professional, and individual. Indigenous forms of midwifery existed amongst Aboriginal communities in Canada for thousands of years prior to contact. Aboriginal midwives provided much-needed services for early Canadian settlers. At the same time these settlers also brought with them their own ideas of how maternity care should be delivered. Once numbers warranted, these settlers began to more firmly establish systems of maternity care that reflected their country of origin as well as the practices found in their new homeland. In New France, for example, midwives were numerous and well organized prior to the English conquest. There were the *entretenues*, who were trained in Paris and paid by the king to serve in the colonies; the *maîtresses sages-femmes*, who were responsible for quality control; *jurés*, who were recognized as experts in the courts; and the local *sage-femme approuvée*, who was either chosen by the priest or elected by the women of the community (Laforce 1990). Along with the waves of other immigrant groups also came their systems of maternity care. Local forms of "neighbour" midwifery emerged in particular locations, especially where immigrant women had few options for other forms of care. Viewed from a different angle, however, for the most part the history of midwifery in Canada is a story of the demise of the midwife – however configured – or at best of the lack of her official recognition and the rise of medicalized childbirth.

The roots of the new midwifery that has emerged in Canada can be traced to these historical systems but emerge most directly from the efforts to keep midwifery alive – i.e., the nurse-midwifery movement – and from the efforts to reinvigorate alternatives to medicalized childbirth, which sparked a rebirth of lay midwifery. Nurse-midwifery practices in rural and remote areas of the country date back to the 1920s and 1930s with the establishment of nursing outposts by the Red Cross in Ontario and the efforts of the United Farm Women and United Farm Men of Alberta to lobby their government to supply midwives to remote areas of the province. These needs were originally met by British-trained midwives but in some cases local institutions responded with training programs. In Alberta, for example, a nurse-midwifery training program entitled "Advanced Practical Obstetrics Course for District Nurses" was established in Edmonton in 1944, the first of its kind in Canada (Hurlburt 1981). Other educational programs were developed in Halifax, Nova Scotia in 1967 for nurse practitioners and in St Johns, Newfoundland in 1978, boldly titled "Nurse-Midwifery" (for a discussion of an earlier course of instruction for Newfoundland midwives, see Benoit and Davis-Floyd, chapter 8). The establishment of these latter two programs reflected the development of nurse-midwifery practice opportunities in rural and remote Canada.

During the late 1950s and early 1960s, the federal agency, Health and Welfare Canada, established networks of nursing stations across the north and expanded nurse-midwifery services. Though not officially granted the title of "midwife," many of the nurses staffing these stations were British-trained nurse-midwives. Others were graduates from the newly developed Canadian schools or from the "Clinical Training for Northern Nurses" program established in six medical schools across Canada in 1969.

In a similar fashion, the philanthropic former International Grenfell Association (later renamed Grenfell Regional Health Services [GRHS]) located in western regions of Newfoundland and parts of Labrador relied heavily on the expertise of immigrant midwives to care for birthing women in these sparsely populated and medically underserviced regions. Similar to the Health and Welfare Canada midwives, the immigrant midwives hired by the GRHS were recruited from Britain, with a few from a small number of other countries. Likewise, most of the Canadian-born midwives employed by the GRHS received their formal midwifery training in Britain, though a small number also attended nurse-midwifery programs in the U.S. and some as far abroad as Australia. In fact, to this day the GRHS formally recruits nurse-midwives from abroad or Canadian midwives with formal midwifery training (which until recently was also typically attained abroad) to work on its maternity wards.

The positive contribution made by immigrant and native-born midwives to these regions is evident in the research conducted by Pat Kaufert and John O'Neil (1993) among Inuit women in the Keewatin region of northern Manitoba. They state, "[The midwife] was a positive figure when at the centre of the stories women told about their experiences of childbirth in the nursing stations, but midwives were also recalled as representatives of government, as authority figures. Despite this ambivalence, women complained bitterly about the disappearance of the midwife, seeing her as the key to the returning of birth to the community setting" (39–40). Indeed, "station" midwives' comprehensive knowledge of pregnancy and childbirth had proved very useful in separating birthing women at genuine medical risk who needed to be transported to southern urban hospitals from those who could deliver their babies in their own home communities. One Scottish-trained midwife recalls her initiation into a northern Ontario Native community:

The woman had only contractions when they called for me. She had several babies before and I had seen her at the nursing station. So when I arrived at her home I said: "Well, where do you want to have the baby?" I knew that they had cleaned a [seal] skin especially for her to have the baby on it. So I asked, "You got some skin?" "Oh yes, I got plenty of sealskin, clean and wiped." So I asked, "Where do you want to be, on the bed?" She said, "Well, no, I want to be on the floor." They used the floor to press against, you see. One of the other women sat behind her to give support … So, anyway, I ended up delivering the baby. Everything I did was all commented upon. I didn't know the dialect enough to really understand it all. But what I did was approved 'cause after that I got called for just about all deliveries.

Despite these positive outcomes, a change in Health and Welfare Canada policy in the late 1970s and early 1980s required all pregnant women residing in isolated and underpopulated northern areas of Canada to travel to urban hospitals located in the south, sometimes several weeks prior to their delivery date. This resulted in fewer opportunities for nurse-midwives to practise, as well as a decline in their confidence in handling uncomplicated births. These trends, accompanied by tighter immigration policies, led to an overall reduction in the number of nurse-midwives practising in rural and remote areas of Canada.

Despite this decline in practice opportunities for midwives located in outlying areas of the country, interest in the concept of nurse-midwifery in non-remote areas of the country began to peak (Hurlburt 1981). For example, Hays (1971) argued in an article in *The Canadian Nurse* that nurse-midwives could function effectively in urban as well as rural and remote settings. Several regional nurse-midwifery associations began to discuss the idea of promoting the integration of nurse-midwives as members of the obstetrical care team (Hurlburt 1981). In Ontario, a group of nurse-midwives presented a statement to their provincial association in 1973 outlining how they might be integrated into the mainstream maternity care system in Canada. A catalyst for these early efforts was the attendance of British-trained midwife May Toth at the International Confederation of Midwives (ICM) conference in Washington, D.C. the year prior. As most of the members of what became known as the Ontario Nurse-Midwives Association (ONMA) were British-trained, the preferred model of care was the British independent midwifery model. Concerns about political expediency, however, led them to pursue a less contentious and less independent American nurse-midwifery model where attendance at birth was limited to institutional settings. Nurse-midwives in B.C., Alberta, Saskatchewan, N.W.T., and the Yukon also adopted the Ontario statement and established the Western Nurse-Midwives Association. Subsequently, a Canadian National Committee on nurse-midwives was formed to nationally promote the nurse-midwifery concept.

These efforts were supported by the larger nursing profession through the Canadian Nurses' Association (CNA). In 1974 the CNA proposed its own statement on nurse-midwifery, recommending that nurse-midwives be recognized as "the health professional best equipped to met the growing needs for counselling services and for greater continuity of care within this area of the health system" (as cited in Hurlburt 1981, 31). In Ontario, the Registered Nurses Association of Ontario (RNAO) made an official statement prior to the CNA supporting the development of nurse-midwifery as a complementary element in the provincial maternity care system. The RNAO's statement followed the ONMA's efforts but also the recommendation of the government-appointed Committee on the Healing Arts (1970) to integrate nurse-midwifery into the health care system. The committee conceived integration as a potential strategy to address the perceived physician shortage and foster cost-effective maternity care. The RNAO subsequently proposed negotiations with the College of Nurses of Ontario, provincial medical organizations, and the Ontario government to draft enabling legislation. These negotiations, however, never came to fruition, due in large part to medical opposition or indifference.

Concurrent with these largely British-influenced developments in nurse-midwifery came a "rebirth" of lay midwifery stemming from the influx of ideas and advocates from the U.S. The idea of lay midwifery was most strongly promoted by the home birth and women's health movements. The cultural milieu of the late 1960s and early 1970s was marked by a general lessening of trust in professional authority, an unprecedented decline in respect for medicine, and a growing recognition of the emotional, social, and spiritual components of life and healing in particular (Barrington 1985; Rooks 1990). Many men and women became aware of different childbirth processes and began to question whether institutionalized birth should be the only option available (Hosford 1976). Many couples chose to redefine birth as a natural process that should take place at home without medical intervention and as a social or community occasion to take place in the company of friends (McCool and McCool 1989; Reid 1989). As Barrington noted, "The West Coast back-to-the-land movement of the 1960s promoted a self-sufficient daring that allowed a few committed idealists to take

birth into their own hands. Their premium on independence and ab-
horrence of institutional power structures suggested home birth even
when there was no doctor available. They began to go it alone" (1985,
32). This movement first occurred among counter-culture groups, but
soon spread to segments of mainstream society as well.

Emerging from the home birth movement were several small yet vocal childbirth groups formed by consumers and their midwives in the
U.S. and later in Canada. These groups challenged the necessity of
"routine" obstetrical practice and questioned the effectiveness and possible iatrogenic effects of intervention. Many instead pushed for "family-
centred" maternity care, which included childbirth education and assistance for home birth parents (Mathews and Zadak 1991; O'Connor
1993; Rooks 1990; Teasley 1983). A number of organized lobbies were
formed, including the Home Oriented Maternity Experience (HOME),
the Association of Childbirth at Home, International (ACHI), the National Association for Parents and Professionals for Safe Alternatives in
Childbirth (NAPSAC), and the International Childbirth Education Association (ICEA). Many of these largely U.S.-based groups had and continue to have Canadian members and Canadian chapters, including
NAPSAC Ontario, CAPSAC in Calgary, and APSAC in Edmonton and in
Nova Scotia (Barrington 1985). Other local groups also formed, such
as Naissance Renaissance in Quebec and Choices in Childbirth in Ontario. Mounting research evidence criticizing the supposed safety of
traditional obstetrical procedures and supporting changes in these
practices lent credibility to these groups (Sullivan and Weitz 1988).

An equally important source of support came from the broader international women's health movement. The primary focus of the women's
health movement, which emerged at a similar time as the home birth
movement, was for women to achieve greater control over their health
and reproductive care (Ruzek 1978). Members of the women's health
movement sought to change consciousness around health issues, struggled to change established health institutions, and organized to provide
health-related services to women (Fruchter et al. 1977). Advocates also
argued that care should be deinstitutionalized, deprofessionalized, and
put back into the hands of women. In line with these demands, several
grassroots women's health organizations developed promoting female
and lay control over health care services (Langton 1991; Ruzek 1978).

Women's health advocates were to a certain extent natural allies of
home birth advocates (Mathews and Zadak 1991). At issue for both
movements was women's control over their bodies and active role in
decision-making about their health care. Several books, which crossed
both movements, were published in the U.S. but read widely in Canada. These included Doris Haire's *The Cultural Warping of Childbirth*

(1972), Raven Lang's *The Birth Book* (1972), Suzanne Arms' *Immaculate Deception* (1975), Gena Corea's *The Hidden Malpractice* (1977), and Ina May Gaskin's *Spiritual Midwifery* (1977). These books all discussed the mistreatment of birthing women due to oppressive obstetrical practices and the viable option that midwifery entailed. The authors, however, did not necessarily agree on precisely where control ought to lie. Rothman (1981), for example, pointed out that traditionalist supporters of home birth who argue for "family involvement" do not challenge the idea of patriarchal control within the family, whereas feminist supporters argue against patriarchal control in favour of women's control over their lives. Nevertheless, the intermingling of both movements served to create fertile ground for the re-emergence of lay midwifery as a means for women and their families to achieve greater control over the birth process.

Lay midwifery in Canada developed out of this juxtaposition of ideas promulgated by the home birth and women's health movements. In the "back-to-the-land" movement, the reappearance of neighbour helping neighbour during birth was a natural part of this new attempt to live in more self-sufficient ways (Edwards and Waldorf 1984). Midwifery also came to typify the struggle of the women's movement. Canadian feminist Mary O'Brien, for example, asserted that "Midwifery is integral to the women's movement. Its revival is a triumphant affirmation of women's right to choose" (cited in Barrington 1984, 7). In both cases, the influx of ideas and advocates from the U.S. was particularly influential, although other commentators, such as Sheila Kitzinger and Ann Oakley from Britain, also had a strong impact.

Canadian midwifery originated on the west coast in the early 1970s in large part because it was the counter-culture centre of Canada. One of the main U.S. influences on west coast midwifery was a midwife from Santa Cruz, California, Raven Lang. In 1972, the same year that her *Birth Book* was published, Lang was invited to help establish a medical program providing care for residents in the B.C. interior (Edwards and Waldorf 1984). There she met Cheryl Anderson, lay midwife-to-be. Anderson had worked at the Vancouver Free Childbirth Education Centre, which had opened one year earlier. Funded by the federal government to provide free prenatal education to transient youths on the west coast, the centre marked the first organized attempt in Canada to meet the needs of a growing population that was opting out of the formal maternity care system by giving birth at home (Barrington 1985). When Lang returned home to California after this short placement in B.C., Anderson went with her to learn more about midwifery. The following year, Anderson, with the help of Lang and others, founded the Vancouver Birth Centre (Barrington 1985; Edwards and

Waldorf 1984). Activities at the birth centre included workshops, conferences, and midwifery classes for the growing number of apprentices.
Lang also helped foster lay midwifery on Vancouver Island when she
moved there in 1974. Throughout the 1970s and 1980s, other communities of lay midwives became established across Canada.

Thus, midwifery in Canada today can be traced back to pre-colonial
Aboriginal birthing systems in the first instance, which were in colonial
times influenced by and combined with midwifery practices carried to
this country by various waves of immigrants from, initially, France and
Britain and then from other countries in Europe and the Far East. As
we moved to the twentieth century, the influence of Britain loomed
largest in the developments of nurse-midwifery, though Canadian-
developed educational programs were also instrumental in helping address the needs of rural and remote populations. The arrival of new
ideas and influential individuals from the U.S., sparking a rebirth of lay
midwifery, later overshadowed the British influence. Eventually, other
models were also to have an impact on the reshaping of midwifery in
Canada – the Dutch model in particular – as Canadian midwives
searched abroad for further inspiration in how to shape their practices.
By the mid-1990s, Canadian-made midwifery models began to emerge
and receive legitimacy in the eyes of government officials and members
of the larger public. As will become evident in the following chapters,
these emerging models of midwifery care are complex blends of indigenous, local, provincial, national, and international models of how best
to provide maternity care for Canadian childbearing women. It is because of this turn of events that the eyes of the international midwifery
community are now on Canada. The new Canadian midwifery is now
the source of ideas and inspiration about how to improve maternity
care in other locations.

It is at this nexus where many of the papers in this book begin. Collectively, the book addresses how midwifery has been reconceived
across Canada to produce unique models of integration, education,
and practice, with all of their provincial and territorial variations. *Reconceiving Midwifery* is designed to provide a systematic account of
the local, historical, and cultural roots of the profession, its evolving
regulatory status, the degree of integration into the mainstream health
care system, the nature of midwifery training and its accessibility across
ethnic and socio-economic groups, while at the same time reflecting on
regional differences. The chapters present an assortment of perspectives
with authors from the social and health sciences, from midwifery, and
from health care activist communities (in fact some authors fit all criteria). Each author, regardless of background, engages in a critical and
reflective analysis of midwifery's development and integration in the

Canadian context. Together the chapters highlight the key issues of power, identity, and social change facing the profession before, during, and immediately following integration.

The volume is organized thematically into four broad sections. The first part situates Canadian midwifery in a historical and cultural context. Part II addresses the key issues of legislation and integration and their challenges across the country. In Part III, the authors reflect upon the models of education and training of midwives within the Canadian context. The consequences of integration for equity and accessibility are discussed in Part IV. The volume concludes by highlighting how the collection as a whole moves the discourse on the new midwifery in Canada to a higher plane of social science analysis. At the same time, the editors note the gaps in research on midwifery that warrant further investigation. As such, the book represents a snapshot in a continuing dialogue – by social scientists and also by midwives themselves – about the shaping and reconceiving of midwifery in Canada, a female-dominated profession that is both very old and yet still so very new in this country.

REFERENCES

Arms, Suzanne. 1975. *Immaculate Deception: A New Look at Women and Childbirth in America*. San Francisco: San Francisco Book Company.
Barrington, Eleanor. 1984. *The Legalization of Midwifery in Canada*. National Action Committee on the Status of Women.
– 1985. *Midwifery is Catching*. Toronto: NC Press.
Benoit, Cecilia. 1989a. Traditional Midwifery Practice: The Limits of Occupational Autonomy. *The Canadian Review of Sociology and Anthropology* 26, no. 4: 633–49.
– 1989b. The Professional Socialization of Midwives: Balancing Art and Science. *Sociology of Health and Illness* 11, no. 2: 160–80.
– 1991. *Midwives in Passage*. St John's, Nfld.: Institute of Social and Economic Research.
– 1994. Paradigm Conflict in the Sociology of the Professions. *Canadian Journal of Sociology* 19, no. 3: 303–29.
– 1996/97. Midwifery in Canada and Sweden: A Cross-National Comparison. *Health and Canadian Society/Santé et Société Canadienne* 4, no. 2: 195–224.
– 1997. Professionalising Canadian Midwifery: Sociological Perspectives. In *The New Midwifery: Reflections on Renaissance and Regulation*, edited by Farah Shroff, 93–114. Toronto: The Women's Press.
Benoit, Cecilia, and Alena Heitlinger. 1998. Women's Health Caring Work in Comparative Perspective: Canada, Sweden and Czechoslovakia/Czech Republic as Case Examples. *Social Science and Medicine* 47, no. 8: 1101–11.

Bourgeault, Ivy. 1996. Delivering Midwifery: An Examination of the Process and Outcome of the Incorporation of Midwifery in Ontario. Ph.D. dissertation, University of Toronto.

– 2000. Delivering the "New" Canadian Midwifery: The Impact on Midwifery of Integration into the Ontario Health Care System. *Sociology of Health and Illness* 23 no. 5: 633–53.

Bourgeault, Ivy, and Mary Fynes. 1996/97. Delivering Midwifery in Ontario: How and Why Midwifery was Integrated into the Provincial Health Care System. *Health and Canadian Society* 4, no. 1: 227–60.

Bourgeault, Ivy L., and Mary T. Fynes. 1997. The Integration of Nurse- and Lay Midwives in the U.S. and Canada. *Social Science and Medicine* 44, no. 7: 1051–63.

Burtch, Brian. 1994. *Trials of Labour: The Re-emergence of Midwifery*. Montreal and Kingston: McGill-Queen's University Press.

Corea, Gena. 1977. *The Hidden Malpractice: How American Medicine Mistreats Women*. Updated ed. New York: Harper Colophon Books.

Edwards, Margot, and Mary Waldorf. 1984. *Reclaiming Birth: History and Heroines of American Childbirth Reform*. Trumansburg, New York: The Crossing Press.

Fruchter, Racheal Gillett, Naomi Fatt, Pamela Booth, and Diana Leidel. 1977. The Women's Health Movement: Where Are They Now? In *Seizing Our Bodies: The Politics of Women's Health*, edited by C. Dreifus. New York: Vintage Books.

Gaskin, Ina May. 1977. *Spiritual Midwifery*. Summertown: The Book Publishing Company.

Haire, Doris. 1972. *The Cultural Warping of Childbirth*. Washington, D.C.: International Childbirth Education Association.

Hays, Pat. 1971. Midwives? In Canada? Let's hope so! *Canadian Nurse* (July): 17–19.

Hosford, Elizabeth. 1976. The Home Birth Movement. *Journal of Nurse-Midwifery* 21, no. 3: 27–30.

Hurlburt, Jane. 1981. Midwifery in Canada: A Capsule in History. *Canadian Nurse* (February): 30–1.

Kaufert, Pat, and John O'Neil. 1993. Analysis of a Dialogue on Risks in Childbirth: Clinicians, Epidemiologists, and Inuit Women. In *Knowledge, Power and Practice*, edited by S. Lindenbaum and M. Lock, 32–54. Berkeley: University of California Press.

Laforce, Hélène. 1990. The Different Stages of the Elimination of Midwives in Québec. In *Delivering Motherhood: Maternal Ideologies and Practices in the 19th and 20th Centuries*, edited by Katherine Arnup, Andrée Levesque, and Ruth Roach Pierson, 36–50. London and New York: Routledge.

Lang, Raven. 1972. *The Birth Book*. Ben Lomond, CA: Genesis.

Langton, Phyllis. A. 1991. Competing Occupational Ideologies, Identities, and the Practice of Nurse-Midwifery. *Research on Occupations and Professions* 6: 149–77.

Mason, Jutta. 1987. A History of Midwifery in Canada. In *Report of the Task Force on the Implementation of Midwifery in Ontario*, edited by M. Eberts, A. Schwartz, R. Edney, and K. Kaufman. Toronto: Queen's Park Printer.

– 1988. Midwifery in Canada. In *The Midwife Challenge*, edited by Sheila Kitzinger, 99–133. London: Pandora.

Mathews, Joan J., and Kathleen Zadak. 1991. The Alternative Birth Movement in the United States: History and Current Status. *Women & Health* 17, no. 1: 39–56.

McCool, William F., and Sandi J. McCool. 1989. Feminism and Nurse-Midwifery: Historical Overview and Current issues. *Journal of Nurse-Midwifery* 34, no. 6: 323–34.

O'Connor, Bonnie Blair. 1993. The Home Birth Movement in the United States. *The Journal of Medicine and Philosophy* 18: 147–74.

Ontario Committee on the Healing Arts. 1970. *Report of the Committee on the Healing Arts*. Toronto: Queen's Park Printers.

Page, Lesley, and Patricia Percival. 2000. *The New Midwifery: Science and Sensitivity in Practice*. New York: Churchill Livingstone.

Reid, Margaret. 1989. Sisterhood and Professionalization: A Case Study of the American Lay Midwife. In *Women as Healers: Cross-Cultural Perspectives*, edited by C. Shepherd McClain, 219–38. London: Rutgers University Press.

Rooks, Judith P. 1990. Nurse-Midwifery: The Window is Wide Open. *American Journal of Nursing* (December): 30–6.

Rothman, Barbara Katz. 1981. Awake and Aware, or False Consciousness: The Cooptation of Childbirth Reform in America. In *Childbirth: Alternatives to Medical Control*, edited by S. Romalis, 150–80. Austin: University of Texas Press.

Ruzek, Sheryl Burt. 1978. *The Women's Health Movement: Feminist Alternatives to Medical Control*. New York: Praeger Publishers.

Shroff, Farah, ed. 1997. *The New Midwifery: Reflections on Renaissance and Regulation*. Toronto: The Women's Press.

Sullivan, Deborah A., and Rose Weitz. 1988. *Labor Pains: Modern Midwives and Home Birth*. New Haven: Yale University Press.

Task Force on the Implementation of Midwifery in Ontario. 1987. *Report of the Task Force on the Implementation of Midwifery in Ontario*.

Teasley, Regi. 1983. Birth and the Division of Labor: The Movement to Professionalize Nurse-Midwifery, and Its Relationship to the Movement for Home Birth and Lay Midwifery: A Case Study of Vermont. Ph.D. dissertation, Michigan State University.

PART ONE

Canadian Midwifery in Context

INTRODUCTION

To best understand the stories that make up the process of reconceiving midwifery in Canada in the contemporary era, it is important to situate midwifery within a historical as well as cultural context. Our first chapter in this section is by sociologist Lesley Biggs, entitled "Rethinking the History of Midwifery in Canada." In this paper, Biggs questions the universality of the "neighbour midwife," which emerged as the dominant motif that many scholars and the popular press have drawn upon to articulate the history of midwifery in Canada. She argues that, rather than being a universal form, the neighbour midwife emerged within a particular historical and geographical context, and in other parts of Canada, different midwifery trajectories emerge from the historical records. Based on these other case studies, it becomes clear that a host of factors (network of professional relations, race, class, gender, culture, colonization, and regionalism) shaped the contours of the midwife's practice, her skill level, her working conditions, her professional and personal achievements, as well as her ultimate demise. Rather than one type of midwife dominating the historical record, then, the fragments of Canadian midwifery presented in Biggs' chapter illustrate that considerable variation existed in both the history and cultural understandings of the midwife across Canada.

A similar theme is presented in the cultural analysis of the re-emergence of midwifery undertaken by Margaret MacDonald in chapter 2. Drawing on her anthropological background, MacDonald reflects on the role that "tradition" has played as a key political symbol in the new Canadian midwifery and in the process expands upon the issues raised by Biggs. Based on ethnographic fieldwork with midwives and their clients in Ontario in 1996–97, MacDonald explores how midwives and their clients see themselves in relation to "traditional" midwifery in Canada and other places. She also considers recent debates in anthropology that posit tradition as a flexible human invention constructed in the present. MacDonald problematizes the notion of traditional midwifery while highlighting midwives' agency in the cultural (re)construction of their work and place in society.

Rethinking the History of Midwifery in Canada[1]

Lesley Biggs

INTRODUCTION

Beginning in the 1970s, feminist historians and social scientists turned their attention to the history of midwifery and childbirth. Inspired by critiques emanating from the women's health movement and from a resurgence of midwifery and natural childbirth, feminist scholars strived to uncover the work of women who were formally trained as midwives or who offered assistance as neighbours and relatives of labouring women. Little was known about midwives or the practices of childbirth. The received knowledge was based on the history of obstetrics, in which physicians armed with scientific knowledge and new technologies were portrayed as champions of women's health overcoming the dark forces of superstition and ignorance (see, for example, Shorter 1982).

In response to this Whiggish approach to the history of midwifery, obstetrics, and childbirth, feminist historians and social scientists have written counter-narratives that challenge many of the myths and assumptions underlying the "official" histories of obstetrics. These studies highlight the confluence of social, cultural, economic, and political factors leading to the decline of female midwifery and the ascendance of male medical control over obstetrics. In addition, feminist scholars have been engaged in a recovery project, resulting in a spate of studies about the history of childbirth, midwifery, and maternity care more generally.[2]

My own work (Biggs 1983) was part of this initial surge of interest in the history of midwifery and childbirth. I argued that the decline of midwifery in Ontario from 1795 to 1900 was intimately tied to allopathic

medicine's attempts to gain a monopoly over health care and that female midwives were a source of unwanted competition. But, in rereading my early work in light of the many developments that have taken
place within feminist scholarship, I have become aware of the *absence*
of the stories of different groups of women. That is, I have become concerned not so much about what I said but more about what I didn't say.
There is, for example, in my article no mention of Aboriginal midwifery; it is as if the history of midwifery began with the arrival of the
settlers. In addition, almost all of the sources cited are by commentators
of English origin. What were the views of Irish immigrants who settled
during this time period, or of other European immigrants who came
later?

In this chapter, I retell the story of the history of midwifery in Canada, but with the hindsight of twenty years of debate within feminist
historiography and feminist theorizing more generally. In particular, I
revisit the concept of the "neighbour midwife" (Mason 1987), an image that has dominated Canadian midwifery history. I argue that the
evidence suggests that rather than being a universal form of midwifery
practice, the neighbour midwife emerged within a particular historical
context, namely the settlement of Upper Canada throughout the nineteenth century and the first wave of immigration on the prairies in the
twentieth century. The fragments of evidence culled in my research reveal a myriad of cultural understandings of the figure of the midwife,
as is evident in the differences in the naming of midwives. The evidence
also shows that not all women who attended births were called midwives; rather the title of midwife, more often, was reserved for those
women who had acquired a specialized set of skills either formally or
through years of experience and was conferred by the Crown, Church,
or by a community under specific circumstances. Finally, I examine the
demise of midwifery, which has been equated often with the elimination of midwifery by male physicians. While it is true that in Ontario
physicians actively sought to eradicate female midwifery and the status
of female midwifery was the subject of a lively public debate, in other
places in Canada, female midwifery was either endorsed or ignored.
Support for midwifery in New France (Laforce 1990), the persistence
of midwifery in Newfoundland (Benoit 1990, 1991; McNaughton
1989), and the survival of Aboriginal midwifery, particularly in northern areas until the 1960s (Benoit and Carroll 1995; O'Neil and Kaufert
1995, 1996), suggests that the trajectories for the decline of midwifery
took place at different times for varied groups of women within Canada (as well as between and within other Western, industrialized countries). These stories remind us that many models of midwifery have
existed in both pre- and post-Confederation Canada, and their demise
was intimately tied to particular configurations of professional inter-

ests, race, colonialism, class, industrial development, and regional politics. Thus no singular history of midwifery exists but rather many.

FEMINIST THEORY, GENDER, AND MIDWIFERY

In recent years, the universal and essentializing features of the category
"woman" have been destabilized (Barrett and Phillips 1992); women
who have been marginalized both within and outside the feminist movement and the academy have insisted that women experience gendered
oppression through a nexus of social relations across and through race,
ethnicity, class, heterosexism, ability, geography, and age. Thus, many of
the concepts and theories of second-wave feminism[3] have been shown
to represent the interests and goals of white, middle-class, heterosexual
women rather than all women, as was first assumed.

What are the implications of the new feminist theorizing in the retell-
ing of the history of midwifery in Canada? For activists and theorists
working in the areas of childbirth and midwifery, the shift in feminist
theorizing has caused some unease, in part because many midwifery advocates and supporters (both within and outside the academy) position
themselves as "progressives" and understand the struggle for midwifery
to be part of the larger feminist health agenda, presumed to be beneficial
to all women. The suggestion, then, that midwifery researchers (such as
myself) and activists have been guilty of systemic discrimination, no matter how unintentional, is difficult to accept. In part, this discomfort can
be attributed also to the universalizing tendencies in many of the earlier
analyses of midwifery, pregnancy and childbirth,[4] and which are embodied in the concept of the neighbour midwife. By virtue of the fact that
midwifery, maternity care, and childbirth centre on women's reproductive and biological status, it is all too easy to fall into the essentialist trap
of assuming commonalities among women rather than examining their
experiences in socio-cultural and historical contexts.

Very recently, feminists working in the area of midwifery and childbirth have begun to re-theorize gender. Sheryl Nestel (1994/95; 1996/
97; see also this volume for further detail), in her study of the legalization of midwifery in Ontario, examines a variety of exclusionary practices that contributed to the monoracial profile (i.e. white) within the
Ontario midwifery movement. These strategies included the privileging
of Ontario practice experience for entry into the new profession, the reliance on the baccalaureate degree or its equivalent, the construction of
immigrant and refugee women's needs in terms almost solely as clients
rather than as practising midwives, and the dependence of Ontario midwives on racialized[5] women's bodies to meet the requirements of preceptorship.[6] Nestel persuasively argues that the homogeneity of social
identities within the midwifery movements in Canada and elsewhere

provided a common ground for lobbying for midwifery legislation, but that the unintended effects were to exclude many racialized women from practising midwifery.

While Nestel's study is important because it analyses the exclusionary strategies mediated through gender and race, Tess Cosslett's 1994 study draws our attention to the construction of "official" narratives governing childbirth practices and experiences. Her analysis of the sexist and objectifying features of medical discourse offers no surprises to feminist critics of the medical model of childbirth, but her discussion of primitivism embedded within the "natural" childbirth discourse is more likely to cause discomfort. She argues that writers such as Sheila Kitzinger, the doyen of the "natural" childbirth movement in Britain, while critical of male constructs of the female primitive, have fallen into the same essentialist trap. To be fair, Kitzinger has written extensively on sexuality, birthing, and parenting and has drawn attention to the diversity of women's experiences including lesbian mothers and women of colour. Noting the shifts and tensions in Kitzinger's discourse from deeming motherhood as women's "natural" role to presenting childbirth as an "art," Cosslett concludes that "[Kitzinger] still needs [the primitive woman] in the background as a validation for what she is doing, as a goal towards which her women strive. All their techniques and information are directed towards attaining the primitive woman's 'flowing presence in their own bodies" (21). The main problem with the official stories of childbirth – whether they belong to the natural childbirth movement or to the medical profession – is that they present a unifying image of "woman" that many women do not fit.[7] Cosslett resurrects the notion of "old wives' tales" to capture the birth stories of "other women" that highlight the multiple meanings of maternity and motherhood as experienced by women from different classes and races (7).

REVISITING THE CONCEPTS OF THE "POPULAR BIRTH CULTURE" AND THE "NEIGHBOUR MIDWIFE"

Much of our knowledge about the practice of midwifery and the experience of childbirth is based on nineteenth- and twentieth-century accounts found in physicians' casebooks and journal articles, newspaper articles, diaries, and letters by settlers in pre- and post-Confederation Canada. Based on these accounts, Jutta Mason has argued that the practice of midwifery consisted of a neighbourhood network of women assisting each other during their labour and delivery and in the postpartum period (1987, 1988, 201). Knowledge about maternity care was acquired informally, based on women sharing information with one another; often one or two women in a community would be seen as having special skills. In some cases such women may have had formal midwifery or nursing training in their country of origin or may have apprenticed with another, more experienced, woman.

This local knowledge of birth was informally transmitted; that is, it formed part of a popular birth culture, which women learned by participating at births or by giving birth themselves. As a result, women did not attend "prenatal classes" but would exchange information about diet, restrictions, and taboos through neighbourly chats. While the midwife appears to have played a minimal role during pregnancy, and a pregnant woman often saw her midwife for the first time when she went into labour, the midwife would provide continuous care throughout labour and delivery and often assisted the mother and her family once the baby was born. By all accounts, one of the major strengths of the neighbourhood network was the material aid (meals, quilts, assistance with housework and other children) given in the postpartum period, especially during the first ten days. Midwives were rarely paid, although they frequently received gifts in kind; as part of the neighbourhood network, it was expected that women would reciprocate when other women gave birth.

Mason does not paint an idyllic picture of the practice of midwifery in the nineteenth and early twentieth centuries. The historical evidence indicates that the provision of midwifery care was uneven at best. The further away a pregnant woman was from a city, town, or village, the less likely she was guaranteed of having any kind of assistance during labour and delivery. Many women often laboured alone while their husbands went to fetch a midwife, nurse, or doctor. In many cases, the birth attendant simply did not arrive on time, or in cases where someone could come, many families could not afford to give anything. In other cases, women refused to pay the physician's fee and chose to rely solely on their husbands to attend them.

Nor does Mason overlook the differences among midwives in terms of skills, class, and ethnic background (a point to which I will return). Nevertheless, her main strategy is to emphasize the commonalities in experience among women in English Canada throughout the nineteenth and the earlier decades of the twentieth century.

The main positive elements of this birth culture can be summarized as follows:

constant companionship by familiar women, who had also borne children; direct or indirect assistance from the woman's husband; gifts of food, clothing and housework from the community; a postpartum rest period for the mother; a community fund of birth knowledge, including a small number of remedies in times of trouble; and the consideration of such help as part of a network of "turn about" help rather than a service requiring payment (Mason 1987, 206).

This image of the neighbour midwife now circulates as a dominant motif in the writing of the history of Canadian midwifery (Baker 1989; Barrington 1985; Biggs 1983; Burtch 1994; Rushing 1991). By stressing the commonality of experience through the concept of the neighbour midwife, a seamless narrative is created in which one overarching theme – the male take-over[8] of midwifery – provides a common thread. However, one of the consequences of the neighbour midwife motif is it tends to elide differences among women and masks the particular configurations of professional (medical, nursing, and public health) interests, regional politics, level of industrialization, class, race, and imperialist agendas that structured the practice and cultural understandings of midwifery. Moreover, the concept of the neighbour midwife has become part of the folklore that has developed with the resurgence of midwifery in Canada and functions as cultural icon onto which the professional midwifery project is mapped. In establishing lineage between the neighbour midwife and the new midwifery, contemporary midwives are able to draw upon the image of reciprocity, denoting equality in status between midwife and client to advance their own professional project. At the same time, they are able to eschew a professional (read hierarchical) model of interaction, which has been a central feature of the midwifery professionalization project. A careful rereading of the Canadian literature suggests that the concept of the neighbour midwife not only needs to be contextualized, but its deployment in the present day context also needs to be carefully scrutinized. As Margaret MacDonald so elegantly argues in the next chapter, tradition has functioned as a political symbol for the contemporary midwifery movement and has been used as an historical resource to create (partially) a distinct occupational identity. At the same time, MacDonald reminds us that "tradition" does not have a fixed meaning but can be interpreted in a variety of ways that can inform and constrain midwives' professional project.

RETELLING THE HISTORY OF MIDWIFERY IN CANADA

Midwives, Neighbours, Birth Attendants? What's in a Name?

The concepts of "popular birth culture" and "neighbour midwife" tend to homogenize a range of birth attendants under one general rubric. Mason's own description of the popular birth culture includes the assistance offered by neighbours, husbands, midwives, country practitioners, and nurses in providing maternity care. However, the available evidence suggests women could and did discriminate between the help of a neighbour and that of a skilled midwife. In her study of the experiences of childbirth on the prairies, Nancy Langford argues that homestead mothers relied on experienced midwives, while others called on inexperienced neighbours (1995, 284) – some of whom (often reluctantly) became lay midwives. For example, Mrs Elizabeth Akitt of Edmonton, Alberta, who was attended by a doctor and a nurse with midwifery training, indicated that "I know that what lots of women have gone through childbirth by not having a doctor. Sometimes, there was just a neighbour: no midwife" (cited in Rasmussen et al. 1976, 78). At the same time, women who acquired skills could also gain recognition as a midwife. In recalling the beginning of labour, a first-generation settler in Alberta indicated to Eliane Leslau Silverman that "Some good friends were with us; one of them wasn't exactly a midwife, but people used to call her that" (1984, 66). This difference in naming suggests that a midwife occupied a different position from the neighbour midwife and acknowledges that midwives had a unique set of skills. Even the neighbour midwife, one who had no training initially, could earn community recognition as a midwife, having acquired experience while attending births.

The "granny midwife" in Newfoundland would, on the surface at least, most closely fit the model of the neighbour midwife described by Mason. Although knowledge about midwifery was informally transmitted, granny midwives drew upon "a community fund of birth knowledge" (Mason 1987, 206) or everyday knowledge that was acquired through a long period of apprenticeship. Thus, unlike the range in skills possessed by the neighbour midwife most granny midwives acquired a great deal of experience and skill. Hence, the epithet of "granny" signalled the wisdom and skill of midwives and denoted the respect with which granny women were held within outport communities[9] (Benoit 1991, 48–58; McNaughton 1989, 323).

One common thread among birth attendants (whether neighbour midwives, granny midwives, nurses, or doctors) serving primarily Anglo-European women seems to be that midwifery was understood as a form of work (for which they may have been remunerated, but more often not) rather than a spiritual or religious calling. For example, Hélène Laforce argues that midwifery was recognized as a distinct occupation in New France. The model of midwifery established was transplanted from France and organized within a hierarchical structure according to the kind of work performed and the kind of training. Each town in the French colonies had its own *entretenue* midwife, who trained at Hôtel-Dieu de Paris and was paid by the king; its *matrones* and *maitresses-sage-femmes*, who were responsible for quality control; or *jurés*, who alone were allowed to give expert opinion in court. Each village also had its *approuvée* midwife,[10] who trained by apprenticeship and often worked with assistants, and *accoucheuses*, who represented the new generation of obstetrical practitioners in the eighteenth century (1990, 37).

Similarly, in their studies of granny midwives in Newfoundland, both McNaughton (1989) and Benoit (1991) conceptualize midwifery primarily as an occupation. McNaughton distinguishes between the neighbour midwife, who worked without pay, and the "entrepreneur midwife," who financially supported herself and her family by working as a midwife. Benoit identifies four types of midwives who were differentiated by the type of training and place of practice: the traditional lay or granny midwife, who, as noted above, was trained informally and provided care to women in their homes; rural clinic midwives, who were primarily British-trained nurse-midwives working in outport clinics; cottage hospital midwives, who were formally trained local women working in a regionalized hospital system; and ward practitioners, or academically trained nurses working in hospitals. Regardless of training or place of practice, "midwifery [in Newfoundland] was a skill rather than a power and midwives were definitely not regarded as supernatural practitioners" (McNaughton 1989, 324). At the same, granny midwives participated in the religious rites associated with welcoming a new child into the community, or with its death resulting from complications during childbirth.

Aboriginal Midwifery

Although the concept of midwifery-as-an-occupation appears to be an apt description of midwifery practice in Anglo-European communities, this model does not apply to the Aboriginal midwifery on the Pacific Coast. The nations of Aboriginal peoples in British Columbia regarded birth as "part of a natural and creative process ... Birth, as well as death, were (and continue to be) part of the cycle of life within the sacred realm" (Benoit and Carroll 1995, 25; for more detail, see this volume). Drawing on oral traditions based on focus groups of Aboriginal women, Benoit and Carroll found that midwives occupied a position of high status within British Columbian Aboriginal communities in the pre-contact period, not only because she/he possessed a wealth of knowledge that was acquired during a long period of apprenticeship but also because the midwife played an integral role as keeper of indigenous cultural traditions. Moreover, unlike the Anglo-European traditions, in which midwifery was seen as a solely female activity, both men and women could provide skilled midwifery care – although women usually served as the primary attendant. In general, Pacific Coast Aboriginal women and men were taught about the birthing process, and they had intimate knowledge of anatomy, physiology, and herbal medicines.

Similar findings can be inferred from O'Neil and Kaufert's (1995, 1996) work with the Inuit in northern Manitoba. Although less detailed, the themes that emerged in their interviews stressed the safety of birth in the pre-contact period, the competency of midwives, which was linked to the possession of knowledge, and the control that birthing women exercised in labour (for example, being able to choose the birth position). Unlike the model of Aboriginal midwifery found on the west coast, O'Neil and Kaufert found among the Inuit "no one model of traditional birthing, in the sense of a set of prescribed procedures which define where birth should be, who should be present, and how it should be managed" (1996, 420–1). O'Neil and Kaufert attribute this lack of uniformity to the nomadism of the Inuit, making it difficult to predict where a birth might take place and who would be available to assist.

Little attention has been paid to the history of midwifery as practised by Aboriginal women. It is, as Benoit and Carroll (1995) observe, "a narrative untold." What little information exists suggests that the cultural meaning of midwife in Aboriginal communities differed significantly from Anglo-European models. In their study of Aboriginal communities in British Columbia, Benoit and Carroll found that there is no equivalent of the term "midwife" among the different tribes and nations along the Pacific Northwest Coast. "Rather, linguistic translations tend to reflect the various roles midwives played. For example, among the Nuu-cha-nulth, the term midwife carries the meaning of 'she can do everything'; among the Coast Salish, 'to watch – to care'; among the Chilcotin, 'women's helper'" (232). In the 1950s, Saladin D'Anglure found that in northern Quebec,

the midwife (*sanaji*, "she who makes") occupied an essential place in the kinship system, as the cultural mother responsible for the role and for settling the sex of the infant (it was believed that male babies could transform themselves into girls at birth, and sometimes the reverse) and for presiding overall at the important rites of passage accompanying the first performances of the child, receiving important presents on such occasions. Terms derived from or resembling kinship terms accompanied the relations between the midwife and the children she delivered, and between the children delivered by the same midwife; thus *uitsiaq* "husband-in-law" and *nuliatsiaq* "wife-in-law" were used reciprocally by a boy and a girl with the same midwife (cited in O'Neil and Kaufert 1995, 60–1).

Similarly, O'Neil and Kaufert found in their study of the Inuit in northern Manitoba that the midwife was like a godparent to the infant that she helped birth. Like the *sanaji* of northern Quebec, the midwife was responsible for making the sex of the child, as denoted by the phrase "I made a boy" or "I made a girl" (1995, 61).

While these examples of Aboriginal midwives' relationship to labouring women and their children illustrate the distinctiveness of Aboriginal from Anglo-European midwifery traditions, they also highlight the difficulties in developing a singular history of Aboriginal midwifery, which would elide the differences among tribes, nations, and linguistic groups. Just as variation in the meaning and role of the midwife exists among Anglo-European communities, there are notable differences among Aboriginal communities. In addition, the reliance on oral histories for knowledge about midwifery in the pre-contact period raises as many questions as it answers. In collecting oral narratives about Inuit birthing practices in the pre-contact period, O'Neil and Kaufert argue that these oral traditions are being used to justify contemporary Inuit demands for control over childbirth:

For the Inuit, the belief that 'traditional' (i.e., pre-contact) birth was safe is basic to their demand for control over childbirth. The distinction between pre-contact and pre-settlement is an imposed one, for the current discourse blends both periods and reconstructs historical memory to fit ideological needs. The preservation of traditional beliefs in relation to pregnancy and childbirth is part of the reaffirmation of Inuit culture, but it is also a political act. As such, memories of the past are being collected, redefined and shaped to meet the political and symbolic needs of the present community (1996, 420).

While it is beyond the scope of this paper to consider the historiographic debate on the interpretation of oral histories,[11] suffice it to say, the relationship between contemporary needs and the reconstruction of historical events is the focus of much discussion among historians, anthropologists, ethnographers, and folklorists (see von Gernet 1996 and Cruikshank 1996 for reviews of these issues). This debate applies not only to the collection of oral narratives among Aboriginal peoples but also to the interpretation of oral narratives more generally. However, the emerging consensus seems to be that "oral tradition anchors the present in the past" (Cruikshank 1996, 5). Oral traditions should be treated as "living texts"; their meanings are not fixed but are culturally mediated. There is a process of selection in which some materials are discarded, some are retained, and some are re-interpreted. But, despite the infinite variability in oral traditions, von Gernet argues that they will always be constrained by previous traditions (1996, 11).

The Skills of Birth Attendants

The title of midwife implies a special set of skills either acquired through formal training or conferred by a community. The question arises, "Under what conditions was the specialized role of the midwife more likely to emerge?" Mason's account of childbirth and midwifery in Canada, Mitchinson's 1991 study of women and their doctors in Victorian Canada, and Langford's 1995 analysis of childbirth on the prairies in the first decades of the twentieth century indicate that there was considerable variation in "the community fund of birth knowledge," ranging from virtually no knowledge of birth to a wealth of knowledge utilized by highly skilled midwives. What is striking about the recollections of first-generation settlers – mostly of Anglo-European origin – in pre-industrial Canada in the first half of the nineteenth century and on the prairies in the first decades of the twentieth century was their lack of knowledge about birth control and childbirth. This ignorance can be attributed to the experience of immigration and settlement. Many settlers were young; they were separated from their families of origin and lived in isolated areas. They did not come to Ontario (previously known as Canada West and Upper Canada) or the prairies with "a community fund of birth knowledge"; nor did they have ready access to trained birth attendants of any kind.

The variation in knowledge about midwifery appears to be dependent upon the level of cohesion within a community. As we have seen in the case of Aboriginal women and women living in the outports of Newfoundland, these communities were able to sustain a long tradition of midwifery while they remained isolated from modern, industrial societies. Other anecdotal evidence suggests that women who settled in communities formed along ethnic and cultural lines were more likely to have been served by women who were recognized as midwives. Midwives played integral roles, for example, in Mennonite communities in Manitoba and first-generation Japanese-Canadian communities in the lower mainland of British Columbia (Mason 1987, 1988; Burtch 1994). Rushing cites a letter from a Japanese physician who requested "federal regulations for the control of the Japanese midwives who [were] practising in almost one hundred percent of all Japanese obstetrical cases without any co-operation with the medical profession" (Rushing 1991, 22). Silverman refers to the case of a black midwife who served " 'all of the coloured people there in Amber Valley [Alberta]. She went north of us too, to the white people' " (1984, 68). Mason (1988) also argues that throughout the 1950s and 1960s, midwives continued with little fanfare to provide services to traditional religious families, especially among orthodox Jews, Roman Catholics, and Jehovah's Witnesses, as well as among Mennonites in Ontario and Hutterites in Saskatchewan.

The diversity of experiences represented even in these tantalizing fragments suggests that the reasons for the persistence of midwifery in some communities can be attributed to a preference for a birth attendant who

spoke the native language of the birthing mother and who had an understanding of her cultural and religious traditions (Rushing 1991, 22). The
isolation of these communities (either by choice or enforced) suggests
that "a community fund of birth knowledge" would have accumulated
and that these midwives were probably highly skilled. Retaining midwives from the same culture may have been one strategy used by a community to mark its cultural and religious distinctiveness from the
dominant white, Anglo culture; alternatively, the persistence of midwifery within certain ethnic and racialized communities may be a result
of the xenophobic and racist attitudes of the dominant white, Anglo society. Only further study will provide some answers to these questions.

The experience of a midwife described in Walter (Valdimar) Jacobson
Lindal's history of Icelandic settlements in Saskatchewan is particularly
instructive for expanding our understanding of the historiographic issues surrounding Canadian midwifery. Lindal noted that "Each of the
early Icelandic settlements in Saskatchewan was blessed with a midwife
of highest quality and devotion to duty" (1955, 114); some were formally trained, "others [were] taught in the school of experience ..."
(69). While Lindal lavished praise on all of the Icelandic midwives, he
singled out the courage and initiative of Gudrun Goodman, who, although unable to save the life of a mother who had been gored by an
ox, administered an anaesthetic and chloroform, operated, and saved
the child (69–70; cited also in Rasmussen et al. 1976, 76). Gudrun
Goodman then raised the child, Gudbjorg Eyjolfson, as her own.[12]

The details of this extraordinary case suggest that we need to be
more cautious in our construction of histories of midwifery. In the first
instance, the skills possessed by Gudrun Goodman do not fit the model
of the neighbour midwife; rather this story indicates that some immigrant groups contained highly trained midwives. (Subsequent research
revealed that Gudrun Goodman[13] studied midwifery in a formal program in Iceland and was highly esteemed for her skills in both Iceland
and Saskatchewan.) Second, and equally important, stories such as this
one are generally not accessible to the professionally trained historian
unless she/he speaks the language of the immigrant group. The details
of this case were recorded in the 1922 *Almanak*, an annual journal
published in Icelandic for the Icelandic communities living on the prairies. This information would not have been available to me without the
assistance of Stella Stephanson and Nelson Gerrard (who translated
passages from the *Almanak*) – both are members of the Icelandic communities in Saskatchewan and Manitoba respectively.

The absence of information about these midwives can, in part, be attributed to the biases inherent in histories based on written records,
most of which are written in English and which therefore reflect the ex-

periences of women of British origin. At the same time, we cannot assume that midwives from northern and eastern Europe and Russia were uniformly "uneducated." Settlers from northern Europe (Sweden, Norway, and Iceland) have traditionally valued literacy and therefore may have kept records of their midwifery practices, but these midwives would have recorded their accounts in their mother tongue. Their descendants, however, may not have considered these records worthy of keeping and thrown them away because they were no longer accessible to subsequent generations; some may have found their way into archives across the country but are available only to bilingual researchers.

Gudrun Goodman's story underscores the fact that we have only limited knowledge about the midwives living in non-Anglo-European and/or religious communities, and most of what we have is based on anecdotal evidence culled from secondary sources or interviews of first- and second-generation, English-speaking homestead settlers. To date, no systematic study of midwives living in racialized, ethnic, and/or religious communities in Canada has been conducted.

Where is the Story Taking Place? The Decline of Midwifery in Canada

Often the history of midwifery in Canada as a whole is equated with the history of midwifery in Ontario. In part, events in central Canada have captured historians' attention because the debate there over female midwifery was highly charged (Biggs 1983; Connor 1994; Mitchinson 1991; Rushing 1991; Strong-Boag 1980) and female midwifery was eclipsed by the male obstetrical system relatively early on (i.e. by the end of the nineteenth century). Rushing's analysis of the demise of midwifery offers a good starting place for understanding the different trajectories for the history of midwifery in Canada. She persuasively argues that market forces had a major impact on the occupational power of physicians, nurses, and midwives. Rather than view the decline of midwifery simply as an example of occupational imperialism, Rushing's analysis focuses our attention on the supply of the producers, the demand for services, inter-occupational conflicts, and producer-client relationships. Similarly, Connor (1994) and Mitchinson (1991) offer important correctives to my own work of 1983, which focused almost exclusively on the professional project of male physicians and the rise of scientific medicine in the last quarter of the nineteenth century. They argue that "no one factor accounts for the decline of midwifery, rather a congruence of social, economic, and political factors [occurred]" (Mitchinson 1991, 164). While not discounting the role of competition between midwives and physicians, Mitchinson and Connor each emphasize other factors, such as a decline in physicians' respect for women's intellectual ability (including a range of sexist and misogynist beliefs); physicians' concerns about midwives' lack of formal training (although it is clear that physicians were on weak ground until the ascendancy of the germ theory in the 1880s); the superiority of physicians' knowledge and skill, particularly with the introduction of anaesthesia; the failure of midwives to organize and lobby for professional status as a result of class, linguistic, and geographic barriers; the inability to recruit younger women into midwifery; and finally, women's demand for physician services, which, no doubt, represented a mixture of accepting the propaganda about midwives and desiring "the new, modern way of birth."

Important as these forces were, however, they need to be placed within a larger context. The persistence of and demise of midwifery within different regions in Canada and between different groups of women need to be explained. The available evidence suggests the uneven decline of midwifery across Canada is intimately tied to the level of industrialization in each province/region and to colonial and nationalist agendas. In turn, these social, cultural, and political forces shaped the market for maternity care services. Colonial agendas operated very differently depending upon the goals of the colonizing agents. During French rule of North America, from 1650 to 1763, to encourage population growth the king of France established a birthing system in which a network of midwives served the French colonies, including New France and Isle Royale (Laforce 1990). After the conquest of New France in 1763, the profession of midwifery remained relatively intact in Quebec until the end of the nineteenth century, serving both the francophone and anglophone communities.[14] The longevity of midwifery practice in anglophone hospitals was made possible because British-trained doctors were used to working with midwives, but as a new, indigenously trained Corporation of Doctors emerged, this understanding was lost. Midwifery continued to be practised in francophone hospitals because "the Church encouraged midwifery and defended the rights of midwives to attend births" (Naissance-Renaissance, cited in Rushing 1991, 13). In contrast, no tradition of midwifery was established in Upper Canada,[15] and most women relied upon the neighbourhood network.[16] Despite these two very different models of midwifery, its practice by women in both Quebec and Ontario had been eclipsed by the male obstetrical system by the end of the nineteenth century. This eclipse was possible because the level of industrialization and urbanization in these two provinces could support a market for health services, including maternity care. Rushing argues that physician attacks on midwives in Ontario were most pronounced during the period from 1871 to 1911,[17] when "cut-throat" competition existed in maternity care services (Gibb, cited in Rushing 1991, 13). During these years, an oversupply of physicians existed in Ontario, leading to intense competition for clients among physicians and between physicians and female midwives. Consequently, physicians attempted to regulate the market in maternity care and eliminate female competitors through licensure, thus leading to the highly charged debate around the regulation of female midwives.

Hélène Laforce makes similar observations about the regulation of midwifery in Quebec. She attributes the demise of midwives to periodic surpluses of doctors (41). Early attempts (1790 to 1840) to control midwifery through certification were virtually unenforceable, but by 1870, when physicians were able to consolidate their position, they sought to eliminate the competition including midwives. In addition, Laforce attributes the decline of midwifery to the influence of the various types of international medicine (1990, 41), which shaped not only the content of medical knowledge (toward a scientific model) but also its organization. Laforce points to the concentration of medical knowledge in large faculties of medicine that "allowed for better control by the government as well as by the Corporation of these institutions and of their curricula" (44). As a result of this centralization of health services and knowledge, midwives, and particularly nuns, eventually lost control over their institutions.

Changing colonial relations had a direct impact upon the provision of maternity care services between Aboriginal and Anglo-European women. At the time of European contact, Aboriginal women's ability to give birth in an apparently easy and stoic manner was noted by missionaries, physicians, and other representatives of the colonial project. Mason cites two such examples.

In 1830, in her travels throughout Upper Canada, Anna Jameson wrote that birth was "in general a very easy matter among the Indian women, cases of danger or death being exceedingly rare ..." A physician reminiscing about the natives of the Maritimes reported that: "The Indian women were well built, lived an outdoor life, were healthy, strong, very patient, and bore children well, a very large proportion of women were normal. She [sic] walked or stood up until the last stage of labour. Delivery took place while the woman was squatting on her knees or her hands and knees or elbows, only occasionally lying down. She might hold on to an attendant, usually another woman, or a sash, strap, or stick which was fastened nearby for the purpose. Pressure was made on the abdomen by kneading with the hands or with a binder. After birth the perineum was washed. She rested one day and was up on the second day." (Cited in Mason 1987, 199)

While it may be the case that Aboriginal women had little difficulty in giving birth, we need to interrogate the selection of this information for public consumption. Why did these writers comment on the birthing practices of Aboriginal women? Was it because these practices sharply contrasted with those of Anglo-European women? Was it a way in which "difference" was established between the two cultures?

In her compelling study of the images of Aboriginal and white women in western Canada during the period of the fur trade, Sarah Carter draws our attention to the ways in which race functioned in co-lonial discourse, creating boundaries between white British identities – both male and female – and the colonized "Other." Carter's analysis demonstrates that the construction of Aboriginal and white feminini-ties were created in tandem; the construction of the "One" depended upon the construction of the "Other." Carter persuasively argues that the portrayal of white women as "civilizers" of society, embodying "virtue, domesticity and ennobling influences" (1997, 205), was predi-cated on the image of Aboriginal femininity as "immoral, and licen-tious." These categories of difference, affirming the "superiority" of white women and reinforcing the subordinate position of Native women, ensured that the worlds of white and Native women remained apart. It is not surprising, then, to learn that by the first wave of immi-gration to the prairies from 1901 to 1910, homestead women did not rely on the assistance of Native women (Langford 1995, 286–7).

However, these representations of white and Aboriginal femininities do not explain the fact that initially, during the early period of immi-gration to the prairies, white female settlers accepted assistance from Aboriginal midwives. Carter herself indicates that the memoirs of early white women settlers frequently mention the assistance provided by Native women;[18] "Aboriginal women played a positive role in main-taining the health of many of the new arrivals" (1997, 185) by serving as midwives and through their knowledge of edible plants. How, then, do we explain the shift from a situation where white women accepted, indeed depended upon, the assistance of Aboriginal midwives to one where Aboriginal and white women were isolated from one another not only geographically through the reserve system but also socially?

The example cited above suggests that a counter-narrative of Aborig-inal women also operated – one grounded in discourses of primitivism that evoked images of the "Noble Savage," uncorrupted by civiliza-tion. (However, based on archaeological evidence, Waldram, Herring, and Young [1995] point to considerable variation in the health status of Aboriginal peoples in the pre-contact period depending upon time and region.) Such a stereotype may have been operative at the period of contact when white fur traders depended upon Aboriginal peoples for their very survival. The discourse, then, of the Noble Savage provided an ideological mechanism that enabled white women to accept the services offered by Aboriginal midwives because it neither challenged the superiority of the white women nor tarnished the image of Aboriginal people (at least from the colonial point of view). But by the mid- to late nineteenth century, when tensions between whites and Aboriginals had intensified, Aboriginal women were increasingly regarded as morally inferior to white women; white colonial men saw Aboriginal women as "immoral and sinister" while white women were seen as "chaste and pure" (Carter 1997, 18). Viewed through these mutually exclusive images, the colonizing gaze ensured that little contact occurred between Aboriginal and white women.

The image of the Noble Savage can also be found in the north as late as the 1950s and 1960s, again when sustained contact between whites and the Inuit had taken place. In their study of northern obstetrical practice O'Neil and Kaufert found that nurses and physicians percieved "Inuit women [as] highly efficient birthing machines" (1995, 63) and variations on this theme were often repeated by nurses and physicians in the north. But in order to account for the evacuation of Inuit women to hospitals in the south and the need for interventions during labour and delivery beginning in the 1970s, physicians and nurses resorted to a reversal in the primitivist discourse that emphasized the corruption of the Noble Savage by "civilization." They blamed intermarriages with white men, contact with (white) civilization resulting in changes in diet, and the use of alcohol and drugs. In the view of many nurses and doctors, these changes in "lifestyle" led to more complicated births, in part the result of larger babies, which required the assistance of the obstetric system at the time of delivery (O'Neil and Kaufert 1995, 63). This explanation was sharply contested by Inuit women, who blamed obstetrical interventions in labour for the increase in complicated births.

The demise of Aboriginal midwifery was tied to the expansion of Anglo-European colonial power, and thus occurred at different times and in different places. Benoit and Carroll reported that Aboriginal midwifery on the Pacific Northwest Coast was not banned until 1949, but "long before this date, however, government medical personnel had labelled Aboriginal midwives as charlatans, and dismissed their original birthing practices as outdated and harmful" (1995, 239). In the Arctic, missionaries and traders did not arrive until the 1940s and 1950s (O'Neil and Kaufert 1996), while the evacuation of birthing Inuit women from the north, as mentioned above, did not begin in earnest until the 1970s.

Efforts to introduce institutionalized support for midwifery on the prairies and among the poor in the cities were championed by white middle-class women. But concerns for the newly arrived immigrants from eastern, central, and southern Europe, who had virtually no access to health care services on the prairies, and impoverished, urban industrial workers were articulated within the context of imperialist and national agendas. The Anglo-Saxon middle class strove to create a vision of Canada based on its own image and values, and these ideals were often framed through popular eugenics that asserted the superiority of those of "British stock."

The impetus for trained childbirth helpers came from women living on the margins (i.e. those living on the prairies, British Columbia, and the outposts of northern Ontario), who decried the scarcity of health services. Looking for a cause, the National Council of Women (at the suggestion of its Local Council of Women in Vancouver and supported by the Montreal, Ottawa, and Toronto councils) passed a resolution in 1896 calling for the establishment of the Victorian Order of Home Helpers (for more detail, see Buckley 1976 and Mason 1987). The aim of the order was to provide assistance in nursing the sick, especially for mothers and children, midwifery care, housekeeping, and household sanitation to those who otherwise could not afford it.

These efforts to implement a system of midwifery by the National Council of Women failed, as has been well documented (see, for example, Buckley 1976, Dodd, 1994 and Mason 1987). Canadian doctors were opposed to the establishment of formally trained midwives as proposed by the National Council. Physicians, "having a tentative hold, or the beginning of a hold, on the market for birth attendance," refused to approve "the introduction of sanctioned competitors" (Rushing 1991, 17) and, as Suzanne Buckley observed, "the middle-class women demurred" (1976, 149). Canadian doctors, however, were not the only opponents to formally trained midwives; the emerging nursing profession also objected. Rather than alienate physicians, whose support the nursing profession believed they needed, the nurses accepted a subordinate position to medicine in return for protection of their newly emerging occupational status. In response to these professional interests, the National Council created the Victorian Order of Nurses (VON), which would provide nursing services to the indigent and the isolated; midwifery was eliminated from its responsibilities, and only women "who were thoroughly trained in hospital and district nursing" could practise as a VON.

While women living in central Canada spearheaded the campaign for the VON, prairie women also developed a local campaign to establish midwifery services. Concerned about the alarmingly high rates of infant and maternal mortality and morbidity, as well as recognizing the need for Saskatchewan midwives to be paid for their services (Taylor 1997, 413), the Women's Grain Growers (WGG) began in 1916 to lobby for a midwifery act. Georgina Taylor (1997) persuasively argues that the provision of midwifery services was part of a larger campaign to provide "medical aid within the reach of all" championed by Violet McNaughton, president of the WGG, who worked tirelessly to provide affordable (read publicly funded) medical aid to farm families.[19] But McNaughton and the WGG failed in their efforts to secure midwifery or maternity services more generally for childbearing women.

Although individual physicians did support midwifery, like the National Council of Women, McNaughton and the WGG encountered opposition from powerful members of the medical community, most notably from Dr Maurice Seymour, the commissioner of public health in Saskatchewan, who had strong support from George Langley, the minister of municipal affairs. Seymour was not only a founding member of the Medical Council of Saskatchewan but was also in the process of establishing public health within the government bureaucracy. Drawing on his professional and bureaucratic statuses, as well as the power of medicine that by this time was well ensconced, Seymour easily brushed aside McNaughton and the WGG's demands. But, according to Taylor, "the greatest stumbling block" to McNaughton and the WGG's proposal was from the Canadian Graduate Nurses' Association. It too was engaged in its own professional project, which McNaughton "saw as standing for 'full class protection, and (to the poor farmer) impossible rates'" (cited in Taylor 1997, 428). Disappointed but undaunted, McNaughton turned her attention to securing the employment of nurses in rural municipalities as well as to the plight of "ordinary nurses" who, while performing invaluable services to rural communities, had poor working conditions and low rates of pay.

The story of midwifery in Newfoundland proceeded on quite a different trajectory than in Ontario or Quebec, for Aboriginal peoples, or on the prairies. Unlike the situations in these provinces, where the status of midwifery was controversial and advocates encountered opposition from the medical establishment, midwifery in Newfoundland was legalized in 1931 and the law regulating midwives remained in effect until 1970 (Benoit 1990; McNaughton 1989). In response to the high infant and maternal mortality rates and to the relative isolation of childbearing women in outport communities, the Newfoundland government paid for the services of rural clinic midwives, the majority of whom were recruits from Britain. While granny midwives continued to work until the 1950s, the majority of maternity care services were provided by the cottage hospital midwives, who were employed in small hospitals (eighteen in total) dotting the island and Labrador. According to Benoit (1991), the cottage hospital system represented a transitional stage between premodern maternity care and the contemporary obstetric system, but it was an institutional arrangement that afforded the most autonomy to the vocationally trained midwife while providing her with job security, regular hours, and a salary.

As in other parts of Canada, however, the trend in Newfoundland since the 1970s has been toward the regionalization of health services, including maternity care. Yet midwifery continues to be practised, albeit in a truncated form, through the establishment of an academic program based at Memorial University. According to Benoit, the results of this program are mixed because many of its graduates work as managers, instructors, or researchers but few serve in health stations or in the remaining cottage hospitals – and those that do stay for only a short period of time. "One reason for this abysmal showing," Benoit argues, "has been the students' lack of both *practical* and *socio-cultural* knowledge of the types of clients served by the cottage hospitals" (1991, 89).

This brief review of these case studies reveals that the demise of midwifery was shaped by a confluence of factors including professional (medical, nursing, and public health), race, class, imperial, and colonial politics, which took on particular contours in specific times and places. While the overall effect has been the elimination of autonomous female midwifery, there is no singular history of midwifery, contradicting the official feminist narrative of "a male medical take-over." To be sure, strong medical opposition was evident when female midwives represented (real or imagined) serious competition to the emergent medical profession (as was the case in Ontario and Quebec), and this, in turn, was tied to the level of industrialization and the amount of disposable income for health services. But, as we see in the situation in Newfoundland, midwifery was established with the assent of the medical profession when the profession was unable to meet the health care needs of women in the outport communities. These case studies also reveal that the fate of midwifery was tied to the emergent public health agenda, which sometimes coalesced with midwifery interests (as in Newfoundland) and other times did not (as in Saskatchewan); likewise, public health interests sometimes converged with medical interests, but in other cases they did not (Dodd 1994). It is also apparent that the nascent nursing profession played a significant role in thwarting the establishment of midwifery. Finally, it is apparent that the fate of Aboriginal midwifery was intimately tied to colonial agendas. When the early white settlers were in a situation of dependency, Aboriginal midwifery flourished. As Aboriginal peoples became subordinated, they were more vulnerable to the imposition of a foreign health care system, which operated as a mechanism of colonization.

CONCLUSION: THE STORIES AREN'T FINISHED

In this chapter, I have argued that the concept of the neighbour midwife, so widely accepted within Canadian historiography, needs to be historicized. Rather than representing a universal experience, the neighbour midwife existed only within specific geographic and historical contexts, namely the settlement of Ontario from the 1830s to the 1880s and on the prairies during the first decades of the twentieth century. Moreover, the existing evidence – based almost exclusively on written, English-language materials – suggests that the neighbour midwife came into being to serve the needs of Anglo-European women who had few other resources at their disposal. Many of these women, but not all, who assisted women during the birthing process performed ably, often admirably, under extremely trying circumstances. Our judgment of these women's skills (or lack thereof) then also needs to be framed within the historical conditions under which they practised. The image of the dirty, gin-soaked harridan of Sary Gamp, so frequently deployed in official medical histories, lacks a sensitivity to the historical context in which the midwife emerged. Gamp is trotted out as an example of the ineptitude of midwives (at best) or the danger that they posed to childbearing women (at worst), thereby providing a justification for medical intervention and allopathic medicine's monopoly over childbirth. But, just as medical constructs of the historical midwife function as an icon onto which medical, political, and professional interests were mapped, so too does the concept of the neighbour midwife; and just as O'Neil and Kaufert concluded that the resurrection of traditional birthing knowledge by the Inuit functions to meet "the symbolic and political needs of the present community," so too does the symbol of the neighbour midwife for contemporary scholarly and midwifery narratives. In establishing a lineage between the neighbour midwife of yesteryear and the contemporary, professional midwife, and by calling for a woman-centred approach that harkens back to a golden age when women assisted other women, the contemporary midwifery movement has created a competing "official" narrative to that offered by allopathic medicine. This new narrative has been a powerful tool in counteracting many of allopathic medicine's claims on and about childbirth and has no doubt contributed to the creation of the new midwifery profession.

The concept of the neighbour midwife not only conjures up images of the benevolent neighbour helping other women (which contrasts sharply to the avarice of the male medical practitioner), it also denotes equality between and among women based on their shared experience of childbirth. As I have argued, one of the effects of uncritically examining the concept of the neighbour midwife is that it has erased or elided the stories of "Other" women who practised as midwives or attendants during the birthing process. The fragments of history presented in this chapter illustrate that considerable variation existed in cultural understandings of the midwife, and that these understandings emerged in relationship to the childbearing woman, her family, and the local community. In all of the cases cited in this paper, it becomes clear that a host of factors (professional, race, class, gender, culture, colonization, and regionalism) shaped the figure of the midwife, the level of her skills, the conditions under which she practised, and her ultimate demise (and resurrection). Rather than one model of midwife being present, then, in Canadian history, we can point to many.

It seems to me that we are at a turning point in the Canadian historiography of midwifery. We can no longer rely on the neighbour midwife as the dominant motif to interpret the past, precisely because it creates a linear narrative of history that excludes the experiences and contributions of many other women. As an alternative way of thinking about the writing of history, Elsa Barkley Brown, drawing on jazz as an analogy, writes that

History also is everybody talking at once, multiple rhythms being played simultaneously. The events and people we write about did not occur in isolation but in dialogue with a myriad of other people and events. In fact, at any given moment millions of people are all talking at once. As historians we try to isolate one conversation and to explore it, but the trick is then how to put that conversation in context which makes evident its dialogue with so many others – how to make this one lyric stand alone and at the same time in connection with all the other lyrics being sung. (1997, 274)

Brown offers a new approach to doing the history of women and gender – one that does not privilege the experiences of one group over another. In the case of the history of midwifery in Canada, the neighbour midwife was created in response to a configuration of people and events. In the rewriting of the history of Canadian midwifery, we do not necessarily have to reject the concept of the neighbour midwife outright, since she too represents a set of experiences, but they are only part of the story. We need, then, to research and write the stories of the many other women from different racial, cultural, ethnic, and class positions, drawing these lyrics together, celebrating the multiple rhythms and accepting the discordant beats.

NOTES

1 I would like to thank Ivy Bourgeault, Cecilia Benoit, and Robbie Davis-Floyd for their invitation to write this paper and for their helpful comments. I'd also like to thank the participants in the conference "Midwifery North" for their feedback on an earlier draft on this paper, as well as my colleagues Larry Stewart, Valerie Korinek, David Coburn, and Jim

Waldram. Special thanks to Raymond Stephanson, who provided much support and encouragement for my writing over the years. The paper is dedicated to Ruth Roach Pierson, who inspired my love of history and mentored me through my first article on midwifery!

2 For histories of maternity care in Canada, see Arnup 1994; Arnup, Levesque, and Pierson 1990; Barrington 1985; Benoit 1990, 1991; Biggs 1983; Bourgeault 1996, Bourgeault and Fynes, 1996/97, 1997; Buckley 1976; Burtch 1988, 1994; Connor 1994; Dodd 1994; Laforce 1990; Langford 1995;
McNaughton 1989; Mason 1987, 1988; McKendry 1996/97; Mitchinson 1991; Oppenheimer 1983; Taylor 1997. In Britain, see Donnison 1977; Lewis 1980; Oakley 1976, 1984. In the United States, see Davis-Floyd 1992; De Vries 1985; Donegan 1978; Ehrenreich and English 1979; Leavitt 1986; Litoff 1978; Wertz and Wertz 1977; and in Australia, see Robinson 1996–97; Willis 1983.

3 Second-wave feminism refers to the resurgence of political activism around women's issues that began in the 1960s and extended to the mid-1980s. This movement focused on the universality of women's oppression.

4 There are a few notable exceptions here, namely Brigitte Jordan's study of birth in four cultures, published in 1978, which documented tremendous variation in the cultural meanings and practices among the Yucatan, Holland, Sweden, and the United States. In addition, Emily Martin's 1987 study illustrates that there are significant differences in the meanings of pregnancy and childbirth across race and class in the United States.

5 Racialization refers to the active and ongoing process by which one group, based on physical characteristics such as skin colour, is identified by the dominant group as having a "race." In Canadian society, members of the dominant group, who are, inter alia, white, rarely see themselves as having a racial identity.

6 Preceptorship refers to that part of training where students gain hands-on experience (in this case in midwifery) under the supervision and guidance of a qualified teacher.

7 Pat Kaufert (1988) makes a parallel argument with respect to both feminist and biomedical constructions of menopause – neither of which match women's realities of menopause.

8 The elimination of midwifery can refer either to the active measures taken by physicians or to the gradual decline in interest in midwifery-attended births, but this process is understood generally to refer to the former connotation. However, as Mitchinson (1991, 168) rightfully points out, "although the historiography on midwifery suggests hostility on the part of doctors towards midwives, the reality was not as clear cut."

9 One example of the high esteem in which "granny midwives" were held is a photograph of gravestone erected by the people of Carmanville "in loving memory" of Nora Ellsworth (displayed in Benoit 1991, 58).

10 "For example, in February, 1712, the women of Boucherville elected Catherine Guertin, who was approximately forty-six years old. She had to take
an oath before the priest, as decreed by the Bishop of Quebec" (cited in Clio
Collective 1987, 79).

11 The main source of disagreement in assessing the contribution of oral traditions to historical analysis lies in determining their "truth value." In her review, Julie Cruikshank (1996) argues that it is a mistake to ascertain the
"accuracy" of oral traditions in positivist terms; oral traditions are not, in
her view, repositories of "facts." Rather, the guiding question should be
"how are oral traditions used by contemporary storytellers?" Drawing on
cross-cultural comparisons, Cruikshank urges researchers to study oral traditions in practice; that is, researchers need to attend to the context in
which the oral traditions are told, who is telling the story, and the words
with which the story is told. In contrast, von Gernet asserts that oral narratives can indeed be used as evidence in the Western historical sense, using
conventional internal and external tests. Von Gernet concludes that "there
is sufficient evidence to warrant *a priori* an assumption that Aboriginal oral
traditions *may* contain evidence of 'actual' past events (in the western
sense) which occurred centuries ago" (1996, 13).

12 Adoption of children was an accepted practice among Canadian Icelanders.
It often occurred when a family had a large number of children for whom
they could not adequately provide; the care of the child was transferred to
another family with fewer or no children.

13 Gudrun Goodman was born in 1853 in Iceland. She lost her mother at the
age of eleven. She worked her way through a women's academy (which appears to be the equivalent of high school), and then studied midwifery in a
formal program. Goodman came to Canada in 1886 and homesteaded by
herself in Churchbridge, Saskatchewan, and then moved to Theordore,
Saskatchewan, in 1894. She worked in the post office and as a midwife until she retired to Foam Lake. Goodman was about forty years old when she
performed the Caesarean section. (Helga Arnason, 1922. *Almanak*. Winnipeg: Olafur S. Thorgeirson.) Nelson Gerrard, a historian of Icelandic
culture living in Winnipeg, translated this information for me. I greatly
appreciate his contribution to this paper, and that of Stella Stephanson, my
mother-in-law, who tracked down some of the details about Goodman.

14 For a fascinating first-hand account of the experiences of Charlotte Fuhrer,
a working-class midwife working in Montreal from the 1860s to the end of
the nineteenth century, see Ward (1984). For an ethnographic profile of
Henriette Blier Pelletier, a Quebec-born midwife who practised in French-
ville, Maine, from 1885 to 1935, see Paradis (1981).

15 With regard to the Maritimes, Rushing reports that "In 1755, the women of
Lunenburg, Nova Scotia, requested Colonel Sutherland to pay two women as
midwives. In response the Board of Trade appointed two midwives, and two
midwives were still found on the civil lists nine years later" (1991, 10).

16 This is not to say that no formally trained midwives practised in Canada West. In 1848, the Toronto General Dispensary and Lying-In Hospital was established to serve the needs of destitute women and to train midwives (Mitchinson 1991, 167).

17 Mitchinson (1991, 175) argues that "the most vociferous attacks came at mid-century" and that physician interest in midwifery had declined by the end of the century, notwithstanding the spark of interest generated by the National Council of Women's proposal to introduce the Victorian Order of Helpers. My own analysis suggests that the debate began in mid-century, reached its zenith in the 1870s, and began to wane thereafter, as medical dominance was established.

18 For example, Carter cites the recollections of a woman settler in the Qu'Appelle district. " 'Whenever the stork visited us, a nice old Cree lady, Mrs Fisher, from across the lake, acted as both doctor and nurse for the neighbourhood. She couldn't speak a word of English and often told us long yarns in Cree, then laughed heartily because we couldn't understand her' " (1997, 186). In addition, Carter cites the example of " 'Madame Chat-Chat' or Elise Boyer, an Ojibway woman who married a Metis farmer and lived east of Fort Ellice in Manitoba, and [who] was midwife and traditional medicine woman … Although she never gave birth to her own children, she raised many of her friends' and relatives' children, and was a stepmother to her husband's children … At the age of ninety-nine, Elise Boyer was presented with the Manitoba centennial corporation Order of the Crocus in 1967 in honour of contribution to the development of Canada" (1997, 203).

19 By forging alliances with the Homemakers' Clubs, the Saskatchewan Grain Growers' Association, and the Saskatchewan Association of Rural Municipalities, McNaughton and the WGG forced the provincial government to amend the Rural Municipalities' Act in 1916 to allow municipalities to hire a doctor and nurses. The Rural Municipalities' Act allowed two or more contiguous hospitals to establish a union hospital, while the government provided grants to cover the costs of hospitalization. Georgina Taylor argues that McNaughton's work was "an important early step on the long road to the system of hospital care and extensive public health care system in Saskatchewan. It was also the first step on the road to medicare in Canada" (1997, 393).

REFERENCES

Arnup, Katherine. 1994. *Education for Motherhood: Advice for Mothers in Twentieth Century Canada*. Toronto: University of Toronto Press.

Arnup, Katherine, Andrée Levesque, and Ruth Roach Pierson. 1990. *Delivering Motherhood: Maternal Ideologies and Practices in the 19th and 20th Centuries*. London and New York: Routledge.

Baker, Maureen. 1989. *Midwifery: A New Status*. Ottawa: Research Branch, Library of Parliament, Minister of Supply and Services.

Barrett, Michelle, and Anne Phillips. 1992. *Destabilizing Theory: Contemporary Feminist Debates*. Cambridge: Polity Press.

Barrington, E. 1985, *Midwifery Is Catching*. Toronto: New Canada Publishers.

Benoit, Cecilia. 1990. Mothering in a Newfoundland Community: 1900–1940. In *Delivering Motherhood: Maternal Ideologies and Practices in the 19th and 20th Centuries*, edited by Katherine Arnup, Andrée Levesque, and Ruth Roach Pierson, 173–89. London and New York: Routledge.

– 1991. *Midwives in Passage*. St John's, Nfld.: Institute of Social and Economic Research.

Benoit, Cecilia, and Dena Carroll. 1995. Aboriginal Midwifery in British Columbia: A Narrative Untold. In *A Persistent Spirit: Towards Understanding Aboriginal Health in British Columbia*, edited by Peter H. Stephenson, Susan J. Elliot, Leslie T. Foster, and Jill Harris, 223-48. Victoria: Canadian Western Geographical Series. Vol. 31.

Biggs, Catherine L. 1983. The Case of the Missing Midwives: A History of Midwifery in Ontario from 1795–1900. *Ontario History* 65, no. 2: 21–35. Reprinted in *Delivering Motherhood: Maternal Ideologies and Practices in the 19th and 20th Centuries*, edited by Katherine Arnup, Andrée Levesque, and Ruth Roach Pierson, 20–36. 1990. London and New York: Routledge.

Bourgeault, Ivy. 1996. Delivering Midwifery: An Examination of the Process and Outcome of the Incorporation of Midwifery in Ontario. Ph.D. dissertation. Department of Behavioural Science, University of Totonto.

Bourgeault, Ivy, and Mary Fynes. 1996/97. Delivering Midwifery in Ontario: How and Why Midwifery Was Integrated into the Provincial Health Care System. *Health and Canadian Society/Santé et Société Canadienne* 4, no. 2: 227-62.

Brown, Elsa Barkley. 1997. What has Happened Here?: The Politics of Difference in Women's History and Feminist Politics. In *The Second Wave: A Reader in Feminist Theory*, edited by Linda Nicholson. New York and London: Routledge.

Buckley, Suzanne. 1976. Ladies or Midwives? Efforts to Reduce Infant and Maternal Mortality. In *A Not Unreasonable Claim: Women and Reform in Canada, 1880s – 1920s*, edited by Linda Kealey, 131–49. Toronto: The Women's Press.

Burtch, Brian. 1988. Midwifery and the State: The New Midwifery in Canada. In *Gender and Society: Creating a Canadian Women's Sociology*, edited by Arlene McLaren, 349–71. Toronto: Pitman.

– 1994. *Trials of Labour: The Re-emergence of Midwifery*. Montreal and Kingston: McGill-Queen's University Press.

Carter, Sarah. 1997. *Capturing Women: The Manipulation of Cultural Imagery in Canada's West*. Montreal and Kingston: McGill-Queen's University Press.

Clio Collective. 1987. *Québec Women: A History*. Translated by Roger Gannon and Rosalind Gill. Toronto: The Women's Press.

Connor, J.T.H. 1994. 'Larger Fish to Catch Here than Midwives': Midwifery and the Medical Profession in Nineteenth-Century Ontario. In *Caring and Curing: Historical Perspectives on Women and Healing in Canada*, edited by Dianne Dodd and Deborah Gorham, 103–34. Ottawa: University of Ottawa Press.

Cosslett, Tess. 1994. *Women Writing Childbirth*. Manchester and New York: Manchester University Press.

Cruikshank, Julie. 1996. Claiming Legitimacy: Oral Tradition and Oral History. Royal Commission on Aboriginal Peoples. CD ROM for Seven Generations: An Information Legacy. Ottawa: Libraxus.

Davis-Floyd, Robbie. 1992. *Birth as an American Rite of Passage*. Berkeley: University of California Press.

De Vries, R. 1985. *Regulating Birth: Midwives, Medicine and the Law*. Philadelphia: Temple University Press.

Dodd, Dianne. 1994. Helen MacMurchy: Popular Midwifery and Maternity Services for Canadian Pioneer Women. In *Caring and Curing: Historical Perspectives on Women and Healing in Canada*, edited by Dianne Dodd and Deborah Gorham, 135–61. Ottawa: University of Ottawa Press.

Donegan, Jane. 1978. *Women and Men Midwives*. Westport: Greenview Press.

Donnison, Jean. 1977. *Midwives and Medical Men*. London: Heinemann.

Ehrenreich, Barbara, and Deirdre English. 1979. *For Her Own Good*. New York: Anchor Press.

Jordan, Brigitte. 1978. *Birth in Four Cultures: A Cross-Cultural Investigation of Childbirth in Yucatan, Holland, Sweden, and the United States*. Montreal: Eden Press.

Kaufert, Patricia. 1988. Menopause as Process or Event. In *Biomedicine Examined*, edited by Margaret Lock and Deborah Gordon, 331–49. Dordecht: Kluwer Academic Publishers.

Laforce, Hélène. 1990. The Different Stages of the Elimination of Midwives in Québec. In *Delivering Motherhood: Maternal Ideologies and Practices in the 19th and 20th Centuries*, edited by Katherine Arnup, Andrée Levesque, and Ruth Roach Pierson, 36–50. London and New York: Routledge.

Langford, Nancy. 1995. Childbirth on the Canadian Prairies, 1880–1930. *Journal of Historical Sociology* 3: 278–302.

Leavitt, Judith. 1986. *Brought to Bed: Birthing Women and Their Physicians in America, 1750*. New York: Oxford University Press.

Lewis, Jane. 1980. *The Politics of Motherhood*. London: Croom Helm.

Lindal, Walter (Valdimar) Jacobson. 1955. *The Saskatchewan Icelanders: A Strand of the Canadian Fabric*. Winnipeg: Columbia Press.

Litoff, Judy Barrett. 1978. *American Midwives*. Westport: Greenview Press.

Mckendry, Rachael. 1996/97. Labour Dispute: Alberta Midwives and Nurses

Battle over Birth Attendance. *Health and Canadian Society/Santé et Société Canadienne.* 4(2): 285–314.

McNaughton, Janet Elizabeth. 1989. The Role of the Newfoundland Midwife in Traditional Care. Ph.D. dissertation, Department of Folklore, Memorial University of Newfoundland.

Martin, Emily. 1987. *The Woman in the Body.* Boston: Beacon Press.

Mason, Jutta. 1987. A History of Midwifery in Canada, Appendix 1. *Task Force on the Implementation of Midwifery.* Mary Eberts, Chairperson. Toronto: Queen's Park Printer. For a shorter version, see Mason, 1988.

– 1988. Midwifery in Canada. In *The Midwife Challenge,* edited by Sheila Kitzinger, 99–133. London, Sydney, Wellington: Pandora.

Mitchinson, Wendy. 1991. *The Nature of Their Bodies: Women and Their Doctors in Victorian Canada.* Toronto: University of Toronto.

Nestel, Sheryl. 1994/95. 'Other Mothers': Race and Representation in Natural Childbirth Discourse. *Resources for Feminist Research/Documentation sur la Récherche Feministe* 23, no. 4: 5–19.

– 1996/97. A New Profession to the White Population in Canada: Ontario Midwifery and the Politics of Race. *Health and Canadian Society/Santé et Société Canadienne* 4, no. 2: 315–42.

Oakley, Ann. 1976. Wisewoman and Medicine Man: Changes in the Management of Childbirth. In *The Rights and Wrongs of Women,* edited by J. Mitchell and A. Oakley. Harmondsworth: Penguin.

– 1984. *The Captured Womb.* Oxford: Basil Blackwell.

Oppenheimer, Jo. 1990. Childbirth in Ontario: The transition from Home to Hospital in the Early Twentieth Century, In *Delivering Motherhood: Maternal Ideologies and Practices in the 19th and 20th Centuries,* edited by Katherine Arnup, Andrée Levesque, and Ruth Roach Pierson, 51–74. London and New York: Routledge.

O'Neil, John, and Patricia Leyland Kaufert. 1995. Irniktakpunga! Sex Determination and the Inuit Struggle for Birthing Rights in Northern Canada. In *Conceiving the New World Order,* edited by Faye D. Ginsburg and Rayna Rapp, 59–73. Berkeley: University of California Press.

– 1996. The Politics of Obstetric Care: The Inuit Experience. In *Canadian Women: A Reader,* edited by Wendy Mitchinson, Paula Bourne, Alison Prentice, Gail Cuthbert Brandt, Beth Light, and Naomi Black, 416–29. Toronto: Harcourt Brace. First published in *Births and Power: Social Change and the Politics of Reproduction,* edited by W. Penn Handwerker et al., 53–68. 1990. Boulder: Westview Press.

Paradis, Roger. 1981. Henriette, la capuche: The Portrait of a Frontier Midwife. *Canadian Folklore Canadien* 3, no. 3: 110–25.

Rasmussen, Linda, Lorna Rasmussen, Candace Savage, and Anne Wheeler, eds. 1976. *A Harvest Yet to Reap: A History of Prairie Women.* Toronto: The Women's Press.

Robinson, Kris. 1996–97. Midwifery: An Australian Perspective. *Health and Canadian Society/Santé et Société Canadienne* 4, no. 2: 343–66.

Rothman, Barbara Katz. 1982. *In Labour: Women and Power in the Birthplace*. New York: W.W. Norton Co.

Rushing, Beth. 1991. Market Explanations for Occupational Power: The Decline of Midwifery in Canada. *American Review of Canadian Studies* 21, no. 1: 7–27.

Shorter, E. 1982. *A History of Women's Bodies*. New York: Basic Books.

Silverman, Eliane Leslau. 1984. *The Last Best West: Women on the Alberta Frontier, 1880-1930*. Montreal and London: Eden Press.

Strong-Boag, Veronica. 1980. *Elizabeth Smith: A Woman With a Purpose: The Diaries of Elizabeth Smith, 1872–1884*. Toronto: University of Toronto Press.

Taylor, Georgina. 1997. Ground for Common Action: Violet McNaughton's Agrarian Feminism and the Origins of the Farm Women's Movement in Canada. Ph.D. dissertation, Department of History, Carleton University.

von Gernet, Alexander. 1996. Oral Narratives and Aboriginal Pasts: An Interdisciplinary Review of the Literatures on Oral Traditions and Oral Histories. Report submitted to the Department of Indian Affairs and Northern Development under contract 95–205: Oral Tradition – Part 2.

Waldram, Jim, D. Ann Herring, and T. Kue Young. 1995. *Aboriginal Health in Canada: Historical, Cultural and Epidemiological Perspectives*. Toronto: University of Toronto Press.

Ward, Peter. 1984. *The Mysteries of Montreal: Memoirs of a Midwife by Charlotte Fuhrer*. Vancouver: University of British Columbia Press.

Wertz, R.W., and Dorothy Wertz. 1977. *Lying-In: A History of Childbirth in America*. New York: Schocken Books.

Willis, Evan. 1983. *Medical Dominance: The Division of Labour in Australian Health Care*. London: George Allen and Unwin.

2

Tradition as a Political Symbol
in the New Midwifery in Canada

Margaret MacDonald

INTRODUCTION

A midwife travels by horse and sleigh and then on snowshoes across a frozen lake to attend a woman in labour at her log cabin home. The baby is delivered by lamplight as the voice-over is heard: "Until well into this century most of us Canadians were born where we lived. And the only professional hands guiding our arrival in the world were theirs: The Midwife." This brief but moving vignette is called "Midwife. A Heritage Minute." It is one of several dozen vignettes broadcast on television across the country that depict important events and characters in Canadian history and culture. According to the vignette's promotional material, it "dramatizes the importance and stature of the midwife in Canadian history: a skilled midwife risks the hazards of a rural winter to deliver a child on an isolated farm. The mother and father depend upon the midwife's calm skill, and the training she probably received from her own mother ..."

Many readers will be familiar with this stereotypical image of the traditional midwife in Canadian history. She was a natural, essential part of every community; she was known as the neighbour midwife, the granny midwife, or the lay midwife. Until 1850, traditional midwives still abounded in all parts of Canada. Most were lay or empirical midwives who had existed for generations in First Nations communities or who had transported their knowledge and skills from intact community midwifery traditions or formal education programs in Europe. The majority of pioneer women were assisted in childbirth by other women recognized and respected in their communities, who were called upon for their expertise. It must also be true that a great many women on the Canadian frontier gave birth alone or assisted only by their husbands. Traditional midwifery in Canada did not exist as a profession in the sense that there were probably few women whose primary work was that of attending women in childbirth; most women who acted as midwives to their neighbours and kin also raised children and did farm work. In parts of Nova Scotia, Quebec, Newfoundland, certain ethnic and Aboriginal communities, as well as in remote parts of the country, however, midwives did work as established professionals appointed• by either the Church or the Crown (Benoit 1991; Biggs 1983; Laforce 1990; Kaufert and O'Neil 1993; Mason 1987).

The Heritage Minute does what many popular, historical, and anthropological representations do; it depicts midwifery as a tradition passed down from generation to generation, the domain of women and the domestic sphere, making the best of things under difficult circumstances. On the one hand, it appears to document a piece of Canadian history in a straightforward manner. On the other hand, it might be read as a timely piece of public relations. "Midwife. A Heritage Minute" reinterprets and revalorizes traditional midwifery – for other versions of history have not been so kind – at precisely the historical moment when midwifery has finally been legalized in several Canadian provinces after more than a century of official absence.

The Heritage Minute midwife also has much in common with valorized depictions of midwives and traditional birth attendants in other times and places. Feminist scholars in particular have sought to combat the invisibility of women as birthers and birth attendants in history (Biggs 1983; James-Chetalet 1989; Mason 1987) and to validate the cultural and clinical logic of indigenous or traditional birth systems in non-Western settings (Cosminsky 1976; Jordan 1978; Laderman 1983; MacCormack 1982; McClain 1981, 1989; Sargent 1989). One of the key differences, however, between portrayals of the activities of traditional midwives in Canada and those of women in other times and places is that they are characterized more as a set of everyday practices rather than as highly specialized knowledge or ritual. As Mason writes,

So the baby was born and the bread was done. Having a baby, while it was seen as a very special occasion, did not involve a radical break from the business of everyday life ... The event of birth was so securely entwined with the other work of women – the preparation of food, the manufacturing of clothing, the maintaining of the home ... The birthing woman was surrounded by other women she knew who shared her life and fate and status in most respects. (1987, 202–3)

Many readers will also be familiar with how the story of midwifery in Canada goes from here. Traditional forms of midwifery were displaced by an interrelated set of social, economic, and cultural changes during the modernization of society. One of the most important factors was the expansion of biomedicine and the rise of medical specialization starting in the late nineteenth century (Sullivan and Weitz 1988; Rushing 1988). Physicians struggling to promote their profession and secure their clientele engaged in a successful campaign to discredit midwives as incompetent, unclean, and outdated (Ehrenreich and English 1973). Integral to the displacement of midwives was the redefinition of childbirth as a medical event, fraught with danger, and in need of intervention by obstetricians. The shift toward industrialization and new relations of production in North America were also influential in redefining birth, providing the metaphor of reproduction as a medical-mechanical event (Susie 1988).[1] While physicians filled the roles of the managers of what they saw as the mechanical process of birth the traditional midwife, in contrast, was more like a craftsperson. In addition, gender ideals of women as frail and dependent (and thus incapable of either giving or attending birth unaided by male experts) began to flourish during this time, especially among the middle and upper classes (James-Chetalet 1989, 421). All of these processes contributed to the growing acceptance of medicalized, physician-attended birth, and hence to the rejection of midwifery as a female profession. Physician-attended childbirth grew steadily throughout the nineteenth century in Canada, particularly among the middle and upper classes. The transition from home to hospital birth accompanied this trend. Obstetric ideology and practice radiated steadily outward from urban centres and after the 1940s lay midwifery was retained only in some Mennonite, Hutterite, and First Nations communities as well as in remote non-urban areas of Canada (Benoit 1991; Biggs 1983; Campanella et al. 1993; Kaufert and O'Neil 1993).

The history of midwifery in Canada has often been read as a tale of loss and endurance. There has been a tendency in both popular and scholarly accounts to romanticize and essentialize traditional midwifery. Lesley Biggs' critical reappraisal of the history of midwifery in Canada in this volume shows that while the image of the neighbour midwife functions as the "dominant motif," it tends to "homogenize a range of birth attendants under one general rubric." Her work points to the variability of birth attendance historically and also suggests that the decline of midwifery in Canada was "uneven" rather than total and deliberate (Biggs 2004). Nevertheless, midwifery underwent serious decline and devaluation and remained without social, legal, or medical status in Canada for more than a century, even as most other industrialized nations maintained formal provisions for the profession.

In the late 1970s and 1980s community midwifery emerged as a social movement devoted to exploring and promoting low-tech, woman-centred alternatives to standard obstetrical care. Ideologically this new midwifery sought to restore the definition of birth as a natural event, to reinvent women as competent birthers and attendants, and to restore the location of birth to the home. The intensification of this movement led to the legal and professional recognition of midwifery in Ontario in January 1994 under the Regulated Health Professions Act.[2] Legislation to regulate midwifery in Ontario and incorporate it into the health care system was a significant moment for birth care in Canada and marks a critical juncture for midwifery as a profession. Midwifery legislation has also been introduced in several other provinces.[3]

To describe and understand this new midwifery in Canada as a meaningful social and cultural phenomenon is the focus of my current work as a medical anthropologist. The data for this chapter is drawn from a much larger ethnographic study of midwifery in Ontario that I conducted in 1996 and 1997. My methods involved participant-observation at midwifery clinics, prenatal classes, and professional meetings, as well as in-depth interviews with both midwives and their clients.[4] I was drawn to explore the meaning of tradition in contemporary midwifery (and to this Heritage Minute vignette in particular) when Maya (a pseudonym), a midwife in my study, complained to me that it perpetuated a mythical version of midwifery that interferes with her own experience of being a young, urban-based midwife who carries a cell phone and drives a sport utility vehicle. And yet the sense that she is participating in a tradition of women helping women in childbirth is very important to her – as it is to most midwives in the province. Maya's ambivalence about the Heritage Minute's romantic portrayal of traditional midwifery is an emerging discourse within the new midwifery as it develops across the country. While contemporary midwifery's direct engagement with and positive evaluation of tradition has often been made to appear self-evident in both popular and scholarly accounts, it is, in fact, complex and contested.[5]

In this chapter I explore contemporary Canadian midwifery's interpretation and engagement with traditional midwifery and argue that the relationship is not as self-evident and uncontested as it may seem. The new midwifery in Canada has been strongly influenced by the trials of midwifery history in this country; by the relationship between traditional forms of midwifery and the predominance of biomedicine; by the official absence of midwifery throughout the twentieth century;

and by the generally wary and sometimes hostile relations between community midwives and formal health care providers over the last several decades. This set of circumstances encouraged the nostalgic sense of having lost the tradition of midwifery in this country and underpinned the sense of triumphal renaissance that was felt in 1994 when midwifery was officially recognized in Ontario.

Yet contemporary Canadian midwifery has not been reclaimed or resurrected from the past so much as it has been reinvented in the present, out of present-day concerns. In addition, while community midwifery in Ontario emerged as a radical challenge to the hegemony of the medical establishment, its new location within the health care system alters its status and meaning in a number of significant ways. My analysis of the new midwifery in Canada endeavours to go beyond familiar analytical oppositions of tradition vs modernity and natural vs biomedical; these are sets of categories that have often been used to "place" midwifery. I approach this task through a re-telling and analysis of midwifery narratives – stories of becoming and being a midwife and stories of seeking out and experiencing midwifery care. It is in these stories that the new midwifery in Canada comes into view as a complex and innovative cultural system in a phase of reinvention. In the ethnographic section of this chapter my observations and analyses are drawn specifically from midwifery clients and midwives practising in Ontario in the mid-1990s. It is important to note that while the midwives in my study may share a notion of traditional midwifery with midwives from other provinces, there are also important areas of difference that remain unexplored.[6]

TRADITION AS A POLITICAL SYMBOL

Tradition, in its literal sense, refers to things passed down from one generation to the next – including knowledge, practices, and material objects, including technologies. But as recent debates in anthropology highlight, "culture" and "tradition" are anything but stable realities handed down from generation to generation. Rather, culture and tradition are flexible human "inventions" constructed in part in the present out of present-day concerns. As Handler and Linnekin insist, tradition is better understood as "an on-going interpretation of the past" (1984, 275). More specifically, Hanson (1989) argues that a group's identification with tradition is often used as a rhetorical strategy in political struggles of the present; or as Keesing (1982) has described it, tradition is often used as a "political symbol." In other words, calling something a tradition creates a sense of authenticity and ownership for the group making that claim. To understand tradition as invented does not invalidate its authenticity, nor the right of the group or culture to claim it, but rather draws analytical attention to the processes of its production and use. How both positive and negative readings of traditional midwifery are employed in Canadian midwifery's professional and ideological struggles exemplify what Janice Boddy refers to as "managing tradition" (1995).

Sociologist Beth Rushing takes a similar analytical approach to understanding contemporary independent midwifery in Canada and the U.S. She explores how ideology contributes to "occupational power" in midwifery, defining ideology as "a set of beliefs by which a social group makes sense of its environment and which these groups manipulate in order to project images of themselves." Ideologies, Rushing continues, are "on-going social processes that are not fixed but are shaped also by the uses to which they are put" (1993, 47). Rushing explores the use of feminism and science as the two major ideologies or ways of defining the boundaries of midwifery and seeking professional legitimacy. While she notes that other notions such as spiritual values and "family values" or ideas of strengthening the family bond (in both conservative and non-conservative strains) are also important to midwifery ideology, Rushing argues that science and feminism are the two most powerful ideologies used in the effort to promote and establish midwifery – especially in public presentations. Her definition of ideology in the context of health professions and occupational power is similar to anthropological definitions of tradition and culture as they are used in analyses of cultural identity formation and practice. Just as ideology is a key factor in the creation and maintenance of occupations and professions, so are notions of culture and tradition factors in the creation and maintenance of group identity. National, ethnic, cultural, and professional groups alike use culture and tradition to define themselves and, significantly, to distinguish themselves from other groups, as do social and political movements.[7]

The content of contemporary midwifery ideology, or "birth culture" as it is sometimes called, gives value and meaning to both midwives and their clients/consumers. One of the key differences between Rushing's focus and the focus in this chapter is that Rushing looks at how ideologies of feminism and science appear as legitimating strategies in *public* representations of midwifery in the U.S. and Canada.[8] In contrast, I am analysing the personal views and feelings of midwives and midwifery clients rather than official representations of midwifery, though these two realms of representation are certainly linked. How close midwives and birthing women in Ontario feel to traditional

midwifery is not necessarily reflected in the legitimizing official representations. Indeed, exploiting midwifery's links to the past may have
ambiguous effects in terms of establishing its legitimacy vis-à-vis the
public, other health professions, and the state, as it cannot be assumed
that a positive evaluation of tradition is understood.

It is important to stress that there is no singular, genuine traditional
midwifery to which all midwives or birthing women in my study refer.
Nor do I intend to imply that there is consensus among midwives about
how close midwifery in Canada really is or really should be to various
versions of traditional midwifery. My central argument is that midwives and birthing women in Canada are fashioning a new professional and cultural identity that incorporates a traditional midwifery of
their own making – foregrounding some aspects of traditional midwifery while distancing themselves from others. I am interested not so
much in whether particular images of midwifery are true but rather in
the production, meaning, and uses of claims based upon them.

WHAT IS TRADITIONAL MIDWIFERY?

The development of midwifery as a social movement and its eventual
recognition as a profession in Canada is, within the midwifery community and in the popular and scholarly imagination, a tale of resto-
ration – of lost status, of lost knowledge, of lost ties between women,
and of loss of control over birth. These themes mark absences in
women's experience of birth in the latter half of the twentieth century
and underpin the prevailing characterization of contemporary midwifery as having reclaimed and resurrected the ancient tradition of
women helping women in childbirth. Indeed, the process to incorporate the very first group of midwives into the health care system in
Ontario was known informally as the "grannying in" process. Also,
the hard-won provision for home birth in the Ontario model of care is
a particularly potent link not only to traditional forms of midwifery
in Canada but also to birth attendants in non-Western places who
work in women's homes. The strong symbolic association of contemporary midwifery in Canada with traditional midwifery – in both historical and anthropological versions – is evident in popular and
scholarly accounts, which frequently employ the images of renaissance, re-emergence, and nature in their titles and analyses. For example, Barrington describes midwifery as having an "interrupted
heritage" (1985, 15). Shroff refers to contemporary midwifery in
Canada as "the re-birth of an ancient calling" (1997, 15). A typical
media report declares midwifery "Childbirth's ancient art reborn as a
profession"(Sarick 1994).

In the social movements devoted to midwifery and home birth across Canada and the United States these compelling themes go hand in hand with a sophisticated critique of medicalized and institutionalized birth in North America. A generation of women's health workers, writers, activists, and scholars helped set up the polemic at play when we think of midwifery as the opposite of obstetrical medicine (Arms 1975; Kitzinger 1980, 1991; Oakley 1984; Rothman 1982; Martin 1987; Davis-Floyd 1992). Anthropologists studying non-Western birthing systems also contributed to the appealing association of midwifery with tradition and nature, as opposed to modernity, progress, and medicalization (Jordan 1978; Laderman 1983; Sargent 1989). The portrayal of midwifery as an ancient tradition – timeless, enduring, universal – is closely related to the problematic notion of midwifery as an extension of women's *natural* birthing and mothering experiences.

Such analyses rightly posit midwifery as a radical critique of "technocratic birth," Robbie Davis-Floyd's term for the constellation of ideas, institutional and clinical practices, and effects that characterize modern obstetrical medicine (1994).[9] Tradition and Nature, posed as essential qualities of midwifery in opposition to modernity and technocracy, have been highly useful and successful political symbols. They may be construed as examples of strategic essentialism, to use Spivak's (1993) term, which condense what midwifery stands for and what it stands against.[10] Yet close examination of the new midwifery in Canada at the level of practice reveals a rich and nuanced space between these neat analytical oppositions. What I mean by practice here is not clinical practice per se, but rather in the sense that Bourdieu (1977) intends. Culture, he observes, is not a set of rules and static meanings but is manifest in everyday human practices. Bourdieu's theory of practice marks the trend in anthropology toward viewing culture in terms of practices rather than essences. When we take this theoretical approach the tensions between tradition and modernity or nature and medicine become a lens through which to view the new midwifery in Canada. Scholarly analyses of midwifery in Canada and the U.S. have noted but not always emphasized tensions between categorically separate realms.[11] Davis-Floyd, for example, even as she identifies and elaborates the technocratic/holistic dichotomy for analytical purposes, points out that it may "overemphasize the polarities, which although real, can obscure some important commonalties" (1994, 1136).[12]

"MANAGING TRADITION" IN THE NEW MIDWIFERY

Most of the midwives in my study were among the first group of midwives to become registered in Ontario.[13] The majority had learned their skills over a number of years through a combination of self-teaching, study groups, formal course work including correspondence courses from accredited midwifery programs in the United States or the United Kingdom, and apprenticeship with more experienced or foreign-trained nurse-midwives. All of the midwives in my study had practised extensively outside the health care system in Ontario prior to legislation. All were committed to midwifery and most had been politically involved in the push for legislation. Though differences between midwives certainly exist, they do share in common the belief that birth is a profound event in a woman's life, not just a physiological process; that maternity care should be low intervention, personalized, and woman-centred; and that women should be supported to "give birth safely with power and with dignity" (CMO 1994, 1).

Many midwives in my study identify strongly with the image of the traditional midwife – particularly with her qualities of individual caring and patience as well as with her location within a community rather than an institution. Those who learned and practised in the pre-legislation era experienced their work very much this way and fear the loss of these traditional aspects of midwifery in the face of new bureaucratic and institutional demands brought on by regulation. Maya, the midwife who first drew my attention to the Heritage Minute, insists that the public image of midwives needs updating, but that midwives should also be wary of becoming too modern, too bureaucratic, too technological:

I don't ever want to see my practice get to the point where I am just checking off boxes and examining test results. I want to be able to continue to give that nurturing that I give … [Unfortunately however], I don't see midwifery even lasting the way it was – taking time to make some bread for the mother while she's in labour, or comb her hair, or nurture her. I see it becoming very professionalized and losing some of those old doula kind of skills, that mothering kind of skill. And that is because we don't have the time … I see midwifery changing, and as hard as we fight to have it not change from that romantic thing of going out in the middle of the night – how can it not? We have cell phones and fax machines and pagers and a heavy caseload and papers and committees and [we are] doing fifteen jobs at once and wearing eighteen different hats.

In addition to identifying strongly with the unique social aspects of traditional midwifery, contemporary professional midwives in Ontario also identify it with a certain clinical autonomy. Since integration into the provincial health care system, some midwives describe the loss of their ability to exercise a special kind of clinical judgment, or what Jordan (1978) calls authoritative knowledge, sometimes expressed as intuition (Davis-Floyd and Davis 1997). Lillian, for example, is a midwife who has worked in northern Ontario most of her career. She began her career as a registered nurse, and as she grew interested in childbirth alternatives, she pursued formal midwifery training at a foreign institution. Finally she perfected her skills in a home birth apprenticeship with a local community midwife. Lillian's eclectic training is typical of her cohort of community midwives in the pre-legislation era. Though not all had nursing backgrounds, most had a combination of formal and informal training and only a very few were entirely apprentice-trained. Lillian is in favour of professionalization because she believes it offers the public greater access to midwives and assurance of their qualifications. At the same time, however, she sometimes strains under the new professional standards:

There was a certain freedom before midwifery was incorporated into the system in the sense that although we had a very strong professional association that had very well-defined standards of practice, the midwives were less bound by medical standards than we are now ... As people outside of the system we could have a little bit more leeway; we could be a little bit more flexible in terms of what this individual woman needs instead of being bound by the medical standard. Now we are a lot more caught into the system. For example, there are circumstances where I may not be able to do what I think is best because I am bound by medical standards.

Community midwives in Ontario, as elsewhere in Canada, argued that apprenticeship provides the best opportunity to learn these subtle, individual skills – clearly associated with traditional midwifery – in contrast to formal, standardized, institutional training.[14] The Midwifery Education Programme in Ontario, a baccalaureate degree-granting program, does combine classroom study with clinical placements; student midwives work with preceptors where the potential for apprentice-like learning is possible.[15] Some midwives, however, feel that standard education will further erode what is left of the connection of midwifery to the past. They fear not only that the historical tradition of midwifery is at stake but that midwifery's more recent past as a social movement will also be lost. Laura, a largely self-trained, urban-based midwife who practised for over ten years in Ontario before legislation, articulates these sentiments in the passage below. On the subject of how midwifery has changed since gaining professional status, she says:

Yes, one can feel proud that one has these skills and that one can order medication and perform certain procedures. These are certainly skills that I'm glad I have. But in terms of my connection with tradition, I feel sad about certain things because I see myself going in that other direction more and more. Especially those [student midwives] who have no background in the tradition of midwifery before legislation, they will not understand its value. They will know nothing of it. Right now it's a matter of degrees. Right now the majority of us practising have that experience. And then you are going to have the midwifery students who, say, had a midwife before legislation or were childbirth educators before legislation – something. They will have some knowledge about it. And then eventually it's all going to disappear. There is going to be nobody who has any experience about what that was. They will only have heard about it in class or whatever, and you see that now.

Midwifery clients also play a significant part in the changing face of midwifery, and are seen in some ways to deepen the tension between tradition and modernity that some midwives find problematic. Many midwives point out that clientele has changed markedly since midwifery became regulated and publicly funded. This has posed some challenges. Specifically, some midwives find it frustrating to encounter women seeking midwifery care without knowing anything about the clinical model of midwifery or believing in midwifery as a social and political movement. When clients approach it as just another consumer choice, it feels to some midwives like a decontextualized understanding and use of midwifery. I have heard it called "midwifery a la mode" or the "midwifery spritzer." Although serious conflicts between midwives and their clients are rare, these kinds of tensions do underscore some of the central challenges for the new midwifery. Midwives would like their clients to understand midwifery not simply as a new consumer option but as the culmination of a significant social and political movement that challenged the status quo. Midwives' interpretation of traditional midwifery, therefore, not only refers to a particular set of knowledge and practices, or model of care, but also stands as political symbol of women's resistance to the medicalization of pregnancy and birth.

Benoit suggests that while a certain critical nostalgia "can be helpful in challenging the many negative aspects of medically dominated maternity care, the accompanying bias towards premodern midwifery remains problematic" (1991, 92). Aware of this pitfall, midwives strive to hold up the notion of midwifery as tradition while at the same time dispelling myths and misconceptions about the new midwifery by distinguishing it from traditional midwifery. Midwives speak of the need to strike a balance between these social and clinical aspects of traditional midwifery and the modern institutions of which midwifery is now a part. Martina, another rural midwife, tells me:

My great grandmother was a midwife ... so I sort of have this idea that there is still a bit of that in my blood. But at the same time – I mean, we don't just get called during labour – it's much more clinical. We are doing blood work that my grandmother wouldn't have done and more lab work and tests. But I want to hold on to some of that. I don't want to become a techno midwife. It's not what I want to do at all. It doesn't mean that we don't use technology or are not willing to – we certainly do, all the time. But I think that one thing that attracts women to midwives and certainly attracts women to become midwives is that sense of the neighbour, the friend, having a cup of tea. It is more friendly. You've got time to spend time with women.

The same association of midwifery with a strong social and cultural tradition and low-tech, woman-centred authoritative knowledge is reflected in the words and experiences of many women choosing midwifery care in Ontario today. Yet, striking a balance between tradition and modernity is a difficult task not only in the context of new and conflicting institutional demands but also in terms of changing public expectations. Indeed, the idea that midwifery in Ontario might be more traditional than scientific or modern is sometimes met with opposition and alarm from the birthing woman's partner, family, and friends. Despite the positive associations of tradition in some consumer sectors – and alternative health care in particular – the symbolic appeal of tradition is not guaranteed in Canadian society. Particularly in the realm of health care, tradition may just as likely be associated with lack of up-to-date information and resources at best and with superstition and quackery at worst. Midwives and midwifery supporters hoped that professional status would correct negative public perceptions and misunderstandings about the profession.

This brings me to the discussion of some important cultural and political strategies embedded in more critical readings of traditional midwifery revealed in the course of my study. Even as midwives hold onto an identification with traditional midwifery that stands for caring and community commitment and stands against the "bureaucratization and scientization" of their knowledge (see Bourgeault 1996), they are also careful to distinguish themselves from cruder notions of midwifery in other times and places. Sonja is a midwife who practises in a rural area. She developed her clinical skills with a practice partner in the 1980s and later spent several months of intensive clinical training in a public midwifery clinic in the United States. She was also active in the political work that led to the professionalization of midwifery in 1994. In the passage below, Sonja expresses the tension between tradition and modernity inherent in newly professional midwifery.

In a third world country or the far north, if you can't possibly get to a hospital within a reasonable time you might as well stay where you are and make the best of things. You can decide that these are limits of what we can do and just sort of hope for the best. In this part of the country where we have access to the hospital, we have access to emergency service, we have access to lots of technology. There isn't a defensible way to not use it. [There are] the parts of the traditional holistic approach that we can't continue on with, or refuse to give up. We can't just sit there and watch things happen. We have to intervene ... We can't step back and decide that we'll go back to the way things were at the turn of the century when we just sort of let nature take its course.

Sonja's position rejects the perceived naturalism and fatalism of traditional midwifery and welcomes the chance to (in her words) "move midwifery into the twenty-first century." Her words betray a frustration with erroneous public perceptions of midwifery as backwards and wilfully ignorant of medical science. Her rejection of certain aspects of traditional midwifery may also be construed as a feminist strategy to embrace technology as a route to women's empowerment (Haraway 1991). It is an important, if somewhat polarizing, critique. Gaining access to modern medical technology and to institutional spaces has certainly been an important part of the political fight to gain professional status for midwives and choices for birthing women. To the extent that the new midwifery embraces medical technology, it is not, in Sonja's view, a case of selling out, but rather a case of making use of technology and pharmacology for midwifery's and birthing women's own pragmatic ends.[16]

Finally, midwives in my study pointed out several other dissimilarities between contemporary and traditional midwifery. One midwife suggested that there would probably have been more shame about the female body historically; she did not consider this aspect of tradition desirable for the new midwifery, which strives to promote pride and comfort in one's body. Another midwife noted that children and husbands may not have been involved in traditional births as they are encouraged to be in midwife-attended births in Ontario today. In these small but significant ways, contemporary midwifery is seen to be an improvement over traditional midwifery.

CONCLUSION

One of the most vivid stories from my fieldwork is one that a rural midwife named Katherine recounted. I had been to visit her practice earlier in the year and had met and interviewed several of her clients. Our last conversation, in contrast, took place in the lobby of a hotel in the city where she had been staying for some meetings. I asked her for her thoughts on traditional midwifery. How close did she feel to that image? What value did she attach to it? "I certainly can say that I get to play the pioneer a lot," she responded, echoing the sentiments and stories of many other midwives in the province. "I often do births with no phones and no power, and in places where we have to stoke the stove ourselves." One particularly memorable night she was called to a home birth during a severe snowstorm. The roads were closed. Katherine drove her car as far as she could and then skied the rest of the way to the house carrying all her equipment on her back. "I was the only help [this woman] had! So I went in on my skis and was not fearful at all. I just did the pioneer thing." The birth went smoothly and both mother and baby were fine.

This midwifery story is so compelling because it is evocative – in precisely the same way as the Heritage Minute version of traditional midwifery – of a Canadian national identity rooted in the histories of European settlement: the pioneering spirit, strong and capable men and women helping each other, struggling against the elements. In this way midwifery is highly appropriate, indeed ideal, heritage minute material. Even as I sat across from Katherine soaking up the images of this marvellous story she moved on quickly to say that midwifery is not really about such memorable exceptions, and no longer about making the best of things in difficult or dire circumstances. The new midwifery, she insists, is about making a unique model of low intervention, woman-centred maternity care work in a practice with other midwives and in a larger network of trained professionals and public health services. Of the emergence of midwifery and its foray into the public system in the late twentieth century, Katherine carefully extends the familiar metaphor, concluding: "We truly are pioneering for women's health."

If a new vignette about midwifery in Canada were to be made, Katherine would still like to see a home birth scene. The key difference in Katherine's vignette would show two midwives and some of their clinical gear. In Maya's version, the midwife would be under forty and not necessarily a mother. The story could unfold the same way except this time the midwife would get a phone call or her pager would go off. "There's no little girl knocking at her log cabin door. And she would take off in her four-wheel drive in a snowstorm and she would do some pretty horrible roads out there. And she would be doing a home birth; maybe there's a fire going but there could be also beautiful classical music in the background ..."

In this chapter I have shown some of the ways in which tradition is imagined and "managed" in midwifery in Ontario. Looking to the history of midwifery in this country or to birthing practices in other cultures in search of an authentic traditional midwifery tends to provide not certainties but rather a multiplicity of beliefs, practices, experiences, and interpretations. Midwives in Ontario manage traditional midwifery by being selective and strategic in their interpretation, identification, and evaluation of it. They draw positive connections between themselves and traditional midwives in terms of the personalized, patient, continuous, and low-tech care they offer their clients. They also seek to maintain strong links with midwifery as a social movement prior to legislation, which explicitly employed tradition as a political symbol to define itself in opposition to biomedicine. Meanwhile, they are careful to distance themselves from certain negative and fatalistic aspects of tradition in order to establish their status as legitimate professionals in the formal health care system and to maintain access to modern technology and institutions, and thus secure choices for birthing women.

While my analytical approach breaks up the possibility of a genuine traditional midwifery to which we might all refer, it does not break up the power of tradition as a political symbol. My attention to tradition as a political symbol highlights midwives' agency in the cultural (re)construction of their work, and the contributions of birthing women as well. To this end, tradition in contemporary midwifery in Ontario stands as a compelling political symbol of how the care of birthing women "once was" and how it might be. The interpretation of tradition in the new midwifery in Ontario is not blindly romantic; nor, even in the case of strong personal identification, is it exclusive of a simultaneous identification with modernity, technology, and science.

Recently midwifery in North America, as well as in other parts of the world, has been described as "postmodern" (Davis-Floyd and Davis 1997; Davis-Floyd and Cosminsky 2000). Postmodern midwives, write Davis-Floyd and Davis, "are educated, articulate, organized, highly political, and highly conscious of both their cultural uniqueness and their global importance ..." Furthermore, they are "defenders of traditional ways as well as creative inventors of systems of mutual accommodation" (1997, 242). Sociologist Brian Burtch (1994) made similar observations about community midwives in the interior of British Columbia in the 1980s. Such observations mark an analytic and strategic move away from positing certainties within cultural identities and practices and, in social science studies of midwifery specifically, away from portraying midwifery as fulfilling women's natural or traditional place in the world, or women's natural, traditional relationships to childbearing. Such descriptions also mark increasing awareness among scholars and midwives themselves of midwifery as a global feminist issue.

At a recent conference in Toronto organized in preparation for this book, midwives, scholars, midwifery students, midwifery clients, and women's health activists and writers met to discuss social science perspectives on midwifery in Canada. In the discussion that ensued from an earlier version of this chapter on tradition, as well as from other presentations and discussions throughout the weekend, the relevance of my anthropological inquiry about the culture and tradition of midwifery became clear. Tradition as a political symbol will persist in midwifery discourse and experience because of its power to mark as "midwifery" those clinical practices, places, and ways of caring for pregnant and birthing women that differ from mainstream medical care. Nevertheless, several midwives and midwifery students spoke eloquently about their desire to find and express new political symbols for their profession in an increasingly diverse society. Certainly this particular formulation of traditional midwifery, linked to the pioneering spirit in Canadian history, is not salient to all Canadian midwives or their clients.

A discussion of the role of tradition in Canadian midwifery may seem largely academic. Of what relevance is it to midwives and the women they care for? Exploring issues of ideology and identity politics in contemporary midwifery is important because such cultural processes have implications in practice. How midwives and their clients define the new midwifery in Canada informs the care that midwives provide, the knowledge that gets to count, and ultimately both the gendered identities of women as birth attendants and the embodied experiences of women as birthers.

NOTES

1 See Martin (1987) and Davis-Floyd (1992) for ethnographies of childbirth in North America that elaborate the dominance of the medical-mechanical model of reproduction.

2 For a full description and analysis of the process by which midwives organized and were incorporated into the formal health care system see Bourgeault (1996) and Bourgeault and Fynes (1996/97).

3 At the time of writing Quebec, British Columbia, Alberta, and Manitoba have introduced midwifery legislation. Please see chapters 4, 5, 6, and 10 in this volume.

4 I conducted formal, in-depth interviews with twenty-six midwives and twenty-four women (and sometimes their partners) who had midwifery care in Ontario the 1990s. Research participants were drawn from across the province,

with rural, urban, and northern regions of the province represented. Midwives
and their clients tend to be white, middle class, and well educated, although this
is changing slowly. Thus the demographic profile of my research participants
reflects this. Interviews typically took place at midwifery clinics or women's
homes and lasted between one and one-half and three hours.

5 Space does not permit me to describe in greater detail the ways in which individual midwives and birthing women participating in midwifery as a
social movement in the late twentieth century actually read popular and
scholarly texts that constructed the romantic, essentialized image of the traditional midwife. Such a discussion would serve as a sort of ethnographic
"prequel" to themes I explore in this paper, but it is the subject of a work in
progress.

6 For example, the history of midwifery in Newfoundland and Labrador
(Benoit 1991) with its system of cottage hospitals and granny midwives
who continued to practise well into the twentieth century is quite different
than the history of midwifery in Ontario. Thus Canadian midwives' reflections on the meaning and value of traditional midwifery are geographically
and temporally variable.

7 There is a rich ethnographic literature exploring the use of culture and tradition for social and political ends. See, for example, Boddy (1995). The proliferation of the terms culture and tradition in such instances as birth culture,
gay culture, prison culture, and so on – even by relatively transient, short-
lived social groups, such as "rave culture" – speaks to the currency and utility of this rhetorical strategy in group identity formation and demarcation.

8 Rushing notes the irony in this pairing of science and feminism, given the
history of antagonism between them (1993, 62). She points out that in
practice there are clear difficulties combining these two ideologies. However, recent re-theorizations of women's relationships to science and medical technology point to the "pragmatic" resolution or at least negotiation of
the antagonism between science and feminism (Lock and Kaufert 1998).

9 Midwives and birthing women in my study often referred to "medicalized
birth" and defined midwifery in opposition. My study participants' use of
"medicalized birth" very closely resembles Davis-Floyd's term "technocratic birth."

10 Both scholarly and popular works on midwifery may be understood as
"culture-technologies" that, as Boddy (1995, 18) describes, may be used by
a group to articulate and perform their unique characteristics, beliefs, and
practices. Written histories and ethnographies on midwifery and traditional
birth attendance, as well as critical works on standard childbirth practices
in Canada and the U.S., helped to circulate ideas and stories that functioned
to solidify group identity and ideology in the midwifery community in Ontario (see MacDonald 1999).

11 As mentioned above, Rushing identifies the tension between science and feminism in midwifery (1993), Benoit writes of the balancing act between art and science in midwifery (1991), and Burtch notes how midwives in the interior of B.C. distinguish between "spiritual midwifery" and "medical attendance" (1994).

12 Davis-Floyd concludes that both models act as guiding images for giving birth well and contain ideals by which the birth experience will be evaluated. Specifically, both the professional women in her study who had "technocratic" births and those who had "holistic" births reported feeling empowered by their choices of how and where to give birth and which technologies to demand or eschew. In the technocratic model having control over the bodily processes (pain, length of labour) is valued and when this is accomplished, women feel satisfied. In the holistic model, letting go of control or letting the body be in control is valued, and when this happens, women also feel satisfied and empowered.

13 At the time of my study, some community midwives and aspiring midwives who were not included in the pre-registration were protesting the process but in the meantime had been required to stop practising. For largely practical purposes, I focused my study on registered, currently practising midwives, though I did interview a few women who had had to stop practising.

14 See Benoit and Davis-Floyd in this volume for a more detailed description of this argument.

15 See Kaufman and Soderstrom in this volume.

16 See 11 above with regard to recent anthropological theory on women's relationships to technology.

REFERENCES

Arms, Suzanne. 1975. *Immaculate Deception*. New York: Bantam Books.

Barrington, Elizabeth. 1985. *Midwifery is Catching*. Toronto: New Canada Publishers.

Benoit, Cecilia. 1991. *Midwives in Passage*. St John's, Nfld.: Institute of Social and Economic Research.

Biggs, Lesley. 1983. The Case of the Missing Midwives: A History of Midwifery in Ontario from 1795-1900. *Ontario History* 75:21-35.

Boddy, Janice. 1995. Managing Tradition: 'Superstition' and the Making of National Identity among Sudanese Women Refugees. In *The Pursuit of Certainty: Religious and Cultural Formations,* edited by W. James, 17-44. London: Routledge.

Bourdieu, Pierre. 1977. *Outline of a Theory of Practice*. Cambridge: Cambridge University Press.

Bourgeault, Ivy Lynn. 1996. Delivering Midwifery: An Examination of the Process and Outcome of Regulating Midwifery in Ontario. Ph.D. dissertation, University of Toronto.

Bourgeault, Ivy, and Mary Fynes. 1996/97. Delivering Midwifery in Ontario: How and Why Midwifery Was Integrated into the Provincial Health Care System. *Health and Canadian Society/Santé et Société Canadienne* 4, no. 1: 227-60.

Burtch, Brian. 1994. *Trials of Labour.* Montreal and Kingston: McGill-Queen's University Press. College of Midwives of Ontario. 1994. *The Midwifery Model of Practice in Ontario.*

Campanella, Karla, Jill Korbin, and Louise Acheson. 1993. Pregnancy and Childbirth among the Amish. *Social Science and Medicine* 36, no. 3:333-42.

College of Midwives of Ontario (CMO). 1994. *The Midwifery Model of Practice in Ontario.*

Cosminsky, Sheila. 1976. Cross-Cultural Perspectives on Midwifery. In *Medical Anthropology*, edited by X. Francis, S.J. Grollig, and H.B. Hatley. 229-48. The Hague: Mouton.

Davis-Floyd, Robbie. 1992. *Birth as an American Rite of Passage.* Berkeley: University of California Press.

– 1994. The Technocratic Body: American Childbirth as Cultural Expression. *Social Science and Medicine* 38, no. 8: 1125–40.

Davis-Floyd, Robbie, and Sheila Cosminsky. 2000. Introduction to Daughters of Time: The Shifting Identities of Contemporary Midwives. A special issue of *Medical Anthropology* 20, no. 2-3/4 (2001).

Davis-Floyd, Robbie, and Elizabeth Davis. 1997. Intuition as Authoritative Knowledge in Midwifery and Homebirth. In *Childbirth and Authoritative Knowledge*, edited by R. Davis-Floyd and C. Sargent. Berkeley: University of California Press.

Ehrenreich, Barbara, and Deirdre English. 1973. *Witches, Midwives, and Nurses: A History of Women Healers.* Old Westbury, NY: The Feminist Press.

Handler, Richard and Jocelyn Linnekin. 1984. Tradition: Genuine or Spurious? *Journal of American Folklore* 97, no. 385: 273–90.

Hanson, Allan 1989. The Making of the Maori: Culture Invention and its Logic. *American Anthropologist* 9: 890–902.

Haraway, Donna 1991. *Simians, Cyborgs, and Women: The Reinvention of Nature.* London: Free Association Books.

James-Chetalet, Lois. 1989. Reclaiming the Birth Experience: An Analysis of Midwifery in Canada from 1788 to 1987. Ph.D. dissertation, Carleton University, Ottawa, Ontario.

Jordan, Brigitte. 1978. *Birth in Four Cultures.* Re-issued 1993. Prospect Heights: Waveland Press.

Kaufert, Patricia, and John O'Neil. 1993. Analysis of a Dialogue on Risk in Childbirth: Clinicians, Epidemiologists, and Inuit Women. In *Knowledge, Power, and Practice: The Anthropology of Medicine and Everyday Life,* edited by S. Lindenbaum and M. Lock, 32–54. Berkeley: University of California Press.

Keesing, Roger. 1982. Kastom and Anticolonialism on Malaita: "Culture" as Political Symbol. *Mankind* 13, no. 4:357-73.

Kitzinger, Sheila. 1980. *Birth at Home.* New York: Viking Penguin Books.

– ed. 1988. *The Midwife Challenge.* London: Pandora Press.

Laderman, Carol. 1983. *Wives and Midwives.* Berkeley: University of California Press.

Laforce, Hélène. 1990. The Different Stages of the Elimination of Midwives in Quebec. In *Delivering Motherhood: Maternal Ideologies and Practices in the 19th and 20th Centuries,* edited by Katherine Arnup, Andrée Levesque, and Ruth Roach Pierson, 36-50. London: Routledge.

Lock, Margaret, and Patricia Kaufert, eds. 1988. Introduction to *Pragmatic Women and Body Politics.* Cambridge University Press.

McClain, Carol. 1975. Ethno-Obstetrics in Ajijic. *Anthropological Quarterly* 48, no. 1: 38–56.

– 1981. Traditional Midwives and Family Planning. *Medical Anthropology* 5:107-36

McCain, Carol, ed. 1989. *Women as Healers.* New Brunswick, NJ: Rutgers University Press.

MacCormack, Carol. 1982. *Ethnography of Fertility and Birth.* New York: Academic Press.

MacDonald, Margaret. 1999. *Expectations: The Cultural Construction of Nature in Midwifery Discourse in Ontario. Ph.D. dissertation, York University.*

Mason, Jutta. 1987. A History of Midwifery in Canada. In *Report of the Task Force on the Implementation of Midwifery in Ontario,* edited by M. Eberts, A. Schwartz, R. Edney, and K. Kaufman. Toronto: Queen's Park Printers.

Martin, Emily. 1987. *The Woman in the Body.* Boston: Beacon Press.

Oakley, Ann. 1984. *The Captured Womb: A History of the Medical Care of Pregnant Women.* Oxford: Basil Blackwell.

Rothman, Barbara Katz. 1982. *In Labour: Women and Power in the Birthplace.* New York: W.W. Norton.

Rushing, Beth. 1988. *Midwifery and the Sources of Occupational Autonomy.* Ph.D. dissertation, Duke University.

– 1993. Ideology in the Re-emergence of North American Midwifery. *Work and Occupations* 20, no. 4: 46–67.

Sargent, Carolyn. 1989. *Maternity, Medicine, and Power: Reproductive Decisions in Urban Benin.* Berkeley: University of California Press.

Sarick, Lila. 1994. Childbirth's Ancient Art Reborn as a Profession. *Globe and Mail*, 14 May, A1.

Shroff, Farah, ed. 1997. *The New Midwifery in Canada: Reflections on Renaissance and Regulation*. Toronto: The Women's Press.

Spivak, Gayatri Chakravorty. 1993. *Outside in the Teaching Machine*. London: Routledge.

Sullivan, Deborah, and Rose Weitz. 1988. *Labor Pains: Modern Midwives and Home Birth*. New Haven: Yale University Press.

Susie, Debra. 1988. *In the Way of Our Grandmothers: A Cultural View of Twentieth Century Midwifery in Florida*. Athens: University of Georgia Press.

PART TWO

Legislation, Integration, and Its Challenges

INTRODUCTION

Following on the heels of the critical and reflective analyses of the historical context and notion of tradition presented by Biggs and MacDonald respectively, the chapters in Part II address the key contemporary issues of legislation and integration and the challenges that these both pose for midwifery as a social movement, for the way that midwives practise, and for the manner in which midwives are compensated for services rendered to clients. We begin with practising midwife, midwifery educator, and social scientist Vicki Van Wagner, who writes on the complicated decision to seek legal regulation of midwifery in Ontario in the early 1980s. She begins by situating this decision within the context of a lively debate in the North American midwifery community about the role of midwifery legislation and professionalization. Despite its acknowledged risks, Van Wagner argues that there were good reasons why midwives and their supporters in Ontario chose to actively pursue legislation. She explores the argument that state regulation and funding are vital to the survival of midwifery and shows how an awareness of the dangers of regulation has helped the midwifery movement to craft regulation that arguably strengthens midwifery and at the same time expands birthing women's choices.

The unique situation that emerged in Quebec when the government decided first to *experiment* with the practice of midwifery before announcing its intention to legalize it in 1999 is the focus of chapter 4. Author and health care researcher Hélène Vadeboncoeur attempts to answer the pivotal question as to why this alternative path was taken by giving the reader a detailed description of the process and outcome of the midwifery evaluation study in Quebec and the reactions to its outcomes by various stakeholders. She argues that several factors influenced the Quebec decision to experiment despite the unanimous recommendation by women's groups, midwifery organizations, and a government-appointed task force to avoid this step and instead move quickly toward legislation. These factors include the absence of a larger review of health professions in Quebec, disharmony among provincial midwives, and most of all, the fierce opposition to midwifery legislation from medical associations.

In the third chapter in this section, midwifery educators Jude Kornelsen and Elaine Carty expand upon the theme of interprofessional relationships and the challenges they raise to integration once enabling legislation has been passed. They describe how the integration of midwives into the health care system in B.C. has not gone as smoothly as anticipated due in large part to the resistance mounted by some members of the medical community, as well as anxiety expressed on the part of the nursing profession. Through survey and interview data, Kornelsen and Carty explore the relationships between midwives and physicians, and midwives and nurses, comparing professional and interpersonal perspectives across pre- and post-legislation periods. They highlight the key areas of controversy between midwives and the two other professional groups and suggest ways that an improved collegial working environment could be achieved.

The issues of legislation and regulation are teased apart from the issue of public funding in the chapter that follows by practising midwife and midwifery educator Susan James and sociologist Ivy Lynn Bourgeault. Though certification and public funding are often seen as inseparable, the case of the midwifery integration process in Alberta has proven this assumption wrong. The authors outline how this came to be so through the confluence of internal tensions within the Alberta midwifery community, the comparative strength of other health care interest groups, the reluctance of other state actors and agencies to support midwifery, and the broader influence of the structure of the health care system. Together these factors helped to tip the scale in the direction of not publicly funding midwifery services. By way of contrast, the authors discuss how different circumstances in other provinces, most notably Ontario, worked in the opposite direction – coverage of midwifery services within the public health care system. James and Bourgeault conclude by highlighting the critical implications this decision has had on the midwifery community in Alberta.

Our final chapter in this section is a self-reflective piece on midwifery integration by practising midwife and midwifery educator Mary Sharpe. She explores the evolution of midwifery through the lens of sociologist Dorothy Smith's theory on texts, relations of ruling, and ideo-logical practices. Through interviews with newly legislated midwives and her own personal reflections of twenty years of midwifery practice in Ontario (first as a lay midwife, then as a registered midwife), Sharpe argues that the "texts" midwives draw upon frame women's experiences in ways that may limit some types of midwifery care while at the same time support other styles of practices, offering protection to birthing women, midwives, and the profession of midwifery in different ways. Sharpe then draws out how these "relations of ruling" were revealed in a personal way when she acted as midwife to her daughter.

Taken together, these insightful and partly reflective pieces help introduce the reader to the dynamic process midwifery integration entails across Canada and the critical factors and key decisions that have had and continue to have an impact on the profession as it evolves in its new provincial regulatory environments.

3

Why Legislation?: Using Regulation to Strengthen Midwifery

Vicki Van Wagner

PREFACE

This paper was originally written in 1994, just months after the legal recognition of midwifery in Ontario, to explore and explain the reasons why midwives like myself became strong advocates for midwifery legislation. The idea of including the paper in this book has given me the opportunity to reflect on the paper from the perspective provided both by the years that have passed since the passing of the Midwifery Act in Ontario and through discussion with other Canadian midwives who have worked towards midwifery legislation in their provinces.

INTRODUCTION

In the late 1970s I was a young and idealistic pregnant woman, living in rural southern Ontario and hoping to have a home birth. I searched for a caregiver. I could not discover any midwives in my community or in any other part of the province. I was very relieved to find a physician who still attended home births in Toronto and I made plans to travel into the city to give birth in a friend's home. As I awaited my due date, I struggled with the fact that there were no midwives to attend me in my own community and that the legal status of midwifery in Canada was at best unclear and at worst illegal. My family background is, in part, Dutch, and I knew that midwives and home birth were common in the Netherlands. I also knew that there were midwives practising underground in some parts of the U.S., that midwives were seen as a respected part of the health care system in Europe, and that midwives were delivering babies in most parts of the world. As my interest grew,

I learned that two of my great-grandmothers had worked as midwives, one informally in Ontario, the other in England prior to immigration. My father and his siblings had been born at home on Sheridan Avenue in the west end of Toronto, with my great-grandmother in attendance. It didn't make any sense to me that midwives were not part of our health care system.

By 1980, I was an apprentice midwife in the small "lay" midwifery community in Toronto. What has come to be known as "the midwifery movement" in North America had just begun to organize. The women who sought out midwives found care within the traditional system authoritarian, restrictive, and impersonal. They wanted choices and control over the way they gave birth. We were sceptical about the ability of the government or of institutions to respond to women's needs. If we did not ensure that we could continue to provide a different kind of maternity care, then who would? As midwives, we decided to answer the need for care that focused on the woman rather than on medical procedures and hospital routines, despite our unclear legal status.

At meetings of the newly formed Ontario Association of Midwives (OAM) we began to discuss the pros and cons of establishing standards and regulations for our own practice and about whether midwifery should be "legal." We were aware of a lively debate in the U.S. about what was being called "the pros and cons of licensure" (Solares 1977). The concepts of shared standards of practice, or even voluntary regulation, were looked at with a degree of suspicion by most within our group. We were a mixture of those who had trained by apprenticeship or in formal programs in other countries, some who had nursing backgrounds and some who did not. We had all chosen to practise outside the system without legal protection because we held strong convictions about the need to create alternatives to conventional maternity care.

In this context, my initial response to the debate about legislation was to favour staying outside of formal regulation and training. It seemed to many of us that involvement with regulation could create pressure for midwifery to conform to medical standards of practice and create hierarchical models of training and practice that would undermine women's choices. Professionalization, we argued, could lead us away from our roots as advocates for, and partners with, women. We were also aware that in many countries where midwifery was the norm women critiqued midwifery care in some of the same terms that we had critiqued obstetrics, i.e. that care was increasingly technological, that women were not seen as active participants in their care, that choices about where and how to give birth were restricted. Midwifery, like obstetrics, had become medicalized and impersonal and had simultaneously lost autonomy, status, and an ability to respond to women's needs. Midwives who worked within the health care system, it seemed, were increasingly put in the position of being assistants to physicians or physician extenders rather than using their skills to preserve and promote birth as a healthy process and a significant emotional and social event in women's lives. We feared that working toward midwifery legislation and toward the integration of midwives into the health care system could create a new care provider but not meet the needs of the women who were demanding a different kind of care.

Many of us felt that women and midwives together were creating a kind of care that could only grow outside of institutions. The basic principles of this care – respect for birth as a normal physiologic process and for women as decision makers – were nurtured by what we called continuity of care, i.e., care by a midwife whom the woman knew. These basic principles seemed at the time antithetical to a system that was often authoritarian, fragmented, and routinized. Regulation, institutionalization, and medicalization seemed inextricably intertwined, and like many feminist projects of the time, the midwifery movement tended to see both medicine and government as patriarchal monoliths.[1] Regulation, we feared, could interfere with the growth of midwifery as a real alternative, restricting the autonomy of the midwife by imposing regulated standards of practice, limiting opportunities for midwifery training by moving control of education into institutions, and interfering with the partnership of midwives and women that put women at the centre of childbearing. There was a sense of purity about keeping our project outside of the system that we wanted to preserve.

Alternatives to regulation, voluntary credentialing and decriminalization, were posed in order to allow and recognize midwifery practice without imposing regulation. These systems avoided both regulation by others, i.e. another profession or health body, or regulation by peers, i.e., "self-regulation." They offered protection from legal harassment and the opportunity to remain outside the system. These alternatives had appeal, yet as the debate continued, many in our group began to be uncomfortable about maintaining a position that advocated staying outside the health care system. Some of us began to feel restricted by elements of lay midwifery ideology that seemed to prescribe a narrow view of how women should give birth, raise children, and construct their families. Midwives who had worked as part of the health care system in other countries spoke about how beneficial it could be for midwives to work both inside the hospital and continue to attend home births. They spoke of serving a much more diverse community and

offering choices to women that were not open to unregulated midwives. Some of us increasingly saw lack of legal recognition as a lack of
respect for both midwives and the women who wanted midwifery care.
We began to focus on issues like autonomous practice, women's
choices, choice of birth place, and continuity of care as keys to the kind
of midwifery we advocated rather than remaining outside the system.

By 1983, with the announcement of the Health Professions Legislative Review (HPLR) in Ontario, our young community was plunged
into making decisions about whether to participate and seek legislation
to recognize midwifery as a regulated health profession. Many of us
saw the HPLR as an opportunity that might come only once in our life-
times. As the debate heated up, I was surprised to find myself increasingly aware of the limitations of avoiding integration of midwifery into
the health care system and of the potential benefits of regulation. I was
not alone. A growing number of midwives and childbearing women began to see that the dangers we had identified with regulation were not
inevitable consequences and that some of the benefits of being outside
of the system may have been idealized. Many of us felt that alternatives
such as decriminalization were not viable in the Ontario system[2] as
they meant that although midwifery might not be illegal it would still
remain on the fringe of the maternity care system. This did not seem
adequate as midwifery, unlike some other alternative health systems,
needs to interact with medicine and nursing and the hospital system,
when, for example, complications arise during the birth process. We
began to realize that although we did not want to be controlled by the
system, we wanted to become a part of it.[3]

As we questioned our assumptions about integration into the health
care system as having only a negative effect, it made space for other
questions to arise. Why shouldn't midwifery be respected and available
in a publicly funded system? Why shouldn't governments that funded
medicine and medical education fund midwifery care and education?
Could we create a kind of regulation that would support midwifery
and women's choices in childbirth? We began to think that perhaps we
did not have to choose between being inside (i.e. being co-opted) and
being outside (being limited). Perhaps there were creative alternatives
to explore that would challenge the traditional maternity care system
through midwifery regulation. The debate continued and by 1984 both
midwifery and consumer organizations made regulation of midwifery
central goals.

The advantages of pursing midwifery legislation seemed to fall into
five main themes, which I will explore in this chapter: (1) facing the inevitable and setting the agenda; (2) increasing access to midwifery care;

(3) ensuring the survival of the profession; (4) improving how mid-wives could provide care; and (5) increasing access to practice. The story of how midwifery, despite significant opposition, became part of the health care system in Ontario has been told elsewhere (Van Wagner 1988, 1991; Kaufman 1998; Bourgeault 1996). My goal in this chapter is to describe why midwives in Ontario chose to actively pursue legisla-tion, despite acknowledging its risks, and why many of us continue to believe that without regulation midwifery could not thrive or perhaps even survive. As a midwife who practised outside the health care sys-tem for thirteen years prior to regulation in Ontario and who has con-tinued to practise since, I bring the perspective of having lived through the transition from being a "lay midwife" to a registered midwife and "regulated health professional." I also bring the point of view of some-one who became a strong advocate of midwifery legislation.

WHY LEGISLATION?

Facing the Inevitable and Setting the Agenda

In Ontario, one of the most pressing arguments for legislation came with the launching of the HPLR in 1983. The climate of legal contro-versy over midwifery had stimulated both medical and nursing organi-zations to take positions on the regulation of midwifery. Both made it clear to the HPLR that midwives should be regulated and work only in hospitals. They advocated a model much like that of the U.S., with mid-wifery as a specialty of nursing, taught at the master's degree level and regulated under the College of Nurses (CNO 1983 and OMA 1985).

There were other reasons that some form of midwifery regulation seemed inevitable. Given Canada's anomalous status as the only West-ern country without legislation and given the growing financial crisis in the health care system, midwifery seemed an obvious answer to the overuse of expensive physicians' services in the Canadian health care system (York 1987; Rachlis and Kushner 1989). In addition, the steady decrease in the number of family physicians doing obstetrics in most provinces, particularly Ontario, had left normal childbirth largely in the hands of obstetricians, specialists trained in dealing with pathology and performing surgery (Kaczorowski and Levitt 2000; Loftsky 1996, 1998; McKendry 1999). Midwifery fit in with an emerging discussion of the need to establish alternatives to physician- and hospital-based care, which was reflected in the reports of several committees estab-lished to make recommendations about change in the health care sys-tem (Epp 1986; Evans 1987; Podborski 1987). Midwives seemed the obvious answer, not just to the financial problems of using specialists to provide primary care but to the overuse of technological and pharmaceutical interventions in maternity care.

As these trends emerged in the early 1980s, it became clear to many of us in the Ontario midwifery organizations that some form of midwifery regulation was coming. It seemed of vital importance for midwives and the women whose concerns and demands had created the Ontario model of midwifery care to be involved in defining that regulation. Otherwise, we feared, midwifery would become just another kind of decoration in the hospital labour room, leaving the conditions under which women gave birth largely unchanged.

The Association of Ontario Midwives (AOM) had formed in 1984 from the unification of the OAM and the Ontario Nurse Midwives Association (ONMA), an organization of nurses who were also midwives. The AOM and the consumer organization that formed to support midwives, the Midwifery Task Force of Ontario (MTFO), decided that they would work together toward regulation, but not without clear conditions. They established a set of criteria they felt were critical to creating a system that would not be compromised by legislation. The only form of regulation they supported had to establish midwifery as a self-governing profession separate from medicine and nursing and to allow for direct-entry midwifery education. Regulation was also only desirable if it preserved and strengthened the basic principles of the model of midwifery care, which had evolved in response to women's demands (i.e. childbirth as a normal physiologic process, continuity of care, choice of birth place, and informed choice). Given the context of the Canadian health insurance system, government funding of midwifery services was also a critical aspect of regulation. Regulation can be seen as a necessary step toward the funding of midwifery services, essential but not sufficient to achieve integration into the health care system. Without funding midwives are forced to compete with a fully funded parallel service (see James and Bourgeault, this volume).

At first, given the power of the medical and the nursing professions in the province of Ontario, the obstacles seemed insurmountable. Policy makers and politicians predicted that the plan would not succeed and offered the midwifery organizations various compromises: legal recognition could be worked out if only we would accept that midwives had to be nurses first; if we could agree to work in hospitals only, then self-governing status could be assured. Our organizations refused to compromise. Regulation in itself was not seen as the goal, and it was certainly not sought at any price. We would accept regulation as an inevitable part of continuing to practise in Ontario, but sought to ensure that midwives and the childbearing women they served set the agenda.

Access to Care

In considering the potential risks and benefits of midwifery regulation we realized that there were problems with remaining outside the system that restricted many women's access to midwifery care. Lack of public funding for midwifery care, lack of legal status and therefore credibility of midwives, and lack of access to hospital privileges and therefore the ability to provide primary care in the hospital setting, all worked to narrow the accessibility and the broader appeal of midwifery. Thus, one of the most compelling motivations to seek legislation came from the desire to make midwifery care accessible to a larger and more diverse group of women.

Working outside the system meant having to charge privately for our services. This often made our care inaccessible to poor women and working-class women and to those who could not prioritize their childbirth care as an expense within their family's income. Communities that could not support a "private" practice did not have access to midwifery. Many midwives in Canada made efforts to reduce financial barriers, through using sliding fee scales and sometimes providing free care, a practice that is still common in provinces where midwives practise without government support. This was (and is) an imperfect and at best temporary solution to the access issue. As medical care in Canada is completely covered by government insurance, even with a sliding fee scale, choosing a midwife meant a financial burden that the choice of medical care did not entail. Moreover, given that midwives often report difficulties in earning a living or even covering their costs, without public funding it is difficult for midwives to continue to practise (Kilthei 1989).

Practice outside the system also meant that many women did not know about the option of choosing midwifery care. This was reinforced by the fact that outside regulation, midwives could only provide primary care to women choosing home birth. As a vast majority of Ontario women choose hospital birth this meant that access to the choice of midwifery care was extremely limited. Without regulation many thought midwifery was illegal or an alternative on the fringe of acceptable practice. These factors, combined with the cost of care, meant that the women who sought out midwives tended to be well educated, to be motivated by a critique of the current system, to have the skills and confidence to seek out an alternative caregiver, and to be affluent or committed enough to pay for services (Tyson 1991; DeClercq 1992; Rooks 1997).

This in turn meant that many groups of women who often face barriers in accessing health care, such as immigrant women, Aboriginal

women, and teens, did not have access to midwifery care. Many practising midwives made real efforts to reach out to these groups, but the
barriers of legitimacy and cost were often more than individual midwives could overcome (Cameron and Kilthei 1993; Midwives Collective 1993). This issue of access for marginalized women was a
particularly important issue in the decision to seek regulation. Research
about midwifery care in the U.S. indicates that midwives can make a
real difference when caring for women usually considered to be at high
risk for socio-economic reasons, reducing rates of intervention, prema-
turity, and perinatal mortality (Rooks 1997). We came to see that underground, alternative care excluded those women who might benefit
most from midwifery care (Van Wagner 1988). To avoid regulation and
integration into the health care system began to seem to many midwifery activists, including myself, to be a form of elitism.

Survival of the Midwifery Profession

Altruistic motivations aside, advocates of legal recognition also believed that legislation was critical to the survival of the profession and,
often, to the survival of individual practitioners. Although the movement was vital, it was small and fragile. During the 1970s and 1980s in
North America there were constant and ongoing court battles involving midwives. In Canada, there were highly publicized inquests and
criminal cases in Nova Scotia, Quebec, Ontario, Manitoba, Alberta,
and British Columbia. These cost the parents and the midwives involved, as well as their families and supporters, time, money, and untold stress. Having been involved in a very difficult legal battle myself
in 1985 after the death of a baby whose birth I attended at home, I became even more convinced that professional regulation was essential to
the survival of midwifery. Other health care workers face review within
practice settings and by professional bodies rather than in the courts.
The goal of professional review is mainly to improve practice through
discussion with peers rather than to lay blame. It is important to note
that without legislation, midwives are not free from regulation through
coroner's inquests and the criminal justice system. This form of regulation of midwifery is crude, sensational, punitive, and costly.[4] It is negative not only for the individual parents and caregivers but in its effects
on the public perception of midwifery. Asking midwives to continue to
practise in such an environment seemed unrealistic and unfair.

Across the continent, many midwives were leaving practice just as
they had gained experience and confidence (Sullivan and Weitz 1988).
Some remained involved as vocal advocates of midwifery, writing
books and lecturing, but not practising. Others left midwifery for other

careers. In the U.S., many lay midwives went to nursing school in order to become certified nurse-midwives (CNM), citing the need for legitimacy in order to be able to practise openly and earn a living without the fear of the legal problems that come from lack of status (Nicols 1999). In many provinces, the number of midwives practising declined in the early 1990s, especially in British Columbia, where difficult legal cases and negative publicity dramatically reduced consumer demand.

In Ontario, the promise of imminent legislation created a positive climate and visibility, with a flurry of positive press coverage as the government moved closer to integration and a rivalry between political parties for who was going to take credit for supporting midwifery legislation (Lankin 1994). Yet even in this environment, the number of midwives did not grow and new practitioners often could not find enough clients to establish a viable practice.

Alan Solares, the health policy analyst in California who wrote about the dangers of midwifery professionalization and a passionate advocate of systems other than licensure, made a dramatic turn in 1990, arguing that the profession would not survive without legislation: "Midwifery is in the midst of a quiet crisis. The number of homebirths has declined. The number of midwives practising has declined. Most importantly, midwives are serving a tiny percentage of pregnant women and their families. Midwifery is failing to achieve its extraordinary potential" (1990). When Solares was writing, thirty direct-entry midwives who worked outside the system were in the midst of court battles in California alone, with the profession in a "constant state of crisis." But his article, titled "The Key to Keeping Midwifery Alive in the 1990s," focused on less dramatic reasons for the need for midwifery legislation. Midwives in the U.S., he argued, can't attract enough clients to survive in a system that does not recognize them because they do not have access to third-party insurance or Medicaid payments. The problem of lack of funding was also highlighted by the midwives interviewed by Sullivan and Weitz in their 1988 comparison of unlicensed midwives with licensed midwives in two U.S. states. It is also illustrated by the current situation of midwives in Alberta (see James and Bourgeault, this volume).

Solares also argued that as the baby boomers had reached the end of their childbearing years the demand for midwives as a counter-culture alternative had faded. Younger women, he argued, were not choosing midwifery care. Midwifery needed the credibility that regulation would bring to reach out to the next generation of childbearing women. The system of unofficial regulation he had previously advocated, involving clients taking responsibility for making informed choices about who they wanted to deliver their babies without need for formal evaluation and credentialing, assumed a well-educated and highly motivated client, and in Solares' view, was seriously limiting midwifery's growth and potential contribution.

A decade later there continues to be dispute and debate about whether direct-entry midwifery in the U.S. is growing or declining. Rooks (1997) and Declercq (1992), for example, argue using birth certificate data that direct-entry midwives attend less than one per cent of births in the country. However, as both authors acknowledge, this is very difficult to assess given that direct-entry midwives working in illegal states may not sign birth certificates. Although some direct-entry midwives are regulated, many are not and most are seen as remaining outside the system. Whether or not the research based on birth certificate data is reflective of practice, some direct-entry midwives in the U.S. express concerns about whether without funding or access to hospital practice they can really be accessible to a significant proportion of women. A lively debate on this subject was held at the Summit on the Future of Midwifery held by the Seattle Midwifery School in January 1999.

In Ontario, midwives have moved from serving about 1 per cent of the population to 6 per cent in the first ten years post-legislation. With about 25 per cent of these births taking place at home, more women certainly have access to home birth, but the largest increase in the number of women choosing midwifery in Ontario is among those choosing hospital birth (Kaufman 1999; Katherine 2003). At the current rate of growth, midwives will be serving about 20 per cent of the Ontario population by the year 2020 (AOM, CMO, MEP, 2000). This growth will be through both the government-funded midwifery education program and the registration of midwives from other jurisdictions through the International Midwifery Pre-Registration Programme or the program that preceded it, the College of Midwives of Ontario's (CMO) registration assessment process (Prior Learning and Experience Assessment or PLEA), both of which have been supported by government funds.

Improving Midwifery Care

One of the central arguments of those opposed to legislation is that regulation entails the imposition of restrictive standards of practice (De Vries 1989). Although those of us who were advocates of legislation in Ontario did not accept the imposition of *medical* standards of practice as part of regulation, we saw regulation as helping strengthen *midwifery* standards of practice. We argued that care would be improved by standards defined by midwives in collaboration with childbearing women and other health professionals.

Similar to many other midwives working outside the system, Ontario midwives adopted voluntary standards and complaints procedures prior to regulation. We did this not simply because we wanted to set our own standards before standards were imposed by another profession, though this was certainly the case. We also wanted to provide an opportunity for midwives and their clients to examine and evaluate midwifery practice.

Many Ontario midwives looked to the Netherlands as an example of a country where home birth and midwifery have survived and provided an ongoing alternative to the medicalization of birth that has happened in other industrialized countries. Many Ontario midwives, including myself, travelled to the Netherlands to learn about the system first hand. Dutch midwives and obstetricians argue for a clear set of standards that differentiate normal birth – the province of the midwife – from abnormality – the province of the obstetrician – in order to provide care appropriately. They do not see regulation or standards of practice as a threat to normal birth or to midwives' autonomy. Dutch midwives have fought to maintain regulation that allows midwives rather than physicians to determine the parameters of low and high risk. Ontario midwives saw the Netherlands as living proof of the fact that it is not regulation in and of itself that is problematic but the nature of the regulation.

We hoped that regulation and standards would improve the quality of women's care by helping to establish a more cooperative relationship between medicine and midwifery. Both the regulated and unregulated midwives interviewed by Sullivan and Weitz (1988) saw access to consultation with medicine as one of the most important benefits of regulation. In Ontario, the lengthy process of debate and consultation with medical organizations that was part of the development of the CMO's *Indications for Mandatory Discussion, Consultation and Transfer of Care* is credited with assisting midwives to gain access to hospital privileges and develop positive working relationships with consultants. Although this document helps support safe practice by providing guidelines for midwives about when to consult with, or transfer care to, a physician, these standards are neither prescriptive nor restrictive and expect the midwife to use her clinical judgment to identify the specific situations in which medical care is recommended. For example, prolonged labour and prolonged rupture of membranes are indications for consultation with a physician. But it is the midwife who decides how to define these terms, when to consult an obstetrician, or when to transport to hospital in the case of a home birth. Another example is the CMO's list of contraindications to home birth. The number of contraindications is very small (less than thirty-seven weeks' or more than

forty-three weeks' gestation, breech presentation, and multiple pregnancy), although there are other situations in which a home birth is not
appropriate and transfer of care to a specialist is indicated. Midwives
are expected to use their own judgment and the consultation process to
help the woman determine the appropriate place of birth. The woman
is recognized as the primary decision maker, and the midwife is recognized as an expert at determining when to recommend hospital birth or
medical care.

Midwives and social scientists have expressed concern that access to
working in the hospital may bring added pressure to conform to local
medical standards and can lead to more prescriptive protocols for practice than the CMO outlines for midwives (Kilthei 1989; De Vries 1989;
Bourgeault 1996; Sharpe 1997). The restrictions that come with
awareness of conformity to medical standards of care are not, in my
view, a result of regulation or hospital privileges. Midwives practising
outside the system also need to consult with and possibly transfer care
to physicians. Having practised prior to regulation, I would observe
that unregulated or "illegal" midwives have to be equally aware of,
and are sometimes more vulnerable to, the standards of the local medical community in which they practise. Over and above regulation, developments and trends in medical practice inevitably influence
midwifery. Indeed, pressures on midwives working outside of regulation to recommend testing or treatment based on medical standards
(such as screening for gestational diabetes or screening and treatment
for Group B streptococcus infection) are very similar to regulated midwives. Changes in practice come from changing community standards
more than with regulation.

Those of us who advocated regulation saw that establishing midwifery standards of practice could expand midwives' ability to promote and protect their approach to care. We felt that with regulation
we would be in a better position not only to defend midwifery practices
to medical and nursing colleagues but also to share them with other
practitioners. Integration allows midwives access to hospital committees that develop protocols for care and participation in the teaching of
medical and nursing students. We felt we would have a chance to affect
maternity care in ways that could reach beyond midwives and their clients to the system as a whole.

Access to Practice and Education

Ontario midwifery organizations also saw the establishment of standards of education as a positive feature of regulation. Many of us who
had trained by apprenticeship prior to regulation hoped to build on the

strengths of this approach, but we also wanted to address some of the problems we saw in informal education (see Benoit and Davis-Floyd, this volume). These problems included the lack of any of the financial support usually available to students, lack of a peer group to facilitate academic learning, and in some cases, the lack of a structured curriculum. Access to apprenticeship was very limited and the training often lengthy. We saw that a recognized education program would allow midwifery students exposure to the health care system and opportunities to learn from and work as colleagues with physicians and nurses, in a way that is not possible if midwives are outsiders to the health care system. Learning both in hospital and community settings allows the development of a wide range of skills needed for safe midwifery practice. Access to formal education could also be seen to be fairer, with candidates with appropriate qualifications being considered on an equal basis, rather than in accordance with a particular midwife's demands.

The formal education program developed in Ontario (see Kaufman and Soderstrom, this volume) also places the midwifery student's education in the context of woman-centred care and continuity of care. Although critics of formal education have worried that formal education would become medicalized and distant from women's needs or concerns, it seemed both possible and desirable to integrate some of the characteristics of an apprenticeship system into formal education to protect against this danger of institutionalization. We hoped that the tendencies of formal education to create a distance between the "professional" and the "patient" could be balanced by educating midwives within a model of continuity of care and fostering a strong relationship between the student and the women to whom she is providing care.

The issue of equitable access to midwifery is not just limited to who has access to care but also extends to the issue of who has access to practising as a midwife. Although unregulated midwifery practice seems open, it presents serious barriers. Benoit (1989) points out in her work on traditional midwifery practice in Newfoundland that the benefits of practice outside the system can be overestimated and romanticized. Many women were unwilling to practice in a semi-legal environment, particularly midwives educated in other countries where midwifery was an integral part of the health care system. Those who were new immigrants often stated that they did not want to challenge the established system in a new country (see Nestel and Ford and Van Wagner, this volume). Those from all backgrounds who needed a relatively secure income or who could not risk the chance of an expensive and stressful legal case could not choose midwifery as a career. One of my midwifery teachers, Jude Pustil, was among the first group of practitioners in Ontario's midwifery revival. She stopped practising in the

1980s because she was a single mother and couldn't take the chance of a criminal charge and financial ruin as the sole parent of her children. This is a typical story of unregulated midwifery in North America and contributes to the high turnover in unregulated practice discussed by Solares (1990).

CAN REGULATION STRENGTHEN MIDWIFERY?

Ontario midwives and consumers approached the establishment of regulation with an awareness of the debates about the dangers of institutionalization and professionalization. We came to believe that it was possible to create a form of regulation that would benefit midwifery. Rather than being a threat to the woman-centred model of care that had evolved outside of the health care system, regulation was a strategy for midwifery's growth and development. To date, the debate about midwifery regulation has been largely theoretical. Midwifery policy in Ontario has been seen by some as a model for how a social change movement can work toward feminist goals (Adamson et al. 1988; Armstrong and Armstrong 1996; Shroff 1997). There has also been critique and re-examination of the process from both inside and outside the midwifery community and from many different perspectives (Tyson 2001; Nestel, this volume; Bourgeault 1996; Sharpe, this volume). Over the next few decades, as the impact of midwifery legislation in Canada begins to emerge, we will be able to answer in a very practical way some of the questions raised by this debate.

Some trends are already emerging, leading to new questions and challenges. After a decade of regulation in Ontario, many more women now have access to midwifery care and to home birth. Midwives report that with universal funding, they are serving a more diverse population and practices are expanding and developing around the province. The population of midwives has more than quadrupled and has become increasingly diverse (see Ford and Van Wagner, this volume). Midwifery organizations predict that within twenty years midwives will be serving a significant proportion of the population (20%) and will have become an integral part of the health care system (AOM, CMO, MEP, 2000).

Nearly a decade after the model of choice of birth place, informed choice, and continuity of care was put at the centre of regulation in Ontario, discussions of the need to expand and create flexibility within the model have begun to emerge (Tyson 2001; Cameron 2000). This signals a growing security in the midwifery community that allows a shift in focus from protection to experimentation and change. Midwifery faces the challenges of responding to the needs of an expanding client population, a changing health care system, and the needs of midwives to create sustainable ways to practise in many different communities. How will the midwifery community balance the need to maintain the original principles of the "movement" and the need to change and grow?

Are women's choices restricted or expanded by the formalization of standards of practice? We do know that midwives are providing choice of birth place and continuity of care to their clients and that the number of women choosing both midwifery care and home birth has increased since regulation. Statistics collected by the AOM, the only body presently collecting such data, show that midwives are continuing to provide a low intervention alternative to medical care (Kaufman 1999). Further research is needed to understand in what ways midwives' practice and women's choices are influenced by greater integration with the medical community and how these kinds of influences are perceived by midwives and clients.

Having worked both inside and outside the system, I would argue that integration of midwifery simultaneously allows midwives to provide quality care while supporting autonomous practice. This is illustrated by the example of regulated midwives' access to laboratory testing and prescribing of drugs. Prior to regulation all midwives and their clients had to rely on physicians to fill in the gaps in the "illegal" midwife's ability to provide primary care. We are also more independent in cases where clients choose or need hospital birth. Prior to regulation, there could be a disincentive (for both the woman and the midwife) to transport into the hospital in a situation when hospital birth might offer safer care in that the midwife had to automatically hand over care to a physician. For me, one of the most satisfying aspects of having hospital privileges is in being able to continue to participate in the care of women who have planned home births but need to give birth in the hospital. In the past, like all unregulated midwives, I was relegated to the role of support person once in the hospital and my clients had to receive care from unknown caregivers.

Practising inside the system has also led me to experience the benefits of self-regulation rather than regulation by the courts. Having been involved in the review of cases involving perinatal mortality and morbidity both before and after regulation, I understand quite personally the difference between having my practice scrutinized as non-regulated care provider and as a registered midwife. I have been extremely grateful to participate, post-regulation, in a process of review that focuses on what caregivers can learn to improve care, rather than on whether I had the right to provide midwifery care. A basic acceptance of midwifery and home birth as part of the system allows parents who have lost a baby to focus on grieving rather than on defending their choices and their care-givers. Of course regulation does not mean that midwives will never again face court challenges. Like other health professionals, regulated midwives may be asked to participate in a coroner's inquest or be subject to a civil suit. It is the conditions under which this participation takes place that I would argue are changed for the better by regulation.

The model of practice that has been adopted across Canada, requir-ing midwives to attend women in their choice of birth place and to pro-vide continuity of care and informed choice, is unique in the world and admired internationally. The model is designed to preserve elements of pre-regulation practice, such as the midwifery philosophy of birth as a normal, healthy process, and to safeguard against the dangers seen in regulation and integration into the system – medicalization, fragmenta-tion of the client-caregiver relationship, and restricted client choices. International experience has shown that continuity of care and choice of birth place are vulnerable aspects of the model (Kirkham and Per-kins 1997). Will Canadian midwifery be able to be part of the health care system and maintain these aspects of midwifery care? Will the model of midwifery care as it has been established in Canada be flexi-ble enough for midwifery to meet the needs of childbearing women and the health care system in such a geographically diverse country, and to sustain a growing profession?

There is also, of course, the likelihood that what some of us may see as a loss or gain with regulation, others may see as the opposite. Some opponents of regulation mourn the loss of a small homogenous clien-tele who share the same values and beliefs as the midwife. Others saw "lay midwifery" ideology as restrictive, and welcome a broadening of midwifery's philosophy from what can be seen as a narrow and pre-scriptive "alternative lifestyle" approach to one that is more open to a diversity of women and perspectives on childbirth.

Much has changed and many questions, opportunities, and problems remain. Legal, funded midwifery in Ontario is still in development and any conclusions about its impact must be seen as very preliminary. The profession is in a period of rapid change and development. The major-ity of practitioners in the province have less than five years of experi-ence. It may be far too early to evaluate many of the issues raised and to distinguish between the impact of regulation and the impact of rapid change and growth. Such an analysis deserves much more long-term and detailed research and review. Health policy scholar and activist Pat Armstrong (1999), for example, warns midwives and feminist scholars not to focus on the impact of regulation to the extent of being blinded to many larger social and political forces currently rocking the Canadian health care system.

In my experience as a practitioner in Ontario, there are many ways in which legislation, when combined with government funding of midwifery services, has worked to strengthen midwifery and expand women's choices in childbirth. Regulation, though, is only one part of what is needed for midwifery to thrive and to play an important role in the health care system. It is a necessary but not sufficient step toward the goals of changing childbirth taken on by the underground movement of twenty years ago.

NOTES

1 For an interesting discussion of a similar starting point see Emily Martin's reflections on how her views of medicine changed in "From Reproduction to HIV: Blurring Categories, Shifting Positions" in Ginsburg and Rapp 1995.

2 Another problem with the demand for decriminalization of midwifery comes from examining its origin in the feminist demand for the decriminalization of abortion. The decriminalization of abortion sought to avoid the prosecution of physicians (already regulated health professionals) for performing abortions, which were prohibited under the criminal code. The fight for the decriminalization of abortion was not, for the most part, a fight to allow unregulated abortion. When the abortion law was struck down, it removed only the criminal law prohibiting the procedure. All of the health regulations surrounding the practice of medicine remain and in effect regulate abortion. In this sense the use of the term in the debate about the legislation of midwifery is confusing and misleading.

3 Our struggles with the problems of choosing to work either inside or outside the system are not unlike what Adamson, Briskin, and McPhail (1988) identify as strategies of mainstreaming and disengagement. They argue that the women's movement has been characterized by a polarization between these two positions.

4 A personal note regarding the cost of regulation through the courts. In the 1985 case I was involved in the cost to the parents and midwives was over $100,000. Fundraising by the MTFO and the AOM raised $20,000. The remaining costs were covered personally by the parents and the midwives; through the generosity of our lawyers, who forgave a significant proportion of their fees; and through the Ontario Ombudsman's office, to whom we made a successful appeal to fund part of the costs.

REFERENCES

Adamson, N., L. Briskin, and M. McPhail. 1988. *Feminist Organizing for Change: The Contemporary Women's Movement in Canada.* Don Mills, ON: Oxford University Press.

Association of Ontario Midwives, College of Midwives of Ontario, and Ontario Midwifery Education Programme (ADM, CMO, MEP). 2000. *Midwives and the Future of the Ontario Health Care System.* Association of Ontario Midwives.

Armstrong, Pat. 1999. *Midwives and the Canadian Health Care System.* Presentation to the Professional Issues course of the Ontario Midwifery Education Programme. Toronto: Ryerson University.

Armstrong, Pat, and Hugh Armstrong. 1996. *Wasting Away: The Undermining of Canadian Health Care.* Toronto: Oxford University Press.

Benoit, Cecilia 1989. A Traditional Midwifery Practice: The Limits of Occupational Autonomy. *Canadian Review of Sociology and Anthropology* 26, no. 4.

Bourgeault, Ivy Lynn. 1996. Delivering Midwifery: An Examination of the Process and Outcome of the Incorporation of Midwifery in Ontario. Ph.D. dissertation, Graduate Department of Community Health, University of Toronto.

Cameron, Carol. 2000. *Midwifery in Canada.* The Future of Maternity Care in Canada Conference Proceedings. St Joseph's Health Centre.

Cameron, Carol, and Jane Kilthei. 1993. *Cost Effectiveness of Midwifery.* Association of Ontario Midwives.

College of Midwives of Ontario (CMO). 1994. *Indications for Planned Place of Birth.*

– 1999. *Indications for Mandatory Discussion, Consultation and Transfer of Care.*

College of Nurses of Ontario (CNO). 1983. *Submission to the Health Professions Legislative Review.*

Declercq, Eugene. 1992. The Transformation of American Midwifery: 1975 - 1988. *American Journal of Public Health* 82, no. 2.

De Vries, Raymond. 1989. Caregivers in Pregnancy and Childbirth. In *Effective Care in Pregnancy and Childbirth*, edited by I. Chalmers, M. Enkin, and M. Keirse. Oxford: Oxford University Press.

Epp, Jake. "Achieving Health For All: A Framework for Health Promotion." *Health Promotion* 1, no. 4 (1986).

Evans, J.R. *Toward a Shared Direction for Health in Ontario.* Ontario Health Review Panel, Ontario Ministry of Health, 1987.

Ginsburg, Fay, and Rayna Rapp. 1995. *Conceiving the New World Order: The Global Politics of Reproduction.* Berkeley: University of California Press.

Kaczorowski, J., and C. Levitt. 2000. Intrapartum Care by General Practitioners and Family Physicians: Provincial Trends from 1984–1985 to 1994–1995. *Canadian Family Physician* 46 (March).

Katherine, Wendy (Midwifery Co-ordinator, Ministry of Health and Long Term Care, Ontario). 2003. Personal conversation with author.

Kaufman, Karyn. 1998. A History of Ontario Midwifery. *SOGC Journal* 20, no.10: 976–81.

– 1999. *Outcomes of Midwifery Attended Births 1998.* Presentation to the Association of Ontario Midwives Annual General Meeting.

Kilthei, Jane. 1989. Dangers of Professionalization of Midwifery. *AOM Newsletter* 5, no. 1.

Kirkham, Maris, and E. Perkins, eds. 1997. *Reflections on Midwifery.* London: Bailliere Tindall.

Lankin, Francis. 1994. Presentation to the Relocating Birth Conference, University of Western Ontario, London.

Loftsky, Stan. 1996. Who Will Deliver Ontario's Children. *Ontario Medical Review* (March): 25–7.

– 1998. Obstetric Human Resources in Ontario 1996–97. *Ontario Medical Review* (November): 24–31.

McKendry, Rachel. 1999. Physicians for Ontario. *Report of the Fact Finder on Physician Resources in Ontario.* Ontario Ministry of Health and Long Term Care.

Midwives Collective of Toronto. 1993. *Midwives and Families: Social and Cultural Challenges.* Vancouver: Proceedings of the International Confederation of Midwives Congress.

Nichols, B.P. 1999. Personal communication to author at the Summit on the Future of Maternity Care. Seattle Midwifery School.

Ontario Medical Association (OMA). 1985. *Report of the Reproductive Care Committee.*

Podborski, Steve. *Health Promotion Matters in Ontario: Report of the Advisory Group on Health Promotion.* Ontario Ministry of Health, 1987.

Rachlis, Michael, and Carol Kushner. 1989. *Second Opinion: What's Wrong with Canada's Health System and How to Fix It.* Toronto: Collins.

Rooks, J.P. 1997. *Midwifery and Childbirth in America: The Past, Present and Potential Role of Midwives.* Philadelphia: Temple Hill University Press.

Sharpe, Mary. 1997. Ontario Midwifery in Transition: An Exploration of Midwives Perceptions of the Impact of Midwifery Legislation in its First Year. In *The New Midwifery: Reflections on Renaissance and Regulation,* edited by Farah Shroff. Toronto: The Women's Press.

Shroff, Farah, ed. 1997. *The New Midwifery: Reflections on Renaissance and Regulation.* Toronto: The Women's Press.

Solares, Alan. 1977. In *Safe Alternatives in Childbirth,* edited by D. Stewart and Lee Stewart. Chapel Hill: NAPSAC.

– 1990. The Key to Keeping Midwifery Alive in the 1990s. *Midwifery Today* 14: 30–1, 39.

Sullivan, Deborah, and Rose Weitz. 1988. *Labour Pains: Modern Midwives and Home Birth*. New Haven: Yale University Press.

Tyson, Holiday. 1991. 1001 Midwife Attended Home Births in Toronto 1983–1988. *Birth* 18, no.1: 14-19.

– 2001. The Integrity of Midwifery in Ontario and its Integrity into the Health Care System. *Association of Ontario Midwives Journal* 7, no. 1.

Van Wagner, Vicki 1988. Women Organizing for Midwifery. *Resources for Feminist Research* 17, no. 3: 115–18.

– 1991. With Woman: Community Midwifery. Unpublished master's thesis, York University.

York, Geoffrey. 1987. *The High Price of Health: A Patient's Guide to the Hazards of Medical Politics*. Toronto: Lorimer.

4

Delaying Legislation: The Quebec Experiment

Hélène Vadeboncoeur

Among the provinces that answered women's requests to legally recognize midwives, Quebec is the only one that decided to experiment with the practice of midwifery, in order to see, first, if legalization was indicated and, second, how midwifery could be organized and integrated into the health care system. In this chapter, I describe the experiment and the circumstances that led to this decision, the outcomes of the experimentation, and why the decision to experiment was made and the reactions to its outcomes. I also describe the subsequent announcement by the government to legalize midwifery in 1999 and the terms of this decision. We will see that several factors influenced the Quebec decision to experiment despite the unanimous recommendation of the legalization of midwifery by women's groups and midwifery organizations, as well as a government-appointed task force.

THE RE-EMERGENCE OF MIDWIFERY: FROM HOME BIRTHS TO BIRTH CENTRES

At the end of the 1970s, several events in Quebec revealed a social need to re-evaluate existing obstetrical practices and prompted changes that would accommodate women's demands around childbirth. The movement toward improved obstetrical care resulted in various attempts to transform the practice of obstetrics, including the creation of birthing rooms in some hospitals.

During the 1970s, some Quebec women had started to give birth at home, helped by friends who had given birth themselves and who, slowly, trained as midwives. Midwifery had never been declared illegal, although the conditions allowing the certification of midwives had not been in place for decades.[1] In 1977, for the first time, a group of consumers in Gaspésie, le Collectif de Matane, wrote a *manifeste* asking for the legalization of midwifery. Then, in 1980, the first midwives' associations, the Association des sages-femmes du Québec (ASFQ) was created by non-practising certified midwives, who lobbied the government to establish a College of Midwives (MSSS 1989). The same year, an association of consumer groups from different regions in Quebec in favour of humanizing childbirth called Naissance-renaissance was also born. Also that same year, a milestone event happened: there were simultaneously eleven regional conferences under the Quebec Public Health Association in collaboration with the Ministry of Social Affairs called "Accoucher ou se faire accoucher" (To Give Birth or To Be Delivered), where 10,000 participants, consumers, midwives, nurses, and a few doctors asked for family-centred and humanized childbirth practices, birth rooms, birth centres, and the legal recognition of midwifery (ASPQ 1981).

In 1986, another midwives' association was born: l'Alliance québécoise des sages-femmes praticiennes (AQSFP), formed mainly of lay or community midwives – and a few certified midwives – who had started practising at the end of the 1970s. This association worked in close collaboration with Naissance-Renaissance. It set up standards and an apprenticeship training program and was more active than the ASFQ (Vadeboncoeur et al. 1996). The same year, its members recommended the creation of pilot projects, in order to prepare for legalization (AQSFP 1986). There were around 200 midwives in these two associations, of whom between twenty and thirty were actively practising. There was some division among the midwives, and this played a role in the Quebec government's hesitation to legalize, as we will see later on (Vadeboncoeur et al. 1996).

In the beginning, the nurses' associations were in favour of nurse-midwives only, but in recent years the main union of nurses, the Fédération des infirmières et infirmiers du Québec, has agreed that midwifery should be a profession independent of nursing. All doctors' associations were also against the integration of midwives, despite a slowing down in the practice of obstetrics by doctors in the 1980s (Cohen 1991). They claimed that midwifery was outdated, dangerous (FMSQ and FMOQ 1989; *La Presse* 1989), or at best useless due to the excellent care doctors were providing women, who were, according to them, very satisfied with their services (CPMQ 1985).

Thus, in the 1980s there were two different midwives' associations in Quebec that made moves to obtain the legalization of their profession, there was lobbying by consumers for midwifery services, and there were several positive reports from interested groups. All recommended the legalization of midwifery, except the doctors' associations, although on rare occasions, a few individual doctors reacted differently (Gosselin et al. 1989). Starting in the late 1970s and through the 1980s, several committees were appointed by the government to explore the issues around the legalization of midwifery. One result of the work of one of these committees was a government publication supporting legalization of the practice of midwifery in the province (MSSS 1989), as well as a revised policy, the *Politique de périnatalité* (Québec 1993).

After ten years of lobbying by interested parties and a committee report recommending the integration of midwifery, the Quebec Liberal government decided, with Bill 4 in June 1990, to experiment with the practice of midwifery (Québec 1990). The year before, the minister of health, Thérèse Lavoie-Roux, had tried to convince the College of Physicians to modify the Medical Act in order to allow midwifery practice (see note 1). She was unsuccessful, and so decided to present a bill to the National Assembly. Because of impending elections, it was not adopted until 1990, under a new minister, Marc-Yvan Côté. Bill 4 had two objectives: to determine whether the legalization of midwifery was appropriate and, if so, to recommend how midwives could be integrated into the health care system. This decision to experiment went against the recommendations of the multidisciplinary Provincial Task Force on Midwifery[2] and against a general movement of women's groups and government organizations like the Conseil du statut de la femme, the Commission of Inquiry into Health and Social Services, and the Advisory Council on Social Affairs, all of whom favoured legalization. The decision was largely a compromise to satisfy the medical profession. In the next section I will examine if it succeeded.

DECIDING TO EXPERIMENT: TURNING OFF THE HEAT?

An Act Respecting the Practice of Midwifery within the Framework of Pilot Projects[3]

Bill 4 stated that midwifery would be examined in eight pilot projects for a period of five years. The projects could be administered by hospitals or local community health centres (CLSCs) or by a hospital and a CLSC together. Two provisional bodies were created. The first, the Committee on Admission to the Practice of Midwifery (Comité d'admission à la pratique des sages-femmes), or CAPM, was comprised of representatives of various bodies appointed by the government (among them three European midwives, a doctor, a nurse, and a consumer). It would set up an evaluation process for midwives interested in practising in the projects and certify those who completed it successfully. This involved evaluating their experience and their competencies through a stringent theoretical and clinical exam set up by an expert committee of the Université Laval. The CAPM would also establish a list of obstetrical and neonatal risks. The second committee, the Pilot Project Assessment Board (PPAB) (Conseil d'évaluation des projets-pilotes), would select the projects, monitor their implementation and the quality of the midwifery practice, and make its recommendations to the minister of health after a thorough evaluation study done by university researchers. This committee was comprised of two midwives, two users of midwifery services, one doctor, one nurse, one representative of the Association of Hospitals, one of the Fédération des CLSCs, and three representatives of interested ministries (Québec 1990).

Bill 4 launched the later creation of birthing centres where midwives could practise. In line with what the various studies and groups of women and midwives had identified as being important during the 1980s, the selection criteria for the projects included safety, continuity of care, an autonomous practice of midwifery, humanized care, and support from the community. After a lengthy selection process that took three years, eight pilot projects were chosen, including the already functioning midwifery project in the Puvirnituk Inuit community in northern Quebec. Each project had its own characteristics. Although the pilot projects could take place in hospitals, very few hospitals actually applied because of internal opposition or opposition from medical associations (Blais 1998), and those that did were unable to meet the PPAB criteria.

Apart from the already functioning project in Puvirnituk, in a small hospital, the chosen projects were all administered by CLSCs and were located across Quebec, including Montreal and several small towns. All the funds to first establish these locations and later to pay the midwives came from a protected budget within the Ministry of Health. In each project, a multidisciplinary council (three midwives, two doctors, one nurse, and one consumer) had the responsibility of establishing the protocols of care, monitoring the midwives' practice, and dealing with complaints if need be.

Most often, the coordinator of the birth centres was a midwife, although this was not required by Bill 4. There were no doctors or nurses on the premises, although in the Sherbrooke and Montreal centres, there was a close collaboration between general practitioners and midwives, which had been established years before the projects. The fact that there were no doctors in the birth centres was a point of contention for some, according to Klein (2000). Women whose pregnancy and labour had been "normal" (according to the established list of criteria) could become clients of these birth centres. Staff was comprised of three to six midwives and, in some birthing centres, their assistants: women trained by the midwives to help them or to take care of the women on the premises, a few hours after the birth.

In case of a problem, either during pregnancy or labour or after the birth, the women and/or babies were referred to a physician or transferred to a nearby hospital with which the birth centres usually had signed an agreement protocol.[4] A maximum of 250 births a year were planned in each centre, with each full-time midwife being responsible for forty women and called to act as an assistant on forty additional births. A thorough "authorization to practice" process was undertaken in 1993 and forty-nine midwives were recognized to practice in these centres. These midwives came from a variety of backgrounds: lay or community midwifery with no formal training other than apprenticeship (about half), certified midwifery from abroad, or provincial and international nurse-midwifery programs.[5] Even though the lay midwives had successfully completed the stringent evaluation, doctors' associations repeatedly criticized the fact that they had been authorized to practice.

In this highly politicized and complex context, it took four years between the adoption of Bill 4 and the actual opening of the first birth centres in 1994. This delay was attributed largely to the continuing opposition of medical associations. It manifested itself in the opposition of doctors inside some CLSCs, by orders by medical associations to their members not to collaborate with midwives (Gauthier 1995), and by hospital laboratories refusing to fill midwives' prescriptions (Laurin 1994).

Although the centres in the Montreal area filled up quickly, it took some time for others to build a full clientele. This was due in part to the lack of marketing by the Ministry of Health on the practice of midwifery, in light of this being an experiment. Also, in some areas individual doctors told women that it was dangerous to give birth in the birth centres. One birth centre, in Alma, was forced to close because it had difficulties recruiting midwives and women, a result perhaps of both the previous lack of midwives in the area and the doctors' fierce opposition to midwifery in this region (*La Presse* 1996; *Le Quotidien* 1995).

Evaluation of the Birth Centres[6]

Following the Ministry of Health's call for evaluation proposals, responses came from several individual researchers as well as from a consortium of researchers from universities across Quebec. A committee of experts from two major governmental research funding organizations (Fonds de la recherche en santé du Québec and Conseil québécois de la recherche sociale) evaluated the proposals submitted and accepted the one presented by the consortium. These organizations financed the research, which involved a multi-site study with each pilot project representing a case and a cohort study with matched controls. The case study would examine all the pilot projects and do an in-depth analysis of three centres, including interviews and focus groups with key informants, document analysis, and observation. The aim was to obtain data on the organizational and professional aspects of the study.

In the cohort study, nearly 1,000 women from the birth centres formed half of the sample, being matched retrospectively for several characteristics by the Bureau de la statistique du Québec with an equivalent number of "low-risk" women who had given birth in hospitals around the same time (Fraser et al. 2000). This was done to compare midwifery care with current medical services, in terms of safety (maternal and neonatal mortality and morbidity), "humanization" (individualization and woman-centred care), continuity of care, obstetrical interventions, and cost. Quantitative and qualitative data were gathered from the clientele's obstetrical records, a special perinatal client record made for the study, postnatal questionnaires, unstructured interviews with women, and from the Régie de l'assurance-maladie du Québec (RAMQ). The evaluation study would (1) compare birth centre services with what was offered already in the health care system, and (2) identify which factors (organizational, professional, social) favoured the autonomy of the midwife and were the most conducive to good outcomes (Blais 1998). The evaluation study was descriptive and the recommendations to the government were made not by the research team but by the appointed governmental committee, the PPAB, based on the study results.

The Results of the Study The main findings of the evaluation were as follows: compared to the control, the practice of midwifery was more conducive to humanizing care and ensuring the continuity of care; although both groups were satisfied with the care received, the midwives' clientele appeared to be more "empowered" by the care received (Blais 1998); midwifery care helped prevent premature births and low birth weight; it led to fewer obstetrical interventions (echography, episiotomy, etc.), including cesareans (6 per cent vs 13 per cent), less forceps use and less third- and fourth-degree tears. The transfer rate (25 per cent including pregnancy, childbirth, and postnatal, and 3 per cent emergency transfers) was comparable to other studies. One of the statistics on mortality, the fetal death-in-utero rate (7.3/1000 major fetal malformations excluded) seemed high in comparison with what other studies had shown on obstetrical populations. A comparison between the midwives' clientele and the doctors' clientele on this outcome was impossible, however, in light of the mismanagement of some data by the Bureau de la statistique du Quebec, the agency responsible for the database, where ten months of data on stillbirths in the control group were missing. The relatively small sample of the study for mortality outcomes may also explain this result. Although there were some other variations between pilot projects (number of midwives, protocols, distance between the birth centre and the hospital, involvement of doctors), the results did not vary significantly between them, except regarding the costs involved: some birth centres seemed to generate higher costs because of organizational factors and not enough births. The evaluation, though, had been done early in the life of the birth centres (their second and third year), before they had reached their *vitesse-de-croisière* in terms of clientele. Globally, however, there was a difference in favour of the midwives' group, $2,294 (birth centres) vs $3,020 (hospitals) per birth (Reinharz 1998; Reinharz et al. 2000).

With respect to the integration of midwives in the health care system, the results revealed poor integration during the experimentation. This was due to four main factors: the lack of knowledge about the practice of midwifery of other health care givers; deficiencies in the legal and organizational structures of the centres; competition over professional territories and gaps between the midwives' and other caregivers' cultures (Collin et al. 2000); and significant difficulties in the collaboration with doctors, especially with the specialists (White 1998). A lack of harmonizing with the existing laws that were affected by the practice of this "new" health care professional was also revealed. Other problems were related to a weakness in the collaboration between some of the birth centres and their CLSCs and an overall lack of CLSC mediation with the hospitals (White 1998).

The Recommendations of the PPAB Following the generally positive research results of the evaluation study and other work it had commissioned (i.e., a literature review on the place of birth), the PPAB recommended in December 1997 that the government legalize midwifery as an autonomous profession, allow the practice of midwifery in all birth places after establishing a list of criteria for home birth, and integrate midwifery into the health care system. It also recommended that the practice of midwifery be administered by the CLSCs, that midwives be considered as primary caregivers, and that a direct-entry university training program be established. It also underlined the need to establish clearer consultation and reference mechanisms between professionals in order to establish their respective responsibilities, and to make sure that the midwives would have immediate access to specialized resources at each stage of the follow-up. All of the PPAB's recommendations were reached by consensus except on the matter of the place of birth, in which the obstetrician-gynecologist on the committee expressed his opposition to any birth happening outside of hospitals (Albert 1997).

Reactions to the Experiment A new group of birth centre users who supported choice of birth setting and natural birth – the *Groupe MAMAN* (Mouvement pour l'autonomie dans la maternité et pour l'accouchement naturel) – organized an evaluation in the same year that the PPAB presented its report. Following a suggestion by the midwives, a series of focus groups were arranged in the birth centres in which around 100 couples expressed their views. The parents unanimously recognized the human qualities of the midwives that allowed for an empowering and a family-centred experience. Aspects of "safety" (other than what is usually mentioned around this issue) were underlined: to be listened to, the quality of the encounter with the midwives, their philosophy of practice, the confident (and egalitarian) link established, the global care received. More flexibility in the protocols and rules was asked for as well as a longer postnatal follow-up period. Parents mainly wanted midwifery to be an autonomous profession and wanted to be able to give birth where they wished (Bouffard and Grégoire 1998).

Once the evaluation study was completed, the midwives met at the end of 1997 to share their views regarding the findings. The difficulties expressed included isolation, problems of communication and solidarity, opposition for some from the medical milieu, some negative attitudes of the media, and some of their working conditions. But the midwives said they were generally satisfied with working in the birth centres, though they were worried and tired, underlining the negative impact these years had on their personal lives. Their worries included the possible effects of the system on their practice, the small number of midwives, and bleak prospects of renewing the work force in the near future (Lemay 1997). Another worry was that the opening of the birth centres had a negative impact on home birth, which decreased during the years following the opening of the birth centres. This was because the midwives were either employed full-time in the birth centres or they were more or less forbidden to attend home births while working in the birth centres.

The Reactions of the Interest Groups to the PPAB *Recommendations*[7]
After the PPAB published its report and recommendations, the College
of Physicians of Quebec underlined the necessity of extending the evaluation period before legalizing midwifery for safety reasons, because of
the seemingly high rate of fetal death-in-utero. The government decided to extend the period for data collection and to ask the Conseil
d'évaluation des technologies de la santé to audit the stillbirths more
thoroughly (CETS 1999).[8] The Fédération des omnipraticiens du
Québec (general practitioners) repeated that its organization did not
see why it was necessary to "introduce a new professional in obstetrics" (Dutil 1998).

By way of contrast, midwives were happy about the positive results
of the study and about the recommendations of the PPAB (Tremblay
1998a). Although they were also happy, Groupe MAMAN and a coalition for the legalization of midwifery continued to periodically press
the government to legalize midwifery (Roy 1998), organizing demon-
strations, meetings with ministers, and press conferences from 1997 to
1999 (Trottier 1997; Hachey 1998; *Le Journal de Montréal* 1998).
Groupe MAMAN was particularly worried about what would happen to
home birth.

Translating the Outcomes of the Experimentation into Policy

Following the recommendations of the PPAB, Minister of Health Jean
Rochon announced in early April 1998 that midwifery would be legalized, according to almost all of the PPAB's recommendations. He
stressed the need to first establish norms for home births. A call was
then directed toward universities to submit proposals for a training
program for midwives. According to the media, midwives' reactions
were mixed. Lucie Hamelin, president of the Regroupement les sages-
femmes du Québec (an association created in 1995 following the accreditation of forty-nine midwives), said that they were hoping for a
real collaboration from doctors and were disappointed that home birth
would be delayed. Though happy about the government's adoption of
the international definition of midwifery practice, consumers were similarly disappointed with the delay imposed on home births (Harting
1998). On the other hand, the Fédération des médecins spécialistes du
Québec repeated its opposition to home birth, while the Association
des obstétriciens-gynécologues did not comment. Finally, after decades
of opposition, the College of Physicians reacted positively and promised its collaboration, adding that the pilot projects had proven themselves in Quebec and that a College of Midwives was a good idea

(Tremblay 1998b).[9] The College nevertheless continued to manifest its opposition to home birth and wished that the training of midwives would occur in a Faculty of Medicine (Normand 1998).

The government did not listen to this latter request, and early in 1999 it announced that the school of midwifery would be located at the Université-du-Québec-à-Trois-Rivières – a direct-entry, four-year baccalaureate program inspired by the Ontario program (see Kaufman and Soderstrom, this volume).[10] It was to begin operation in September 1999. The government also announced that midwives would be represented by an autonomous College comprised of six midwives and two persons appointed by the Office des professions (a governmental agency responsible for regulating and monitoring professions in Quebec) and financially supported by the government with $1 million for its first years. For the first four years, the College would also be assisted by a consultative committee (one midwife, one consumer, two doctors, and a nurse). The government also announced that birth centres would continue to operate and that midwives would be able to help women give birth in the place of their choice – after a period of delay for home birth in order to establish the conditions under which it could happen. At last, a bill legalizing midwifery, the Midwives Act (Bill 28), was adopted by the National Assembly in June 1999 (Québec 1999).

Changes Since the Experimentation: Some Obstacles to Legalization Disappear

Thus, the government of Quebec finally legalized midwifery. In the meantime, some of the factors that may have led the government to experiment had changed. First, midwives formed a new association in 1995, the Regroupement les sages-femmes du Québec, that was comprised mainly of the accredited midwives from pre-existing associations. It became the official organization of midwives. One of the two former practising midwives associations, the Association des sages-femmes du Québec, did not dissolve, which led to difficulties among the midwives and may also have delayed legalization. Second, perhaps after they had passed the examination and started to work in the birth centres, the midwives became more credible in the eyes of the public and the government. Third, the consumers' movement, including the coalition for the legalization of midwifery, and the new group of birth centre users, the Groupe MAMAN, became more vigorous in lobbying the government for the legalization of midwifery on its own terms. Fourth, one of the main opponents to the legalization of midwifery, the Collège des médecins du Québec, declared (finally) that it would collaborate.

QUEBEC MIDWIFERY IN CONTEXT:
WHY A DISTINCT ROUTE?

The legal recognition of midwives in Quebec and in other Canadian provinces is an example of professional conflict where the issues were similar at the outset but where one government, Quebec, took a different route. In order to better understand why the Quebec government took a distinct route, we can compare events in this province with those in two other provinces, Ontario[11] and British Columbia.[12]

With regard to what led to some kind of recognition of midwifery, we can observe that Quebec, Ontario, and British Columbia had many similarities. In the three provinces, women and women's groups, along with some of the midwives, had demanded the recognition of midwifery from the end of the 1970s. Organizations of consumers and of midwives in the three provinces lobbied for it. Although it did not have the same legal status, the practice of midwifery in the three provinces was more or less tolerated by the authorities, and midwives had formed associations. There were also coroners' inquests in all three provinces into the deaths of babies born at home with the help of midwives. A common opponent to midwifery legalization was the doctors' associations – at least initially in Ontario – although, paradoxically, Canadian doctors seemed less and less interested in practising obstetrics (Cohen 1991). In the three provinces, nurses initially wanted nursing to be a prerequisite to midwifery. Finally, the general context during these years was one of change and financial cuts in the health care system.

But there were differences between the provinces. An important factor seems to have been that in Quebec, the demand for legalization stood alone whereas in the other two provinces this demand took place amidst a general reform of the health care professions (the Regulated Health Professions Act in Ontario [Ontario 1991] and the Health Professions Act in B.C.). This reform process seemed to have been a window of opportunity (Kingdon 1984) favourable to the adoption of new policies, namely legalizing midwifery. It was structured and provided midwives with specific criteria, enabling them to be more prepared, and it may have diverted the doctors' attention and resources from opposing the midwives, as other professional groups were threatening their territory (Bourgeault and Fynes 1996/97). Another difference is the way the coroners' inquests were managed, i.e. more politically in Ontario and B.C. (in Quebec they were centred on the defence of the midwife), resulting in recommendations by the coroner or the jury to the effect of the importance of regulating midwifery and how it should be done.

With regard to the midwives, although in B.C. they appeared more divided on the issue of legalization than in Ontario, both provinces benefitted from the support of international midwives' associations, namely the Midwives Alliance of North America in Ontario (who held a conference in 1984 in Toronto) and the International Confederation of Midwives (who held a conference in 1993 in Vancouver). In these provinces, there were also pilot projects prior to legalization that had been going on for several years, in which midwives could practice in hospitals (a form of a delegated medical act, under the supervision of a doctor) (Klein 1994; Murphy-Black 1995; Bowen 1991). Nothing like this happened in Quebec except perhaps the midwifery services from 1986 in Puvirnituk. Another difference between the provinces is that Quebec was the first to fund midwifery services (albeit in pilot projects only), while B.C. took time in funding the legalization process (Klein 1994). Additionally, the Quebec consumers' movement lobbying for humanization of childbirth, Naissance-Renaissance, took time before becoming involved in the political process. Not only were its objectives larger than the legal recognition of midwifery (the humanization of perinatal care), it seemed to have acted more sporadically than, for instance, the Midwifery Task Force of Ontario, whose lobbying was carried out in a continuous and structured manner. The mobilization of women that had taken place in the 1980s in Quebec was declining. Some lobbying by women's groups continued periodically, and a coalition in favour of the legalization of midwifery periodically pressed the government to proceed, but the midwifery question did not seem to have priority.

But the strongest factor influencing governmental decisions was probably the difference in the power of the medical associations and how they influenced governments. Almost every Quebec respondent in my earlier work agreed that the decision to experiment was a political move, a compromise to try to satisfy the doctors' associations (Vadeboncoeur et al. 1996/97)[13]. Although there was medical opposition in B.C. until the middle of the 1990s against midwifery, in both B.C. and Ontario the medical associations were less numerous than in Quebec, and not organized in powerful unions (Desrosiers 1995).

So if there was strong medical opposition in Quebec and B.C., but a weaker one in Ontario, with Ontario and B.C. both having relatively less powerful medical organizations, it seems logical that Ontario was the first province to legalize, that Quebec delayed legalization and chose a compromise, and that legalization in B.C. took a longer time to come into effect. The strong medical opposition to home birth in Quebec and B.C may also have led these two provinces, within the legislation, to compromise and give a special status to home birth – delaying authorization in Quebec and doing it within a pilot project structure in

B.C. One can observe also that in the 1990s there were pilot projects with midwives in both Quebec and B.C. (for, respectively, birthing centres and home births) and both may have been established in order to satisfy medical opposition. But the major difference is that in Quebec, the pilot projects occurred before legalization, in birth centres, whereas in B.C. they happened after legalization, concerning solely home births.[14] Another factor that may also have delayed legalization in Quebec and B.C. (where it happened respectively in 1999 and 1997) may have have been the dissension or lack of unity among the midwives in both provinces.

In Quebec, considering the initial refusal of the medical associations to recognize the midwifery profession and their wish to limit births to hospital settings and thus keep midwives under their control (Lemieux 1989), what could the Quebec government do? It wanted the midwifery profession to be autonomous and wished to meet the demands of women, at least to a certain extent. Had there been a more equitable balance of power, as in Ontario or B.C., the government may have insisted on legalizing the midwifery profession. But the Quebec government was faced with pro-midwifery groups that were not as united nor as organized as in Ontario, and the demand for the recognition of midwifery took place outside a context of a review of health care legislation that attracted the undivided attention of the doctors' associations. Considering that its own appointed committees during the 1980s had all shown the benefits of midwifery practice and recommended its legalization, it seems that the government did not want to face the medical opposition and chose to "buy time" through the pilot projects for a few years.

CONCLUSION: WILL LEGALIZATION LEAD TO TRUE INTEGRATION?

So in Quebec the government succeeded, despite medical opposition, in legalizing midwifery as an autonomous profession, in establishing a university training program, and in following the international definition of midwifery practice. But there have been problems in implementing some elements of the legislation. Even though the medical associations have finally resigned themselves to the fact that there will be midwives in the health care system, it will take a while before midwives are really accepted into hospitals: more than four years after the Midwives Act was adopted, there are still no midwives practising in hospitals. At the time this paper was written, a joint committee appointed by the provincial association of CLSCs, the Quebec Hospitals Association, and the Ministry of Health has produced guidelines to help hospitals and CLSCs set up agreements regarding midwifery practice in hospitals (Lavoie 2002). The Midwives Act specifies that it is CLSCs that will hire midwives and it is these institutions that will negotiate with the hospitals the renting of facilities and equipment used by the midwives on the premises, the conditions of collaboration between them and doctors and nurses, and admitting and discharging procedures (Québec 1999). As we have already seen, during the experimentation the CLSCs had limited success in negotiating with hospitals agreements on the transfer of women during or after births. If they lacked power then, how will they do it regarding the midwives' access to hospital facilities? [15]

Proceeding through the CLSCs, in the hopes that the essence of midwifery can be maintained and perhaps to prevent other professional groups from requesting hospital privileges in the future, is different than the way general practitioners practising obstetrics and midwives in other provinces proceed. They negotiate on an individual basis with the hospital and have to follow hospital rules and protocols of care. The path chosen by the Quebec government will probably help the midwives be more autonomous, although it could provoke some reactions among the doctors and their representative bodies working in the hospitals where midwives will practise. It probably also explains the delays in producing the guidelines. Specifically, it could impair the integration of midwives into the health care system if they are seen as "renting space and facilities" and not respecting the same hospital rules and protocols that doctors and nurses have to follow. Similar to what James and Bourgeault describe of Alberta, it will also be up to the Quebec regions to decide whether or not they will fund midwifery and if midwifery is to be implemented in their institutions. Although other regions are presently planning birth centres (Aubry 2000), the Ministry of Health will not fund future centres, except for one located near Trois-Rivières, where future midwives have their university training.

Moreover, there is also still strong opposition in Quebec from the medical associations to births outside the hospital, as the regulation for this has been finalized by the new College of Midwives and has been waiting since the winter of 2002 for approval by the Office des professions. In 2003, a regulation stating the conditions in which a birth could happen at home under the supervision of midwives was published in *La Gazette officielle du Québec*.[16] If everything goes well, Quebec midwives could start helping women giving birth at home by the end of 2004 (if the regulation is adopted by the Quebec government). The experiment has shown, as elsewhere, that medical resistance can be an obstacle to the practice of midwifery. This resistance can also, to a certain degree, impact women's experiences of giving birth and may, according to an editorial in the *Canadian Journal of Public Health*, have influenced some of the study outcomes (Klein 2000).

Although it was not the first choice of midwives and women, the experiment nevertheless had some advantages. First, it allowed, and still allows, thousands of women free access to midwifery services and to an alternative place of birth, the birth centres, a public institution unique in Canada. It is interesting to note that although midwifery services were limited to the experiment and to birth centres, funded midwifery services were available earlier in Quebec than any other Canadian province. The experimentation also allowed midwives from different backgrounds to practise legally and to learn from each other while working together for the first time. It also allowed them to extend the application of a home birth model of practice – a model based on the needs of women – into an officially recognized practice. Quebec is also the only province to have thoroughly evaluated the practice of midwifery, in a study that has increased our knowledge of the advantages of midwifery and the problems associated with the legalization of a "new" profession in the health care system. Finally, the experimentation contributed to opening the way to integrating the practice into the health care system, showing what needed to be done in order to achieve that integration.

But the experimentation did delay legalization for ten years. It also delayed the renewal of the midwifery work force. The first eight midwives graduated in 2003 and will start to practise if home births and hospital births under the midwives' responsibility are authorized. There are also a very small number of student-midwives being trained (sixteen admissions a year up until September 2003). The home birth movement was also seriously impaired by the experimentation, since it is now illegal for a midwife to help a woman give birth at home and will be illegal until the conditions of midwifery practice are sanctioned by the Quebec government. This has unfortunately led some women to give birth alone at home with no professional help at all (Des Rivières 2000; Dutrisac 2000), which is, curiously, what happened thirty or so years ago when Quebec women – in order to prevent this situation – started to help their friends give birth at home and slowly became midwives. In the face of medical opposition to home birth, the resistance in certain hospitals to having midwives practising on their premises, and the delays imposed by the Midwives Act, one has to ask whether the consumers' groups, women's groups, and the midwives will be vocal and strategic enough to influence what happens from now on and how midwifery will be thoroughly integrated into the health care system of Quebec. More than four years after legalization, this does not seem to be the case.

NOTES

1 Article 31 of the Medical Act stated that birth was part of medicine, with an exception for midwifery (article 43).
2 This task force was comprised of representatives from the government and teaching institutions, two Quebec midwives, one nurse, one ob-gyn, one family doctor, one lawyer, and one consumer.
3 The data for this section comes largely from my work as a consultant on the pilot projects dossier in various institutions of the Quebec health care system from 1990 to 1995.
4 There were several problems with this requirement given that many hospitals refused to cooperate.
5 More than a dozen additional midwives were accredited in 1997 and a few more in 2001, for a total of sixty accredited midwives in 2002.
6 The report on the evaluation of the pilot projects can be found in Blais and Joubert 1997. See also the articles published in 2000 in the *Canadian Journal of Public Health* 91, no. 1 by Blais; Fraser et al.; Collin et al.; Reinharz et al.; and Klein.
7 This section is based on a review of what was published in the press in the months following the report of the PPAB (beginning of the year 1998).
8 The report by the Conseil d'évaluation des technologies de la santé established that the number of stillbirths in the birth centres from their opening to August 1998 was 5.6/1000, compared to the rate of the Quebec hospitals of 4.2/1000 in 1995 and 3.9/1000 in 1996. It stated that this difference was not significant if the mother's age was taken into account. The CETS, however, did underline the importance of the collaboration between midwives and obstetricians, stating that in some cases the doctor responded too late to a midwife's concerns and in other instances the midwife took too long to contact an obstetrician or general practitioner (CETS 1999; Derfel 1998).
9 This change of attitude was largely due to a change of the College's president, who replaced one fiercely opposed to midwifery.
10 Three other universities applied to give the midwifery training program: McGill University, Université Laval, and Université de Montréal. The student midwives have been doing their practicum at the Centre hospitalier universitaire de Sherbrooke.
11 Unless otherwise stated, the comparison between Quebec and Ontario is based mainly on interviews that were conducted with nine key informants from the two provinces for my master's degree in Community Health (Université de Montréal). In this exploratory study, I sought to understand why the two governments adopted different solutions when faced with a similar situation (Vadeboncoeur 1995, Vadeboncoeur et al. 1996, 1996/97).
12 Unless otherwise specified, the data on British Columbia comes from Alison Rice's chapter in Shroff's book (1997) and from personal communications

in 1994 with Alison Rice and Dr Michael Klein. A special thanks to social scientist Jude Kornelsen (2000), UBC, for her comments.

13 Whereas in Ontario there is one medical association, the Ontario Medical Association, in Quebec, there are the Fédération des médecins spécialistes du Québec, the Fédération des omnipraticiens du Québec, and the Association des obstétriciens-gynécologues du Québec.

14 In British Columbia, the home birth project was designed to collect data on births at home with a legally certified midwife in order to establish standards of practice for home birth. Done in 1998–99, the study compared home births with hospital births of a similar obstetrical status and revealed fewer interventions in the home birth group (epidurals, induction, episiotomies, and Cesareans). There was also no increased maternal or neonatal risk associated with planned home births (Janssen et al. 2002).

15 In November 2003, the new Liberal government proposed a bill (Bill 25) to merge CLSCs, hospitals, and long-term healthcare facilities. No one knows how this will affect the midwives' integration into hospitals or the existing birth centres administered by the CLSCs. The same month, contrary to what the Midwives Act stated, the Collège des médecins du Québec announced that midwives should request individual hospital privileges, as doctors do.

16 Projet de règlement, Loi sur les sages-femmes L.R.Q., c.S.-o-1. Sages-femmes – Normes de pratique et conditions d'exercice lors d'accouchements à domicile, *La Gazette officielle du Québec*, 4 juin 2003, 135e année, no. 23.

REFERENCES

Albert, Joanne. 1997. *Rapport final et recommandations* – Conseil d'évaluation des projets-pilotes. Québec: Ministère de la santé et des services sociaux du Québec.

Alliance québécoise des sages-femmes praticiennes (AQSFP). 1986. Mémoire présenté à la Commission Rochon.

Association pour la santé publique du Québec (ASPQ). 1981. *Rapport-synthèse des colloques régionaux sur l'humanisation des soins en périnatalité: Accoucher ou se faire accoucher.*

Aubry, M. 2000. Le Centre de naissances à Nicolet. *Le Nouvelliste,* 5 September.

Blais, Régis 1998. De l'expérimentation à la légalisation: la pratique des sages-femmes au Québec. *Interface – la revue de la recherche* 19, no. 3: 26–35.

– 2000. Evaluation of the Midwifery Pilot Projects in Quebec: An Overview. *Canadian Journal of Public Health* 91, no. 1: 1–4.

Blais, Régis and P. Joubert. 1997. *Évaluation des projets-pilotes de la pratique des sages-femmes au Québec.* Équipe d'évaluation des projets-pilotes sages-femmes. Groupe de recherche interdisciplinaire en santé. R97–08. Université de Montréal.

Bouffard, Mireille and Lysane Grégoire. 1998. *Bilan de l'expérience des femmes et des hommes ayant bénéficié des services des sages-femmes dans le cadre des projets-pilotes en maison de naissance.* Groupe MAMAN.

Bourgeault, Ivy and Mary Fynes. 1996/97. Delivering Midwifery in Ontario: How and When Midwifery Was Integrated into the Provincial Health Care System. *Health and Canadian Society/Santé et Société Canadienne* 4, no. 2: 227–62.

Bowen, Alison. (Director of the Riverside Hospital Birth Center). 1991. Personal communication.

Cohen, L. 1991. Looming Manpower Shortage has Canada's Obstetricians Worried. *Canadian Medical Association Journal* 144, no. 4: 478–82.

Collin, Joanne, Régis Blais, Deena White, A. Demers, and F. Desbiens. 2000. Integration of midwives into the Quebec health care System. *Canadian Journal of Public Health* 91, no. 1: 1–16–1–20.

Conseil d'évaluation des technologies de la santé (CETS). 1999. *Les mortinaissances dans le cadre des projets-pilotes de la pratique des sages-femmes au Québec.* Report presented to the Minister of Research, Science and Technology, Québec, July 1999.

Corporation Professionnelle des Médecins du Québec (CPMQ). 1985. *Évaluation de la satisfaction de la parturiente relativement à son expérience vécue dans le système de santé québécois: résultats d'un sondage.* Montréal: Centre de sondage de l'Université de Montréal.

Derfel, Aaron. 1998. Birthing Centers Are Safe: Report. *The Gazette*, 27 August.

Des Rivières, Paule. 2000. Dans la clandestinité. *Le Devoir*, Editorial, 10 November, A8.

Desrosiers, Georges (formerly professor of Public Health at the Université de Montréal, now retired). 1995. Personal communication.

Dutil, Renald. 1998. Sages-femmes: les médecins demeurent sur leurs positions. *La Presse.* 9 January.

Dutrisac, Robert. 2000. La loi compromet la santé des femmes et des bébés. *Le Devoir*, 9 November A2.

Fédération des médecins spécialistes du Québec et Fédération des médecins omnipraticiens du Québec (FMSQ and FMOQ). 1989. *Message important et urgent à tous les médecins du Québec.* Document spécial. 12 May.

Fraser, William, Marie Hatem-Asmar, Ingrid Krauss et al. 2000. Comparison of Midwifery Care to Medical Care in Hospitals in the Quebec Pilot Projects Study: Clinical Indicators. *Canadian Journal of Public Health* 91, no.1: 1–5–1–11.

Gauthier, C. 1995. *Info à tous les obstétriciens-gynécologues* – objet: dossier sages-femmes et les maisons de naissances, Association des obstétriciens-gynécologues.

Gosselin, Pierre, et al. 1989. Oui aux sages-femmes, lettre ouverte. *Le Devoir*, 26 May, 8.

Hachey, Isabelle. 1998. Dans le bureau de Ménard, des mères exigent la reconnaissance des sages-femmes. *La Presse.* 17 March. A18.

Harting, Claire. 1998. Les sages-femmes devront être patientes et vigilantes jusqu'à la légalisation de leur pratique. *Le Journal de Montréal.* 3 April, 9.

Janssen, Patricia A., Shoo K. Lee, Elizabeth M. Ryan, Duncan J. Etches, Duncan F. Ferguharson, Donlim Peacock, Michael C. Klein. 2002. Outcomes of Planned Home Births Versus Planned Hospital Births after Regulation of Midwifery in British Columbia. *Canadian Medical Association Journal* 166, no. 3: 315–23.

Le Journal de Montréal. 1998. Les sages-femmes veulent un engagement ferme. 12 November. A18.

Kingdon, John W. 1984. *Agendas, Alternatives and Public Policies.* New York: HarperCollins.

Klein, Michael. 1994. Personal communication.

– 2000. The Quebec Midwifery Experiment: Lessons for Canada. *Canadian Journal of Public Health* 91, no. 1: 5–6.

Kornelsen, Jude. 2000. Personal communication.

Laurin, Renée. 1994. Le centre hospitalier de Gatineau ne fait plus d'analyses en laboratoire – les sages-femmes encore boycottées. Ottawa *Le Droit.* (29 April).

Lavoie, Gertrude. (Vice-president of the Ordre des Sages-Femmes du Québec). 2002. Personal communication.

Lemay, Céline. 1997. *Bilan des sages-femmes.* Montréal. Unpublished.

Lemieux, Louise. 1989. Le débat sur les sages-femmes force les médecins à se remettre en question. *Le Soleil.* 12 May, A7.

L.R.Q.c. M-9 (Art. 19, 31, 33, and 43). Quebec.

Ministère de la santé et des services sociaux (MSSS). 1989. *La pratique des sages-femmes.* Avis sur la périnatalité # 1. Gouvernement du Québec.

Murphy-Black, Tricia, ed. 1995. *Issues in Midwifery.* London: Churchill Livingstone.

Normand, Gilles. 1998. Les sages-femmes pourront exercer dans les hôpitaux. *La Presse.* 3 April. B1.

Ontario. 1991. *Regulated Health Professions Act.* Toronto: Government of Ontario.

La Presse. 1989. Accepter les sages-femmes serait faire marche arrière. 12 May.

– 1996. Fermeture d'une maison de naissances. 22 May.

Québec. 1990. *Loi sur la pratique sage-femme dans le cadre de projets-pilotes.* Loi 4. Gouvernement du Québec.

– 1993. *Politique de périnatalité.* Québec: Ministère de la Santé et des Services sociaux.

– 1999. Loi 28. *Loi sur les sages-femmes.* ch. 24. Éditeur officiel du Québec.

Le Quotidien. 1995. 19 July.

Reinharz, Daniel. 1998. *Le rapport coût/efficacité de la pratique sage-femme et celui des services médicaux, Évaluation des projets-pilotes de la pratique des*

sages-femmes au Québec. Conference 157. 13 May. 66th ACFAS Annual
Conference.

Reinharz, Daniel, Régis Blais, William Fraser, et al. 2000. Cost-effectiveness of
Midwifery Services vs Medical Services in Canada. *Canadian Journal of Public Health* 91, no.1: 1–12 – 1–15.

Rice, Alison. 1994. Personal communication.

– 1997. Becoming regulated: The Re-emergence of Midwifery in British Columbia. In *The New Midwifery: Reflections on Renaissance and Regulation,*
edited by Farah Shroff. Toronto: The Women's Press.

Roy, Paul. 1998. Inquiétudes de groupes de femmes sur l'avenir des sages-femmes. *La Presse.* 13 February. A13.

Shroff, Farah, ed. 1997. *The New Midwifery: Reflections on Renaissance and
Regulation.* Toronto: The Women's Press.

Tremblay, Karine. 1998a. Le métier de sage-femme est en devenir. *La Tribune,*
1 January, A15.

– 1998b. Reconnaissance légale de la pratique sage-femme: le Collège des médecins promet sa collaboration. *La Tribune.* 4 April, A7.

Trottier, Éric. 1997. Des mères manifestent pour accoucher où bon leur semble.
La Presse, 9 March, A7.

Vadeboncoeur, Hélène. 1995. Pourquoi le gouvernement québécois a-t-il décidé
d'expérimenter la pratique sage-femme tandis que l'Ontario légalisait la profession? Travail dirigé. Médecine sociale et préventive. Université de Montréal. Unpublished document.

Vadeboncoeur, Hélène, Brigitte Maheux, and Régis Blais. 1996. "Pourquoi le
Québec a-t-il décidé d'expérimenter la pratique des sages-femmes tandis que
l'Ontario légalisait la profession? *Ruptures – revue transdisciplinaire en
santé* 3, no. 2: 224–42.

– 1996/97. Why Did Quebec Decide to Experiment with the Practice of Midwifery Rather than Legalise the Profession? *Health and Canadian Society/
Santé et Société Canadienne* 4, no. 2: 447–80.

White, Deena. 1998. *L'organisation des maisons de naissance: les processus
d'ajustement à l'environnement externe. Évaluation des projets-pilotes de la
pratique des sages-femmes au Québec.* Conference 157. 13 May. 66th ACFAS
Annual Conference.

5

Challenges to Midwifery Integration: Interprofessional Relationships in British Columbia[1]

Jude Kornelsen and Elaine Carty

INTRODUCTION

On 1 January 1998 midwives in British Columbia began legalized practice. Regulation was the culmination of an arduous struggle for legitimization by some midwives – through their professional association, the Midwifery Association of B.C. (MABC) – and consumers – through the Midwifery Task Force (MTF) – that began in the mid-1970s. Similar to other provinces in Canada, not all practising midwives supported legalization, and fissures developed within the community between those working for official status and those who preferred to continue to provide care outside of a regulatory system (see also Van Wagner, this volume). Despite this, the move toward state recognition began to accelerate in British Columbia in 1991 when the Royal Commission on Health Care and Costs recommended that midwifery be legalized as an autonomous profession. The subsequent announcement in May 1993 of the government's intention to integrate midwifery into the health care system as an autonomous profession renewed debates by the medical community as to whether its establishment was warranted. Reasons given for not integrating midwifery included the move toward fiscal responsibility in the health care sector and the small numbers of constituents midwives would serve (Burtch 1992). Nevertheless, in 1993 the Ministry of Health formed the Midwifery Implementation Advisory Committee (MIAC), made up of representatives from professional medical and nursing organizations, government, and academia, and in 1994 established the self-regulating College of Midwives of B.C. (CMBC). The B.C. Ministry of Health also announced the availability of government funding for midwifery in April 1996 and the first assessment of potential registrants began in May of the following year. Applicants who successfully completed the assessment process began accepting publicly funded clients on 1 January 1998.

What this seemingly progressive narrative belies is that the integration of midwives into the B.C. health care system has not gone smoothly. The two key professions of medicine and nursing have had an important impact on the midwifery integration process on both professional and interpersonal levels. This chapter explores the interprofessional tensions surrounding the implementation of midwifery in the province and discusses the likely prospects for B.C. midwives.

THE TRAJECTORY OF INTERPROFESSIONAL RELATIONSHIPS IN CANADA

The sometimes acrimonious situation in which physicians and midwives presently find themselves is not without precedent. The roots of this current interprofessional relationship can be found over one hundred years ago, when physicians in Canada began to organize as a profession (see Biggs, this volume, for a historical contextualization of the complex relationship between physicians and midwives and the multiple factors leading to a decline in midwifery in most parts of the country in the early to mid-twentieth century).[2] Although the history between nursing and midwifery is more recent it also influences current tensions between the professions. In an attempt to distinguish themselves, midwives characterized nurses as participants in the "medical model" of birth. This included a critique of nursing education, which was assumed to focus on illness instead of health due in part to nursing training originally being hospital-based. During the 1960s, nursing education programs in B.C. (and Canada) moved en masse from hospitals into colleges and universities. This move reaffirmed nursing's commitment to a broad understanding of health and illness and precipitated a new focus on health promotion and preventive care. This holistic approach may lead perinatal nurses to feel they have more in common with midwives than midwives feel they have with nurses. The strategy of distancing midwifery from nursing was essential to enabling midwives to build an autonomous profession with its own identity. This strategy has, however, had the unintended consequence of contributing to the illusion of radically different philosophies of care and has caused much discord between the professions.

The increasing professionalization of midwifery during the 1980s and 1990s in B.C. did little to shift many physicians' and nurses' overwhelming opposition to midwifery care. In spite of a more general acceptance of hospital-based midwifery care, there was only one place in the province – B.C. Women's (formerly Grace) Hospital – that allowed midwives to be the primary care providers during labour and delivery. Objections put forward to midwifery care during this period included (1) the perceived inherent dangers of home birth; (2) the dangers of having unregulated practitioners provide maternity services; and (3) midwives' lack of standardized training. These objections manifested at the professional level through condemnations of home birth and midwifery by representative bodies of both physicians and nurses. Prior to regulation, however, midwives enjoyed more positive relationships with physicians on an interpersonal level, as they were able to choose the ones who were supportive of midwifery in both practical and philosophical ways. Some physicians showed their support for midwifery by providing concurrent prenatal care to midwifery clients, ordering tests and diagnostics where necessary, and taking over client care in cases of transfer from home to hospital. There were also physicians, called "angel-docs" by the midwives, who actively supported midwives when they did transfer to hospital and forcefully argued the case for midwifery among their peers. This level of support was not common, however, and many midwives had difficulty finding physicians to work with in their community.

The relationships midwives enjoyed with nurses were more random, as, due to the shift work organization of nursing services, midwives had little control over whom they would encounter if a client transferred from home to hospital. Thus, interprofessional relationships between midwives, physicians, and nurses in the pre-regulation period are summarized in table 1.

Below we review the concerns of physicians and nurses pre- and post-regulation to explore the nature of the changes that regulation has precipitated. First, however, sources for the data used in this paper will be presented.

Table 1
Interprofessional Relationships with Midwives Pre-Registration

	Professional	Interpersonal
Physicians	Negative	Positive due to self-selection (when supportive physician found)
Nurses	Negative	Predominantly negative due to random assignment

METHODOLOGY

This paper is part of a larger program of research into the consequences – both intended and unintended – of integrating midwifery into the B.C. health care system. To understand the impact of midwifery on the maternity care environment, we elicited the opinions and perceptions of several groups: maternal-child and community health nurses, family physicians offering maternity care and, registered midwives. We sent out surveys to physicians and nurses designed to help them describe the current perceptions they held. Surveys were sent to a total of 600 nurses (selected through a stratified random sample on the Registered Nurses' Association of B.C.'s membership list) in February 1998. A total of 235 responses were received for a response rate of 40 per cent. The survey design was based on a series of focus groups done with perinatal nurses working in a low-risk delivery suite at a large metropolitan hospital in January – February 1995. The survey set out to answer the following questions:

- What is the level of knowledge of nurses regarding midwifery registration requirements and the model and scope of practice as mandated by the CMBC?
- What are the current perceptions of nurses regarding the impact of midwifery practice on such issues as quality of care, health care costs, nursing employment, nursing practice, and interdisciplinary relationships?
- What are some of the factors associated with nurses' knowledge and perceptions of midwifery?

The questionnaire was subsequently modified for use with physicians and sent out to 1,000 family physicians in February 1999 who had self-identified on the Medical Services Plan registration as having an active maternity practice. A stratified random sample was chosen from across the province. One hundred and fifty-two surveys were returned for a response rate of 15.2 per cent.

Also in 1999, we conducted in-depth interviews with forty-two registered midwives (80 per cent of registered midwives at the time) about their practice experience post-registration. The interviews were semi-structured and lasted an average of ninety minutes.

The nurses' and physicians' questionnaires were subjected to descriptive statistical and qualitative analysis. The midwives' transcripts were transcribed and submitted to a multistaged process to extract relevant and meaningful data. Themes and descriptions were analysed within a framework that honours respondents as an essential part of the knowledge-generating process, values the context from within which the information is taken, and strives to allow respondents to create meaningful categories for analysis as opposed to presenting a framework into which the information must fit (see Reinharz 1992; Lather 1986, 1988, and 1991; Meis 1983; Oakley 1989; Stanley and Wise 1991).

We also drew on documentary data including secondary sources, such as newspaper articles, and primary sources, such as press releases and the position statements of various professional organizations during the time of regulation.

Although it is difficult to generalize from these data, our examination reveals only a slight improvement between pre- and post-registration periods in the relationships between midwives and physicians and midwives and nurses. These findings are summarized in table 2 and discussed more fully below:

Table 2
Interprofessional Relationships with Midwives Post-Registration

	Professional	Interpersonal
Physicians	Fluid	Variable: Self-selection is difficult
Nurses	Improved	Improved but variable

PHYSICIAN CONCERNS PRE-REGISTRATION

Family physicians in B.C. are unique in comparison to their colleagues in other provinces in that more of them offer maternity care. Presently 65 per cent of births are attended by family physicians in the province, whereas in Nova Scotia it is 54 per cent, Quebec 40 per cent (Blais et al. 1999), and in Ontario very few births (28 per cent) are attended by family physicians (Klein 2000). Given these numbers, it is logical that family physicians in B.C. have a greater interest in the nature of the maternity care environment. Prior to regulation the four main areas of concern for family physicians were home birth, midwives' autonomy, midwives' training, and remuneration.

Home Birth

The most heated topic of debate for physicians was – and continues to be – the issue of home birth. The medical community, although frequently supportive of choice and autonomy for birthing women and their families, rejected the legitimization of home birth because of the perceived dangers it posed to the mother and child. Specifically at issue were: (1) the lack of immediate emergency support; (2) questions concerning the efficacy of using ante-partum risk assessment tools to predict intra-partum risk (thus the difficulty in predicting who will be "low risk" during delivery); and (3) whether or not current training for midwives provided them with the competency to handle even non-life threatening pathologies should they arise at home. Taken together, these variables suggested to physicians that home birth was an inherently unsafe undertaking with the risks far outweighing the benefits, despite the 1986 World Health Organization report that concluded that "home is the most appropriate birth setting for most childbearing women. Women (and their attendants) choosing this option must be provided with necessary diagnostic, consultative, emergency and other services as required, regardless of place of birth."[3]

When the provincial government announced their intention to legalize midwifery in 1992, they addressed the controversy over the inclusion of home birth within midwives' scope of practice by creating the "Home Birth Demonstration Project" (HBDP), which was designed to explore how home birth would fit into the health care system and to provide immediate feedback about policies and procedures (the HBDP will be discussed in more detail later).

Midwives' Autonomy

Beyond home birth, the CMBC held firm in their articulation of what autonomous midwifery would look like in B.C. when negotiations on the specifics of the midwifery legislation took place. One area of disagreement was whether or not women would have to see a physician before going to a midwife early on in the pregnancy. The College of Physicians and Surgeons put forth this stipulation during negotiations, and the MABC and MTF opposed it due to the "gate-keeping" role for physicians. They did, however, agree to the compromise whereby midwives must "advise clients to consult a medical practitioner for a medical examination during the first trimester of pregnancy." Similarly, during negotiations midwives proposed to do well-woman gynaecological care, including birth control counselling, fitting diaphragms, and prescribing oral contraceptives, but agreed to a compromise that would limit the time during which they could provide these services. That is, they may provide care for up to three months post-partum (they are funded only for up to six weeks post-partum) and unlike their colleagues in many other countries cannot prescribe oral contraceptives. The list of drugs and diagnostics that could be prescribed by midwives in general was also curtailed; some were eliminated altogether, while others required a physician consult prior to prescribing. Another crucial point in the regulations was the recognition of the "grandparent" clause, whereby midwives who had been practising prior to registration could continue to practise upon demonstration of skills and competencies regardless of the nature of their previous training. Although this is standard practice when existing professions are introduced into the health care system in Canada, being upheld in the context of midwifery legislation was crucial because of the questions by the medical profession that midwives should have compulsory nursing (or other formal) training.

The process of negotiations prior to legalization resulted in a scope of practice and level of autonomy that maintained the integrity of midwives' philosophy of care. It is exactly these regulations that define midwifery practice that have contributed to adversarial interprofessional relationships and made midwives' integration into the health care system challenging. Perhaps part of the resistance by physicians post-registration is due to their perceived alienation (even if self-imposed) from the process leading up to legalization.

Midwives' Training

Prior to registration, physicians expressed concerns over the disparate backgrounds from which midwives came. Many community midwives entered the profession through an apprenticeship model of education, gaining their experience primarily in the home with more experienced midwives. Physicians were sceptical about whether or not all midwives had the clinical skills necessary to practise in a safe and efficient manner. By nature of their marginalized status, midwives also lacked access to the culture of hospital-based care. Consequently they were unable to develop the professional and personal relationships with physicians that nurses enjoyed. This lack of familiarity with midwifery led some physicians to stereotype midwives, casting them as part of a counter-culture with questionable clinical skills.

Remuneration

Prior to registration, remuneration was not an issue between physicians and midwives because the latter contracted privately with their clients on a fee-for-course-of-care basis. Within the medical community, however, physicians were already concerned over the perceived low level of remuneration they received for obstetrical care. It could be anticipated that this concern would ultimately impact the professional relationships between physicians and midwives once midwives became part of B.C.'s publicly funded system (Klein 1988).

PHYSICIAN CONCERNS POST-REGISTRATION

Despite the assumption by many in the midwifery community that regulation addresses some of physicians' concerns, on a professional level, the interpersonal relationships between physicians and midwives since regulation has been rocky. Contention still centres around three of the four issues mentioned above – home birth, remuneration, and training.

Home Birth

At the fifteenth Annual Obstetrics, Antenatal Care and Menopause conference in October 1998, a panel discussion entitled "Midwives and Home Births: Sorting out the Politics and Evidence" was presented by members of the Society of Obstetricians and Gynaecologists of Canada, the B.C. Chapter of the College of Family Physicians, and the College of Physicians and Surgeon of B.C. Statements were posed to determine the attitudes of the approximately 200 physicians in attendance and to generate discussion. One of the statements, to which physicians were asked to agree or disagree with, was "Home birth has always been practiced in Canada and British Columbia prior to the regulation of midwives. As physicians we are not asked to attend home birth. Our role is to be available in hospital for the women and newborns of B.C. when transfer is necessary." There was substantial disagreement amongst audience members and the statement itself was cause for a heated discussion. The issues focused on the perceived inherent danger of home birth and the legal liability of physicians who accept transfers from home.

An important point to note here is that home birth was included under midwives' scope of practice as defined in the Health Professions Act, in spite of widespread opposition by the medical community. This came about due to a confluence of factors, most notably consumer demand for the choice of place of birth combined with the government's general agenda to move health care out of institutions and, where possible, "closer to home."

Along with the announcement that midwifery would be legalized in B.C., the minister of health also announced the Home Birth Demonstration Project (HBDP). The mandate of the project was to see how home birth would "fit" into the health care system (for example, how midwives would interface with the ambulatory services when they needed to transfer clients to the hospital). The project was also designed to provide immediate feedback about home birth policies and procedures. To this end, it required all women giving birth at home (and the midwives attending them) to be part of the study. This study was the first systematic examination of the integration of planned home births in a regulated setting in Canada.

The study report was submitted to the B.C. Ministry of Health in December 2000. Two years of data, from January 1998 to 31 October 2000, on 864 planned home births, were analysed. Fifty-eight midwives were involved in the care of these births. According to the authors of the report, "midwives were able to obtain a consultation with a physician in 98 per cent of requests." As home birth did not increase the risk of adverse maternal and fetal outcomes (within the limits of the sample size), the "evaluation team recommended the continuation of planned home births in B.C. within the guidelines established by the College of Midwives of B.C." (B.C. Ministry of Health 2000).

Associated with the HBDP was a tour, the goal of which was to explain the role midwifery and home birth would have post-regulation. The response to the notion of home birth at the fifteenth Annual Obstetrics, Antenatal Care, and Menopause conference was consistent with the ethnographic observational study of the HBDP tour. Lyons and Carty (1999) argue that fear about the safety of home birth is usually based on physicians being part of or seeing a critical situation in the hospital and then extrapolating it to the home. Others working in hospitals, however, can describe equally grave situations of an iatrogenic nature. It is important to note that the issue of liability is closely associated with the safety issue. As Lyons and Carty noted, "Fear was expressed about the consultation process and in particular about the consultant's liability. Physicians were anxious about being called to consult when they do not support home birth and do not have the support of their regulatory college."

The lack of support of the physicians' regulatory college is an impediment to the support of midwifery. There is a perceived conflict between the official policy of their professional organizations and the legislation permitting home birth in B.C. As one obstetrician attending a HBDP meeting commented, "We are being asked to collaborate where those that guide us say it is not safe." When physicians cannot support a fundamental tenet of midwifery care – the right of women to choose their place of birth – it is difficult for them to develop supportive, respectful, and trusting relationships with midwives.

Remuneration

As soon as the details concerning midwives' remuneration were announced late in 1997 they became a lightning rod for physicians' expression of displeasure with midwives in general. This was due in large part to the nature and timing of the announcement. That is, when the re-muneration was announced, the B.C. Medical Association (BCMA) was nearing the end of its fiscal year and it had overspent its budget. To com-pensate for the shortfall it planned "reduced activity days" rather than working for free. These days had the secondary effect of drawing the at-tention of physicians (and the public) to the perceived provincial under-funding of medical services. The situation was further inflamed when the government chose to present the fee schedule for midwives not in terms of yearly income but in terms of dollars per course of care. This presentation overemphasized midwives' income and led physicians to feel demoralized and undervalued. Consequently, midwifery was unnecessarily drawn into what should have been a matter between the BCMA and the government, a dispute that ultimately called their whole model of care into question. Ten months later, at the antenatal conference discussed above, the effects of the nature of the announcement were still evident. Another statement pre-sented to the audience was "Though I acknowledge that physicians are un-derpaid for the intimate and laborious work that we do in attending births, I am capable of separating the concerns that I have with the funding of midwives from the issues of care and collegiality."

Although there was agreement, it was not unanimous. Further evi-dence of physicians' inability to separate the two issues was expressed through letters to the editor in the local press. Similar frustration was expressed during the HBDP tour, where questions concerning remuner-ation were raised at thirteen of the fourteen sites visited. The researcher observing the tour noted "anger was expressed about the introduction of midwifery into the health care system in the face of cutbacks" (Ly-ons and Carty 1999).

Although in some instances physicians have directed resentment over their fee schedule at midwives, in many others it is clear that physicians can distinguish between the issue of remuneration and their profes-sional relationship to midwives. For example, Dr Nan Schuurmans, past president of the Society of Obstetricians and Gynaecologists of Canada, said, "Obstetricians are not angry at the midwives nor do they oppose public payment to midwives ... The debate over midwives did convince obstetricians that they need a big raise" (*Edmonton Journal*, 2 May 1998, A6).

Midwifery Training

Another issue raised by members of the medical community in their ar-gument against the inclusion of midwives into the health care system is the adequacy of midwifery training. Dr Schuumans points to higher rates of obstetrician referrals from midwives than from family doctors to support the claim of inadequate training (*Hamilton Spectator*, 20 May 1997, A6). In a more comprehensive critique, Dr James Goodwin objects to the assumption that within a baccalaureate program, the graduating midwife should have gained knowledge of all the skills necessary to identify risk and manage obstetrical emergencies (Goodwin 1997). He suggests this is even more unlikely when one considers that the program is intended primarily for direct-entry midwives with no previous formal medical training. Several responses to Goodwin's assertions point out both logical fallacies and factual misinformation, including the confusion between cases transferred from home and those that remained at home. Nevertheless, his views represent those of some practising physicians. Physicians' lack of understanding and knowledge about midwives' training and experience has been an impediment to their consideration of midwives as contributing members of the health care team.

In September 2002, the first midwifery students enrolled in a four-year, baccalaureate program in midwifery at the University of British Columbia. The program, modelled on the Ontario program (see Kaufman and Soderstrom, this volume), is situated in the Division of Midwifery within the Department of Family Practice in the Faculty of Medicine. As an integral part of the program, midwifery students will gain proficiency in maternal/fetal health assessment and become certified to carry out neonatal resuscitation. They will obtain these skills by participating in the nationally recognized programs developed by the B.C. Reproductive Care Program intended for nurses, physicians, and midwives. It is hoped that standardized, university-based training for midwives will quell physician concerns over the adequacy of midwifery training.

PHYSICIAN CONCERNS AND THEIR IMPACT ON INTERPROFESSIONAL AND INTERPERSONAL RELATIONSHIPS POST-REGULATION

On a professional level, the notion of team-based or multidisciplinary care has not characterized physician-midwife relations due to physicians' reluctance to welcome midwives as part of the obstetrical team. On an interpersonal level, however, satisfying relationships have been forged despite the obstacles that home birth, autonomy, funding, and training do to discourage such relations. For example, as part of a larger study into midwifery practice post-registration (Kornelsen and

Carty, forthcoming), we asked registered midwives to describe their relationships with GPs. Most said these relations were "good," "fine," or even "supportive." When the midwives were pressed further, however, we consistently heard that relations are good with a select group of GPs that they have chosen to work with. When asked what the odds were of finding a supportive physician from the community of practising physicians, answers ranged from "1 in 10" to "1 in 2," depending on the community. How does this reluctance – or refusal – to work with midwives manifest in practice?

There are several areas where physicians' negative attitudes may hinder patient care, including discharging patients from care if they chose midwifery or home birth, reluctance or refusal to accept transfers from midwives, lobbying hospital boards to refuse to grant admitting privileges to midwives, and refusing to accept midwifery clients altogether. It is not in a physician's best interests to refuse to accept a midwife's transfer patient as the physician in question may be legally culpable for not following through on a course of care. Such situations appear to be relatively rare. If a transfer is accepted, however, the attitudes and actions of the physicians determine to a large extent the nature of the experience for all those involved. Those who accept transfers with reluctance and a propensity to attribute blame to the midwife increase the tension for the midwife and the client/patient. In a climate where there is a predisposition against home birth and distrust of midwives in general, this scenario is played out frequently. We can see this in the attitude that upon transfers to hospital, physicians are "picking up the pieces" or "cleaning up."

On the HBDP tour, Lyons noted that several physicians said they would discharge a patient if they chose to have a home birth (Lyons and Carty 1999). Not as drastic but equally detrimental is the gatekeeping role that many physicians play with patients who inquire about midwifery care. Often unsupportive physicians express doubts over midwives' competency blatantly through verbal condemnations or in other more subtle ways (such as a raised eyebrow or shift in intonation). Raising the stakes even higher, many physicians across the province (and, in fact, across the country) have opted out of obstetrical care altogether. As Linda Knox, acting president of MABC, said, "To withhold maternity care and limit the alternatives to pregnant women because [doctors] have a fee dispute is untenable" (*Vancouver Province*, 6 March 1998, A7).

Currently in B.C. competition overrides cooperation. Perhaps the answer lies not in reducing the number of physicians providing maternity care but in recasting the debate to focus on woman-centred care as opposed to interprofessional competition over turf. Physicians, however, aren't the only profession vying for territory in the maternity care environment. In our examination of the relationship between nurses and midwives in B.C., we see some similarities to that with physicians, but at the same time some unique issues are also revealed.

NURSES' CONCERNS PRE-REGISTRATION

During the 1970s and 1980s the Registered Nurses Association of British Columbia (RNABC) worked to set up guidelines for the practice of nurse-midwifery. For a variety of reasons, however, the various position statements issued by them never translated into a regulatory framework for nurses who were trained as midwives to practise in British Columbia. The association, however, continued into the 1990s to lobby to have midwifery as part of the practice of nursing. They were successful in influencing the 1991 Royal Commission on Health Care and Costs to recommend that "pending the establishment of a College of Midwives nurse-midwives be granted an appropriate scope of practice under the Nurses (Registered) Act ... and that once the College of Midwives was established, nurses be permitted to be members of both the RNABC and the College of Midwifery" (Rice 1997). Nonetheless, the MTF and MABC submitted an application to the Health Professions Council to have midwifery as an autonomous profession, separate from nursing, from the outset. The announcement in May of 1993 at the International Confederation of Midwives meeting in Vancouver that midwifery would be an autonomous profession and publicly funded amounted to a coup by those who supported midwifery over nurse-midwifery. Nurses who were trained as midwives heard themselves being labelled as subservient to the medical model and interventionist by training. This rhetoric was seen to apply, by extension, to perinatal nurses, who also work extensively with birthing women. Hurt feelings were inevitable and naturally extended into the post-regulation period. In our study some nurses also indicated they had few encounters with midwives prior to registration or that the encounters they had were difficult particularly because when midwives when brought their clients into hospital it was due to complications surrounding home birth.

NURSES' CONCERNS POST-REGISTRATION

Two key concerns about midwifery practice expressed by the nurses in our study included the process of midwifery registration and overlapping scopes of practice.

Registering to be a Midwife

The confusion created by a context of similar but distinct areas of practice has been exacerbated by the lack of professional standing accorded to foreign-trained nurse-midwives, many of whom have rigorous training and extensive practical experience. It should be noted, however, that licensure in other jurisdictions does not guarantee licensure in B.C. Similar to procedures in Ontario (see Ford and Van Wagner, this volume), these practitioners can apply to register with the CMBC. Our research noted several obstacles to registration reported by labour and delivery nurses (some of whom were foreign-trained midwives). They included (1) the philosophical rejection of home birth as a viable option for any birthing women; (2) the perceived discrimination by the CMBC against those practitioners who don't support home birth; and (3) the objection to being part of a group that condones "working beyond the law" (see also Nestel, and Kaufert and Robinson, this volume).

More pragmatic obstacles included (1) the cost of upgrading training to meet the criteria established by the CMBC; (2) the lack of a training facility in B.C. at the time when the survey was administered; (3) geographical isolation; and (4) lack of hospital and professional support. Like the physicians, the nurses surveyed by and large took an adamant stand against home birth, thus also against those midwives who practised in a domiciliary setting and who set the requirements for registration to include home birth (the CMBC). This leads to a situation where many labour and delivery nurses, some of whom are foreign-trained nurse-midwives, perceive preferential treatment being given to colleagues whom they believe to have less training and experience. This has led to hostility and the breakdown of interprofessional relationships.

Overlapping Scopes of Practice

Many nurses also expressed pragmatic concerns relating to job security and satisfaction that the introduction of midwives in the health care system raises: "I can see midwives' practice affecting nursing employment. The type of clients midwives will attract even with hospital births will probably go home very quickly. The days post-partum in the hospital and the early discharge visits made by our staff will be reduced."

Not only did many respondents foresee a shift toward more administrative work, many also feared that when they did participate in patient care, they would be relegated to problematic situations that were out of the domain of midwives. As one respondent said, "We want to see natural deliveries and labours also. We like to coach women in breathing, help her find positions for comfort, encourage her to shower, etc. We do not thrive on being invasive!"

THE IMPACT OF NURSES' CONCERNS ON INTERPROFESSIONAL AND INTERPERSONAL RELATIONSHIPS

Nurses are often described as being on the "front line" of obstetrical care. They work closely with their birthing patients from the time the women arrive at the hospital and after they have given birth. They are the intermediaries between birthing women and other medical practitioners and can influence the nature of the experience. They also provide the most direct interface between midwives and the hospital. Although nurses are perhaps not as politically influential as physicians, the relationship of nurses to midwives is a crucial one in determining the ease with which midwives can integrate into the hospital environment. It also plays a large part in allowing for a positive experience for birthing women when care is shared between midwives and physicians/nurses. Our study found that nurses working in obstetrical care had concerns about the introduction of midwives into the health care system. Generally, the concerns were of a professional nature, focusing on whether or not midwives would have an impact on nurses' job security and satisfaction, what position nurses would be forced to assume in the medical hierarchy, and how it would change their relationship to physicians. Nurses' concerns over midwifery arose in large part from a lack of information – or misinformation – concerning midwives' training, competencies, and scope of practice precipitated by their lack of contact with midwives prior to legalization. Many of the concerns expressed by the nurses have dissipated during the past eighteen months as the two professions have had the opportunity to work alongside each other, exemplifying the ability of personal contact to counteract ideological (professional) positions.

CHANGING STATUS, CHANGING RELATIONS?

We have described interprofessional relationships prior to the legalization of midwifery from a professional and interpersonal perspective. We can now juxtapose these experiences with experiences post-legalization as shown in table 3.

Although relations have only improved slightly from a professional perspective, a shift has taken place on an interpersonal level. The overall relationships between midwives and physicians post-legislation can

Table 3
Interprofessional Relations with Midwives Post-Registration

	Prior to Registration		Post-Registration	
	Professional	Interpersonal	Professional	Interpersonal
Physicians	Negative	Positive due to self-selection	Fluid	Variable: self-selection is difficult
Nurses	Negative	Predominantly negative due to random assignment	Improved	Improved but variable

be described as "variable" because of the lack of discretion of midwives over which physicians they now have contact with. Where previously midwives developed a referral system with physicians who were openly supportive, they must now contend with a wide range of physicians with which their increased (and changing) client load brings them into contact.

When we observe both historical precedence and the present situation we can see that from a professional perspective, neither physicians nor nurses welcome the addition of midwifery into the health care system due in large part to the perceived threat of professional competition in various areas of care. Although relations may be more positive on an interprofessional level – especially between nurses and midwives – they are still strained. Given this reality, perhaps a more useful question to ask may be "What can be done to make the integration of midwives into the health care system in B.C. go more smoothly?"

POLICY IMPLICATIONS

There is a growing literature on interdisciplinary collaboration and its implications for interprofessional relationships in the health care literature (see Fagin 1992; Fahy 1994; Lynch 1981). But what does collaboration mean? In their discussion of the meaning of collaboration, Lindecke and Block write, "collaboration is a process of shared planning and action towards common goals with joint responsibility for outcomes" (1998, 213). Midwives need to collaborate with other maternity care providers in the interests of their clients. For example, if a client becomes high risk and transfer of care to an obstetrician is warranted, it would be hoped that the midwife and obstetrician could each contribute to an optimal experience for the client. Likewise, if a medical situation developed during pregnancy, the midwife and the client's family physician need to communicate with openness and respect to ensure the most satisfactory outcome. However, collaboration is not always easy. Stapleton (1998) notes that many barriers exist among health professionals with different educational backgrounds, different ways of constructing knowledge, and different positions of status in a system that is still hierarchical.

Beyond the fissures between the divergent ways of conceptualizing pregnancy and childbirth, we need to recognize that the health care environment in general is in a state of flux. Government initiatives have been undertaken to respond to both changing notions of health and illness (which includes a general move towards a more holistic model of health care) and fiscal constraints. The medical profession is also responding to these realities. Friction occurs, however, when the responses of the government and the medical profession are incongruent (due to differing articulations of the problem, different ways of addressing the problem, or timing). Within this environment of change, we see shifting professional boundaries that demand a readjustment of professional categories. Physicians no longer have attendance at childbirth as part of their exclusive domain of practice. Likewise, however, no longer do midwives have a monopoly over the "midwifery" model of care, as its adoption has come from progressive physicians, nurse-midwives, and nurses.

Perhaps the most useful point to keep in mind is the most obvious: the government of B.C. has included the profession of midwifery in the Health Professions Act. It is now a legal profession entitled to the same rights and privileges and responsibilities accorded to all other health care professions. Likewise, the government has initiated the Home Birth Demonstration Project not to address questions of the safety of home birth but to determine the best way to integrate it into the health care system. Neither midwifery nor home birth is likely to be rescinded.

If midwifery is to survive, physicians, nurses, and midwives need to recognize that we are in a state of transition that causes disruptions to personal and professional identities and the security of each other's place within the maternity care system. But given that midwifery is a registered profession in B.C., we need to move to revisit concepts that are basic to collaboration but have been lost in the current debate. These include the need for respect and compromise, cooperation, and the need to work collaboratively, all of which are embodied in the notion of professionalism. Ultimately, all practitioners must serve their constituents – birthing women. The desire to fulfill this commitment must motivate their actions and actions deleterious to this notion must be abandoned. We anticipate that as midwifery becomes more entrenched in B.C.'s health care system, these attributes of professionalism will dominate future interprofessional relationships.

NOTES

1 The authors gratefully acknowledge support for this paper from the British Columbia Centre of Excellence for Women's Health.

2 The relationship between the rise of professionalization, the political organization of physicians in Canada, and the demise of midwifery is viewed by the authors of this article as one theme among multiple themes in midwifery's history. It is highlighted in this context because of its relevance to contemporary political debates put forward by some physicians in relation to midwifery.

3 World Health Organization (1986), "North American and European Consulting Groups: WHO Report on Health Promotion and Birth." Geneva, WHO. Although it is beyond the scope of this paper to review the issue of safety in relation to home birth, please see the following for an overview of the literature:

Blais, Régis. 2002. Commentary: Are Home Births Safe? *Canadian Medical Association Journal* 166, no. 3: 35–6.

Campbell, Rona, and Alison Macfarlane. 1994. Where To Be Born? – The Debate and the Evidence 2nd ed. Oxford: National Perinatal Epidemiology Unit.

Damstra-Wijmegnam, S.M.I. 1984. Home confinement: The Positive Results in Holland. *Journal of the College of General Practitioners* 34: 425–3.

Davies, J., E. Hey, W. Reid, and G. Young. 1996. Prospective Regional Study of Planned Home Births. *British Medical Journal* 7068, no. 313: 1302–6.

Durand, M. 1992. The Safety of Home Birth: The Farm Study. *American Journal of Public Health* 82: 450-2.

Janssen, P.A., V.L. Holt, and S.J. Myers. 1994. Licensed Midwife-Attended, Out-of-Hospital Births in Washington State: Are They Safe? *Birth* 21, no. 3: 141–8.

Janssen, P.A., S.K. Lee, E.M. Ryan, D.J. Etches, D.F. Farquharson, D. Peacock, and M.C. Klein. 2002. Outcomes of Planned Home Births Versus Planned Hospital Births after Regulation of Midwifery in British Columbia. *Canadian Medical Association Journal* 166, no. 3: 315–23.

Mehl, L., G. Peterson, N.S. Shaw, and D. Creavy. 1978. Outcomes of 1146 Elective Home Births: A Series of 1146 Cases. *Journal of Reproductive Medicine* 19: 281–90.

Northern Region Perinatal Mortality Survey Coordinating Group. 1996. Collaborative Survey of Perinatal Loss in Planned and Unplanned Home Births. *British Medical Journal* 7068, no. 313: 1306–9.

Olsen, A. 1997. Meta-analysis of the Safety of Home Birth. *Birth* 24, no. 1: 4–13.

Peat, Marwick, Stevenson & Kellog. 1993. Literature Review into the Safety of Home Births. Report to the Registrar – Health Disciplines, Alberta.

Thompson, P. 1982. The Home Birth Alternative to the Medicalization of Childbirth: Safety and Ethical Responsibility. In *The Future of Human Reproduction*, edited by C. Overall. Toronto: The Women's Press.

Tyson, H. 1991. Outcomes of 1001 Midwife-attended Home Births in Toronto, 1983–1988. *Birth* 18, no. 1: 14–19.

van Alten, D., M. Eskes, and P.E. Treffers. 1989. Midwifery in the Netherlands. The Wormerveer Study: Selection, Mode of Delivery, Perinatal Mortality and Infant Mortality. *British J Obstet Gynaeco* 96: 656–62.

Wiegers, T.M., M. J.N.C. Keirse, J. van der Zee, and G.A. Berghs. 1996. Outcome of Planned Home and Planned Hospital Births in Low Risk Pregnancies: Prospective Study in Midwifery Practices in the Netherlands. *British Medical Journal* 313: 1309–13.

Woodcock, H.C., A.W. Read, C. Bower, F.J. Stanley, and D.J. Moore. 1995. A Matched Cohort Study of Planned Home and Hospital Births in Western Australia 1981–1987. *Midwifery* 10, no. 3: 125–35.

REFERENCES

B.C. Ministry of Health. 2000. *Final Report to the Health Transition Fund Home Birth Demonstration Project*. Project # BC 404.

Blais, Regent, Jean Lambert, and Brigitte Maheux. 1999. What Accounts for Physician Options about Midwifery in Canada? *Journal of Nurse-Midwifery* 44: no. 4 (July/August): 39–407.

Burtch, Brian. 1992. Reproduction and Law: Midwifery, Abortion and Family Law Reform. In *The Sociology of Law: Critical Approaches to Social Control*. Toronto: Harcourt Brace Jovanovich.

Edmonton Journal. 1998. 2 May, A6.

Fagin, C. 1992. Collaboration between Nurses and Physicians: No Longer a Choice. *Academic Medicine* 67: 91–9.

Fahy, E. 1994. To Be or Not To Be … the Challenges of Interdisciplinary Education and Collaboration in Health Care. *Nursing Health Care* 15: 283.

Goodwin, James. 1997. Where To Be Born Safely. Professional Midwifery and the Case Against Home Birth. *Journal SOGC* 19, no.11: 1179–88.

Hamilton Spectator. 1997. 20 May, A6.

Klein, Michael. 1988. The Midwife Dossier: Cooperation or competition? *Canadian Medical Association Journal* 150, no. 5: 658.

– 2000. Data presented at the national conference on "The Future of Maternity Care in Canada," November 2000, London, Ontario.

Kornelsen, Jude, and Elaine Carty. *Midwives' Experiences of Practice Post-Registration.* B.C. Centre for Excellence for Women's Health (forthcoming).

Lather, Patti. 1986. Research as Praxis. *Harvard Educational Review* 56, no. 3: 257–77.

– 1988. Feminist Perspectives on Empowering Research Methodologies. *Women's Studies International Forum* 11, no. 6: 569–81.

– 1991. *Getting Smart: Feminist Research and Pedagogy with/in the Postmodern.* New York: Routledge.

Lindecke, L., and D. Block. 1998. Maintaining Professional Integrity in the Midst of Interdisciplinary Collaboration. *Nursing Times* 46: 213–88.

Lynch, B. 1981. Team Building: Will It Work in Health Care? *Journal of Allied Health* 10: 240–7.

Lyons, J., and E. Carty. 1999. *Reality, Opinion and Uncertainty: Views on Midwifery in B.C.'s Health Care System.* Part of the series "Perspectives on Midwifery." Vancouver: British Columbia Centre of Excellence for Women's Health.

Meis, Maria. 1983. Towards a Methodology for Feminist Research. In *Theories of Women's Studies,* edited by Gloria Bowles and Renate Duelli Klein, 88–104. Boston: Routledge and Kegan Paul.

Oakley, Ann. 1989. Who Cares for Women? Science Versus Love in Midwifery Today. *Midwives Chronicles* 102, no.1218: 215.

Reinharz, Schulamit. 1992. *Feminist Methods in Social Research.* Oxford: Oxford University Press.

Rice, A. 1997. Becoming Regulated: The Re-emergence of Midwifery in British Columbia. In *The New Midwifery: Reflections on Renaissance and Regulation,* edited by Farah Shroff, 157. Toronto: The Women's Press.

Stanley, Liz, and Sue Wise. 1991. Feminist Research, Feminist Consciousness and Experiences of Sexism. In *Beyond Methodology: Feminist Scholarship and Lived Research,* edited by Mary Fonow and Judith Cook. Indianapolis: Indiana University Press.

Stapleton, Susan R. 1998. Team-Building: Making Collaborative Practice Work. *Journal of Nurse-Midwifery* 43, no.1: 12.

Vancouver Province. 1998. 6 March, A7.

Weitz, R., and D. Sullivan. 1988. *Labour Pains: Modern Midwives and Home Birth.* New Haven: Yale University Press.

6

To Fund or Not To Fund: The Alberta Decision

Susan James and Ivy Bourgeault

INTRODUCTION

Given the particular organization of health care in Canada, the integration of midwifery has to occur within various, somewhat disparate, provincial health care systems. One of the key issues to be decided, apart from regulation, is whether to include midwifery in the system of public funding for maternity care services. Both are provincial jurisdictions. Public funding is a critical issue in levelling the playing field between midwives and physicians and for fostering greater accessibility to midwifery care. Public funding is one of the prime reasons Van Wagner notes in chapter 3 why legislation was pursued in Ontario. But regulation does not necessarily translate into public funding; the two are separate decisions. Alberta offers an interesting case study regarding the question of funding midwifery services and the consequences this decision entails for midwives and women alike.

CONCEPTUAL FRAMEWORK

We draw upon two main bodies of literature to provide a broad conceptual framework. First, funding midwifery services is in part a policy issue. But midwifery also involves the regulation of a central aspect of women's lives. Hence both health policy and feminist literature on the relations between women and the state provide insights.

Health Policy

We draw upon Kingdon's (1995) four-stage model of the policy-making process, which includes (1) the setting of the policy agenda;

(2) the specification of alternatives from which a choice is to be made; (3) an authoritative choice among those specified choices; and (4) the implementation of the decision. Arguably the most critical stage of the policy-making process is agenda setting, where Kingdon describes how three separate streams – problems, policies, and politics – must come together at a "window of opportunity" for issues to be taken seriously by policy decision makers. Central to the agenda-setting process are organized interest groups who highlight a problem, often using mass media to draw attention to it at "focusing events." Here, we define such organized interests or *interest groups* as organizations of individuals with shared interests in bringing about changes to government or institutional policy (Walt 1994). Two key kinds of interest groups include *insider groups*, who are accepted as respectable by government policy makers and with whom they often have a consultative relationship, and *outsider groups*, who are not perceived as legitimate and may therefore have more difficulty penetrating the process.

The key interest groups involved in health policy have been health care providers, including physicians, nurses, and in this case, midwives. With the rise of the women's health and home birth movements, consumers also became involved in the policy-making process (Bourgeault et al. 2001). In several cases, consumers joined with providers, midwives in particular, to create a kind of *advocacy coalition* (Sabbatier 1991).

Although each of these groups has become involved in maternity care policy, they bring varying degrees of power to the negotiation table. Alford (1972), for example, describes how some health interests are structured into the health care system and because of this, have embedded power over other interests. For example, scholars of the professions draw upon Freidson's (1970) conceptualization of professional dominance to argue that the medical profession wields significant power over other occupations within the health care division of labour.

Women and the State

Power and the relations between interest groups and the state are also salient in other women's policy issues. Some feminist state-directed strategies have been relatively successful in advancing women's health and social justice issues (Fox Piven 1990; Fudge 1996; Gotell 1996; McDermott 1996). In the case of women's health initiatives in Canada, Feldberg and Carlsson argue that "governmental institutions at a variety of levels have seemed to respond to women's organizing around health" (1999, 353). This is no doubt due in part to the increasing election of female politicians as central agents for taking up women's concerns (Conway, Ahern, and Steuernagel 1999), or what could be described as the move from outsider to insider status (Briskin 1999). This is particularly salient in those countries known for "state feminism," such as Sweden (Eduards 1991).

Despite some instances of the emancipatory potential of the state in fostering women's issues, however, one must acknowledge the male bias that continues to exist in many welfare states (Benoit 2000; Phillips 1995). For example, Feldberg and Carlsson (1999) argue that Canadian women's health organizations still tend to fall outside of the domain of established politics and are isolated from standard sources of political power. Some feminist scholars link this lack of power in the political system in terms of women's health issues to the lack of power that women as health care professionals have in the health care division of labour (Conway, Ahern, and Steuernagel 1999). For some issues, the view of many Canadian feminists regarding the efficacy of focusing their efforts on the state have shifted, but they nevertheless continue to make demands of it (Briskin 1999). Indeed, we find that many of these women's policy dilemmas are apparent in the case study of midwifery funding in Alberta.

METHODOLOGY

The data for this paper include documentary data and informal interviews conducted throughout the midwifery lobbying process in the mid-1990s by Susan James, the first author, then a practising midwife in Alberta. Documentary data were collected from a variety of media sources as well as from various professional interest groups, colleges, state-appointed policy-making committees, and government documents from the relevant ministries. Informal interviews were conducted with key informants representing these interests as well as those with policy decision-making power.

In what follows we present the various lobbying efforts both for and against public funding, describe the context of the state as audience and actor in the policy-making process, and highlight the structure of health care system funding arrangements that affected the decision in Alberta. We then discuss some of the specifics of the Alberta case in comparison to another Canadian province that decided to fund midwifery: Ontario.

The Midwifery Lobby

A formal lobby effort was first organized by midwives and their supporters in the province of Alberta to promote legalization of midwifery and home birth in response to the policy statement by the Alberta College of Physicians and Surgeons (CPSA) in 1981 forbidding physicians from attending home births (Barrington 1985). This early lobby was launched at local, regional, and provincial levels by a variety of groups representing a number of interests, e.g., domiciliary midwives, childbirth activists, women's rights groups, nurses, and consumers. While the ideologies of these groups may have differed, the overall motives of the lobby effort were clear. Midwifery needed to be recognized as a legitimate health care profession; women and families needed to feel confident in making choices to have midwives as their primary care provider; home birth needed to remain a choice for birth place; and women and families needed to be able to access midwifery care regardless of financial means.

The very small group of midwives who were actively providing care at the time of the CPSA decision organized into the Alberta Council and Register of Domiciliary Midwives (ACRDMA). Their main objectives were to provide mutual professional support and to lobby for recognition and funding of midwifery. In 1982, this group applied to the Alberta Health Occupations Board, a division of the Ministry of Labour, for designation as a health profession. Midwives asked for recognition of their profession, the option of home birth, and for the privilege to "bill" under the Alberta Health Insurance Plan. This request was supported by two active consumer groups: the Association for Safe Alternatives in Childbirth (ASAC) in Edmonton and the Calgary Association of Parents and Professionals for Safe Alternatives in Childbirth (CAPSAC).

A public debate ensued, primarily because of the reaction of physicians to this application (Tait 1982). This debate served two positive purposes for midwives: it educated the public about the unique contribution midwives make to the care of birthing women, and thus increased public support for the midwifery cause. Nevertheless, the Health Occupations Board declined the midwives' request primarily based on a lack of comfort with the safety of home birth. In addition, the board believed that the Domiciliary Midwives did not represent the larger discipline of midwifery in Alberta and recommended that the association collaborate with other groups of midwives.

The only other formal organization for midwifery at the time was the Western Nurse Midwives Association (WNMA). This was a group of nurses with foreign credentials in midwifery or graduates from the Advanced Practical Obstetrics course (APO) at the University of Alberta who lived in one of the four western Canadian provinces. This group actively opposed the 1982 application of the ACRDMA for designation as a health profession (MSRC 1992).

It took four years for the ACRDMA and the WNMA to merge to form the Alberta Association of Midwives (AAM) in 1986. Even after the merger, some executive members of the WNMA blocked the dispersal of their funds to the various provincial midwifery organizations. The purpose of the AAM group was to lobby for legislation that would provide regulation and universal access to midwifery. Unlike the Domiciliary Association, the majority of AAM members were not practising midwifery, nor had any intention to practise should legislation be achieved.

Concurrent with these tense efforts at unification, a provincial consumer group was formed. While several other local groups included midwifery as part of their mandate, the sole purpose of the Alberta Midwifery Task Force (AMTF) was to lobby for midwifery legislation and public funding.

Following on the coattails of Ontario midwives, who were at this time well into investigations and proposals for midwifery legislation, the AAM and AMTF hired a lawyer to advise and assist them gain legislation. In 1989, the AAM made a formal application to the government of Alberta for designation under the Health Disciplines Act.

Government Negotiations and Dissenting Interests

Following the AAM application, the Alberta Health Disciplines Board invited interested parties to communicate their support or lack of support. On the whole, presenters were supportive of a plan to introduce midwifery into the health care system in Alberta. Nursing and medical organizations, however, supported a physician-controlled, nurse-midwifery model and expressly opposed the inclusion of home birth.

Ultimately, the Health Disciplines Board recommended that midwives be regulated as primary health care professionals in the province. Further recommendations included home and hospital birth, continuity of care, adequate third-party remuneration for midwifery services, liability insurance, and the development of a midwifery education program (Alberta Health 1990). While the decision to recommend the regulation of midwifery was made early in the Health Disciplines Board investigations, the actual announcement was concealed until a legal case where an Alberta midwife was charged with practising medicine without a license was completed, which the judge ruled in favour of the midwife (McKendry and Langford 2001; Williams and Levy 1992; Walker 1999).

As a result of these recommendations, in the fall of 1991 the government struck a Midwifery Services Review Committee (MSRC) to inquire into and provide advice on midwifery regulations, services, standards of practice, education, registration procedures, and integration into the health care system (MSRC 1992). The committee was made up of mid-wives, consumers, government representatives, physicians, nurses, and hospital and community health organization representatives. It is note-worthy that the appointees from nursing and medicine did not block the progress of this committee by upholding their professions' stance on nurse-midwifery under the direct supervision of physicians.

The members, conscious of the need to make midwifery in Alberta compatible with trends in other provinces, examined midwifery legisla-tion and practices in a number of jurisdictions in Canada and abroad. The MSRC recommendations were tabled in the Legislative Assembly in April 1992. As a result, midwifery was added as a recognized profes-sion under the Health Disciplines Act in July 1992.

Six months later, in December 1992, the Midwifery Regulation Advi-sory Committee (MRAC) was struck. The MRAC was made up of a simi-lar group of stakeholders as MSRC, but with a larger representation from the midwifery community. The purpose of this committee was to develop regulation and recommendations for education and for the as-sessment of existing practitioners. At this time, the Ministry of Health hired a midwifery coordinator but no formal committee was struck in that ministry to attend to midwifery implementation issues, including the provision of public funding.

In the spring of 1994, the minister of Health designated $800,000 to be used for the implementation of midwifery. Initially, midwives were informed that this $800,000 represented a "salary" of approximately $40,000 for twenty midwives for one year while permanent remunera-tion arrangements were made. However, the purpose of the $800,000 underwent many metamorphoses over the next four years. Finally, a decision was made to use $200,000 to subsidize liability insurance for midwives in the first one to two years of regulated practice; $200,000 to hire two midwifery implementation coordinators for one to two years; and $400,000 to fund a midwifery implementation pilot project. To date, no permanent plans for universal access to funding for mid-wifery services have been made.

In November 1994, the Midwifery Regulation was accepted by a Standing Policy Committee and went into effect in August of 1995. Midwives were assessed for eligibility for registration in August 1996 and were finally registered in July 1998.

Medicine

The reactions of the medical community to legalized midwifery have been mixed. There are many physicians who individually provided sup-port to midwives, including consultation, facilitating access to labora-tory testing, and prescribing medications. Others have spoken publicly of support, always accompanied by a large *"but"* (AMA 1998). Their reservations include the wisdom of midwives as primary care providers, home birth, hospital privileges, and government funding for midwifery services (Jeffs 1998). Others wonder about women's desire for primary care midwifery (Rowntree et al. 1994).

Discussion about midwifery funding also coincided with a prolonged period of Alberta Medical Association (AMA) negotiation about the Alberta Health Insurance Plan. From the early 1980s to the time of writing, the government has proposed a number of alternative methods of flowing health care funds. These have included the addition of "user fees" as a disincentive to "frivolous" use of the medical care system, de-insuring "non-essential" services, change from a fee-for-service model toward a salary model, giving other health professionals access to the insurance funds, and devolving the funds to regional health authorities (Alberta Health 1997; Alberta Premier's Commission on Future Health Care for Albertans 1989; Taft and Steward 2000). The medical community was highly suspicious of any proposals that could be seen to threaten their nearly exclusive access to the Alberta Health Insurance dollars. Restrictions on "extra billing" and a government imposed "cap" on the total amount in the Health Insurance Plan, in addition to a cap on how much individual physicians and individual specialties were able to bill within the plan, acted as additional incentives for physicians to protect these dollars from other care provider access.

Each time there was media coverage of the issue of funding for midwifery services, the medical community responded with misleading statements about the injustice of a midwife receiving far more money than a physician (e.g., Marner 1997; Vlessides 2000). According to one Alberta obstetrician, "The proposed pay for midwives topped $2000 a delivery and the basic $277.79 delivery fee for obstetricians can't stretch further than $563.09 even if the doctor throws in 10 prenatal office visits and another office visit after the birth. Why are we worth so little?" (Pedersen 1998b). Responses such as this compared the amount that the physician received for attending the birth with the amount the midwife received for providing a full course of care. At times, these responses also furthered the claims of injustice by pointing out the overhead expenses of the physician without acknowledging that the midwife too has operating expenses.

Just as midwives were becoming registered, the Alberta Medical Association released unadjusted perinatal mortality statistics that made it appear as though the risk of having a stillbirth or neonatal death with a midwife-attended home birth was 2.5 times higher than with a physician-attended hospital birth (McLean 1998). When the errors in this conclusion were revealed, the AMA remained silent. Concurrently, Alberta obstetricians initiated job action to protest their level of remuneration under the Alberta Health Insurance Plan. Initially, midwives viewed this as an excellent opportunity to open discussions with the Ministry of Health and the Health Regions about funding for women's health care in the province. However, midwifery funding became used as part of the obstetricians' campaign for increased levels of remuneration. At a moment when it seemed that a united front was possible, midwives found themselves being portrayed as greedy and overpaid (Cowan 1998; Pedersen 1998b).

Nursing

The Alberta Association of Registered Nurses (AARN) was slow to give up their position that midwifery was properly within the scope of nursing. Throughout the period of regulation development, the AARN resisted the idea of direct-entry midwifery, suggesting that midwifery ought to be regulated under a special register of the AARN. An AARN-AAM liaison committee was struck after a particularly adversarial proposal was produced by an AARN perinatal nurses' interest group. This proposal was damaging to trusting relationships within the MRAC because the name of the AARN representative to this committee appeared as one of the authors of the proposal.

The period of midwifery regulation development and implementation also coincided with unprecedented health care cuts. In an effort to find alternate work opportunities and to raise member morale, the AARN launched a "direct access to nurses" project (AARN 1993, 1998). Nurses were encouraged to become entrepreneurial, finding a niche where the public would be willing to pay for services. Clearly the area of maternity care was attractive. Nurses already had a history of acting in a quasi-independent way as lactation consultants, prenatal educators, and public health nurses. The public had shown a willingness to pay for midwives, so why not nurses?

The relationship between midwifery and nursing was further complicated by the high proportion of practising midwives who had a nursing background and the high proportion of maternity nurses who had studied midwifery. When trying to get information about midwifery issues, stakeholders sometimes consulted maternity nurses. It is no wonder that consumers, health care professionals and administrators, government, and the media sometimes received mixed messages about the way that midwives would like to join the health care system.

Voices Fighting within the Community

The work of developing midwifery regulation and planning for implementation of regulated midwifery resulted in a fracturing of the midwifery community itself. By the time the assessment for midwifery registration eligibility was held in 1996, trust and morale were at an all-time low. It was exceedingly difficult to present a unified position on midwifery. At the same time, the consumer lobby was disintegrating. It was almost as though consumers saw the acceptance of midwifery regulation as the end point to their work and moved on to other things.

By this time, Ontario had some experience with government regulated and funded midwifery. According to some consumers, all was not good with this new way of midwifery. Consumer publications warned of the evils of state interference in midwifery. Real midwives, these claimed, did not work for the government, but stayed outside the system and responded to the needs of women. Mixed messages began to likewise appear in consumer publications in Alberta (Ko 1998).

State as Audience and Actor

The 1990s marked a period of particularly strident neo-conservatism within the Alberta government (Taft 1997). The midwives' desire for regulation was fine to a government that wished to develop strong control over independent players within the health care arena. However, this government also preached a message of years of overspending in health care, supported privatization of health services, and promoted a competitive marketplace where private health services delivered by regulated or non-regulated individuals would challenge the exclusive rights of established professionals, mainly in medicine and nursing. The addition of a new government-insured profession was contrary to these directions.

Midwifery philosophy regarding the woman's right to choose may have inadvertently contributed to the government position not to fund midwifery services. At a time when the government was focusing on individual rights and responsibilities (e.g., Alberta Premier's Commission on Future Health Care for Albertans 1989; Taft 1997), it was possible to redefine maternity services provided by a midwife as a consumer choice rather than a health care issue. McKendry and Langford (2001) note "one of the unfortunate ironies of the campaign for midwifery in Alberta is that midwives chose to justify their demand for inclusion using arguments which could later be used to justify midwifery's marginalization outside the public health care system."

A series of changes contributed to the government's lack of support of midwifery funding. Most significant was the change of premier from Don Getty to Ralph Klein. In Getty's *Rainbow Report* (1989), midwifery was mentioned numerous times as an example of a new insured service that could contribute to the improved health of Albertans. The MSRC report recommending universal government funding for midwifery was accepted by the Getty government (MSRC 1992). Under Klein's leadership, however, the government position on midwifery funding was that midwives only wanted regulation, they did not want funding (Geddes 1999; Hansard 1995). A number of circumstances contributed to this separation of funding from regulation. In response to the questions of an opposition member, Marie Laing (NDP), about proposed delays in the funding process after regulation, which she argued would interfere with a midwife's ability to earn a living, the minister of health, Nancy Betkowski, said "Part of the cause of the delay is to get the players together to look at what pregnancies appropriately go to midwifery, how they can be paid for, instead of creating yet another add-on to our health care system" (Alberta Hansard, 5 May 1992). Additionally, when the midwifery regulation was reviewed by the Standing Policy Committee of the Ministry of Labour, some members questioned whether they would be perceived as approving funding for services if they approved the regulation. The MRAC chair, Dan Charlton, assured the members that the request before them was only for regulation.

Another impediment to midwifery funding came with the change of minister of health from Shirley McClellan to Halvar Jonson. Funding discussions with McClellan generally addressed issues of *when* and *how much* (e.g., Alberta Hansard, 28 March 1995) whereas discussions with Jonson addressed issues of *if* and *why*. Ultimately, Jonson's stand on funding was that he saw no reason that health regions should not fund midwifery services, but it was not the responsibility of the province to suggest health care spending decisions to the regions (e.g., Alberta Hansard, 9 February 1998).

In May 1999, when midwives and consumers hoped once again for a gift of funding for International Day of the Midwife, Klein denied any government intention to fund midwifery services. Klein shifted the blame for the decision not to fund their services to the midwives themselves (Geddes 1999).

Discussions about funding were further restricted by the split in midwifery regulation and implementation responsibilities between the Ministries of Labour and Health. Midwives and midwifery stakeholders had a fairly high level of consultation and access via the Ministry of Labour (the regulatory agency) through MRAC. But, without similar access in the Ministry of Health (the funding agency), the midwifery community was often kept uninformed about issues of midwifery implementation, including that of funding. Throughout the process of regulation development, MRAC members asked for decisions about funding to further inform the direction of this committee, particularly in developing guidelines for the assessment of midwives and the initial registration process. And with each request, the committee was informed that the Ministry of Labour could in no way influence the work of the Ministry of Health and that the work of this committee must be seen as completely separate from Ministry of Health responsibilities.

Lack of continuity of appointees to the MRAC was also an issue. For example, the initial chair of the MRAC was misquoted as saying that midwives would be billing for their services under the Alberta Health Insurance Plan. It was not long after this that he was moved within the ministry to have far less time for midwifery responsibilities and was ultimately replaced as the MRAC chair. While the funding outcome may have remained the same under his leadership, it is likely that the atmosphere may have been quite different. He was extremely skilled at negotiating the various interests of the members of MRAC and he had a good relationship with the midwifery coordinator at the Ministry of Health. A number of new government appointments to the committee – two new chairs and a new support staff member – were fraught with misunderstandings and tension. The MRAC began to polarize, practising midwives against the other members of the MRAC. The tone of meetings took on a strong anti-feminist stance. The midwives were told repeatedly to be "good girls" and not to raise questions. Resentment and distrust peaked as the task of the MRAC shifted to the development of the assessment process for registration eligibility. The practising midwife members were supportive of a decision to exclude them from the actual examination development process, but felt that too much power was being given to non-midwives in determining the principles of how the assessment would be accomplished. Their discomfort was magnified by frequent claims by the regional health authorities representative that the consumers on the MRAC knew more about midwifery than the midwives.

While the Ministry of Health appointed a midwifery coordinator, there was an overall lack of leadership in the implementation of midwifery on the part of that ministry. Voluntary assistance was frequently sought from the midwifery community and other stakeholder groups for tasks that were abandoned mid-project. The last of these volunteer advisory groups included several of the non-midwifery members of MRAC. The midwifery coordinator elected to look for midwife volunteers outside the MRAC group, hoping that this would defuse some of the tensions that had developed in MRAC. Unfortunately, her choice to approach midwives directly rather than asking for appointments from the AAM merely fuelled the divisions already started within the midwifery profession. The advisory group also tended to avoid consultation with the membership of the AAM, preferring to tell the midwives what was already done, giving information to limited groups of midwives, or setting a one-day turnaround for feedback. Midwives frequently found themselves in the awkward position of being less informed than the media or stakeholders when asked about the most recent developments in plans to fund and implement midwifery services (Pedersen 1998a).

The Structure of the Health Care System

The establishment of seventeen Regional Health Authorities (RHA) in Alberta further sidetracked funding decisions. In 1994, the tone of funding discussions began to change from province-wide funding to an integration of midwifery funding at a regional level. The RHAs, however, were in no position to address this issue. Their priorities were to establish their management structure and to craft budgets within the constraint of significant health care cuts. The minister of health dictated that particular services, including maternity services, must be provided by every health region. With the exception of medical care, however, no particular health care provider was included in the required services of a RHA.

The RHAs contended that they were being asked to do more with less and that their mandate was to be responsive to community needs overall. How could a new service, with small numbers and proportionately minute demand within any region of the province, even hope to capture the attention of an RHA? Midwives themselves resided in only five of the seventeen RHAs and the number of midwives per RHA (1 – 10) may have been too small to take seriously when the RHA was experiencing so many competing demands for dollars. Moreover, decisions about integrating non-physician practitioners to do work currently done by physicians were not easy. The Alberta Health Insurance Plan would pay the physician but the RHA would have to find the dollars to pay the non-physician (Church and Barker 1998).

In 1997, the Ministry of Health offered a proposal to the RHAs to apply for access to a proportion of the $800,000 as an "incentive" to integrate midwifery into their regional program and budget. This was a time-limited, one-time-only offer. To be eligible for money, the RHA had to commit to a three-year plan of funding for midwives. The amount that would be flowed to a particular RHA would depend on the number of regions that applied. This proposal furthered the tensions within the midwifery community. From the outset, all the RHAs with midwives except Calgary said that they would not apply for the "incentive" funding. Calgary RHA seemed to be moving forward in developing a proposal where they would receive all or nearly all of the

$800,000. The Calgary midwives became involved in their region's proposal development and stopped supporting the AAM actions to attain universal provincial funding. Their rationale was that getting funding in one region would be good for midwifery overall. The fracture line between north and south deepened.

Some RHAS were interested in midwifery, particularly as a solution to social or financial challenges. One RHA thought that introducing midwives to a specific geographic section of their region where the socioeconomic status was particularly low would improve perinatal outcomes in this region. Midwives may have been interested in this, but the RHA did not want to support the midwifery model of practice, which included continuity of care, midwife as primary care provider, and choice of birth place.

Another RHA was investigating innovative programs to justify keeping small hospitals open. Women in their region tended to go to the neighbouring region with larger hospitals and greater choices including epidurals. They proposed adding midwives to these small hospitals as an incentive to keep women in the community. Again, the model of practice was limited to hospital births only and limited continuity of care and primary care responsibilities. Generally these proposals were developed with little or no midwifery input.

Options and Outcomes

At the time of writing, there is no universal coverage of midwifery services in the province of Alberta. Alberta women accessing midwifery care are currently charged a midwifery fee between $2,500 and $3,500. The pilot project that was designed to evaluate the impact of the implementation of midwifery into the health care system upon first registration of midwives was given the go-ahead to start in the spring of 2001 (O'Brien 1999). Nearly 1,000 women applied to be one of the 150 who had their midwifery fee covered. In March 2001, Marsh Canada (the liability insurance broker for Canadian midwives) announced a 350 per cent increase in liability premiums for midwives. The pilot project was delayed until the government decided to subsidize the $15,000 premium (Brooymans 2001; Olsen 2001). All data for the project were collected by July 2002.

Two other projects including midwives but not within the primary care, continuity, and choice of birth place model provide some access to funded midwifery services for women in two communities (Alberta Health and Wellness 2000). To date, it is not clear whether the midwives who have become involved with these projects will continue to be eligible for midwifery registration because the projects do not give them the minimum requirements for ongoing registration.

Some of the elements for fully integrated, fully funded midwifery are in place. The Hospitals Act has been amended to facilitate midwife-admitting privileges. To date, midwives in some communities have been granted privileges, where others were given privileges only for the integration evaluation project (Vlessides 2000). A further increase in Marsh Canada premiums in 2002 led to a change in insurance policy with government subsidy of the midwives' premiums. The subsidy is a one-year only arrangement and the midwives must agree to offer additional public services in exchange for the subsidy (Government of Alberta 2002). The ministry responsible for university education has expressed a strong support for the development of a midwifery education program in Alberta. No funding for a program will be released, however, until there is an ongoing plan for funding of midwifery services. In 2001, midwives provided care for 649 women. Despite these small successes, the total number of registered midwives in the province has decreased from thirty-two to sixteen over the past four years as midwives migrate to provinces where funding is available or stop practising all together.

THE ALBERTA CASE IN CONTEXT

It is revealing to compare midwifery integration in Alberta with that in another province – Ontario. In both cases, the midwifery community organized into lobby/interest groups, first separately for practising home birth midwives and largely non-practising nurse-midwives, and later both groups merged for a more unified front. Similarly, consumer groups were created, both being small but vocal in the two provinces. In both provinces, midwifery integration occurred in the context of a review of all health professions and their regulatory structures.

In terms of dissenting voices, both cases are also similar in terms of the direction of the medical and nursing efforts that favour nurse-midwifery. But one important difference in the dissenting interests within the medical profession in the two provinces may be the relative interest and engagement in the practice of obstetrics. While interest has waned in both provinces, family practitioners in Alberta still have much higher proportion of obstetrical practice than do their counterparts in Ontario (Klein 2000).

Politics also matters. It is no accident that most of the headway that the Ontario midwifery lobby made was against a backdrop of an increasingly midwifery-friendly state – moving from a fairly centrist Conservative to Liberal to left-of-centre New Democratic provincial government through the late 1980s and early 1990s. The Alberta midwifery lobby was not as privileged, with some of their most important challenges being faced during a hard right turn of the provincial Conservative government from Getty to Klein.

In addition to politics, the agency of internal state advocates was relatively absent in Alberta, whereas four successive feminist ministers of health in Ontario helped to champion the cause of midwives and their consumer supporters from within the state. Thus, the temporary *feminization* of the Ministry of Health in Ontario had a strong impact (Bourgeault and Fynes 1996/97). The composition of the Task Force on the Implementation of Midwifery in Ontario was made up of four arguably midwifery-friendly appointees, whereas in Alberta the composition of the MRAC took a more traditional form of including representatives from each of the professional and institutional interest groups, many of whom were not supportive of midwifery integration let alone of public funding for its services. In addition to having midwifery-friendly appointees, advisory committees in Ontario also included several midwives from the provincial association (even if sometimes *ex-officio*). Thus throughout the process it could be argued that midwives as a group evolved from having outsider to insider status (Bourgeault et al. 2001). Where midwifery representatives were included in advisory bodies in Alberta, it was unclear as to how representative they were given they often lacked any official status with the AAM.

The centrality of decision-making authority within the Ministry of Health in Ontario was also immensely helpful in the midwifery community's lobby efforts. Other than the final decision-making about the location of the Ontario Midwifery Education Programme, it was entirely within the Ministry of Health that decisions regarding midwifery integration were to be made. In Alberta, decision-making not only was divided internally within the state between the Ministries of Health and Labour, but was also increasingly diffused amongst the seventeen Regional Health Authorities. This diffusion of decision-making bodies had the unfortunate side effect of creating a great deal of disunity within the Alberta midwifery community and preventing any kind of organized effort that their lobby was attempting to foster.

Finally, the economic context in the two cases also warrants attention. Midwifery made most of its headway in Ontario during the relatively prosperous 1980s. Assumptions of public funding were not inconsistent with social spending during this decade. In Alberta, again, given the process occurred somewhat later – during what was portrayed as the lean 1990s – such assumptions were difficult to make.[1] Indeed, it is intriguing how the issue of *choice* was used against the midwives' case in Alberta, whereas it help bolster midwives' efforts in Ontario.

These factors are not divorced from one other. The lack of sustained interest amongst the generally small consumer groups may have been due in large part to the lack of progress in Alberta and the lack of respect for the integrity of groups formed within the midwifery community and recognition of the importance of their representation. Reflecting upon these processes and outcomes of the quest for public funding for midwifery services from a health policy perspective, one can see how the three separate streams that Kingdon described – problems, policies, and politics – did not come together in Alberta to create a "window of opportunity" for issue of midwifery funding as it has been argued to have been the case in Ontario (Bourgeault et al. 2001).

The Alberta lobby instead remained what is the usual case for women's policy groups – outsiders to the sources of political power and the decision-making process. Some individual "midwives" may have achieved limited insider status in Alberta, but questions were raised about how representative such midwives were of the larger community. Overall there was little organized input from the broader midwifery community – by design or by default. Moreover, taking into consideration the influence of gender and the broader context of women's negotiations with the state, the case of midwifery lobbying for public funding in Alberta reveals the negative capacities the state has had for provincial women's initiatives. This is unlike the positive capacities that a somewhat feminized sector of the provincial Ontario state has had for women's initiatives there, including promoting funding for midwives' services.

NOTES

1 Given the wealth of the province of Alberta compared to many other poorer provinces (e.g., B.C., Quebec, Manitoba) that have decided to publicly fund midwifery in the lean 1990s, this argument may say more about the orientation and different kinds of political machinery and ideology in relation to their public spending agendas than about a provincial funding crisis.

REFERENCES

Alberta Association of Registered Nurses (AARN). 1993. *Position on Increased Direct Access to Services*. Provided by registered nurses. Edmonton.
– 1998. *Barriers to the Implementation of Primary Health Care: A Background Paper*. Edmonton.
Alberta Hansard. 1992. 5 May. Nancy Betkowski.
– 1995. 28 March. Mrs McClellan.

– 1998. 9 February. Mr Jonson.

Alberta Health. 1997. *Reaching an Agreement for Better Health*. Background on discussions with Alberta's doctors.

– 1990. *A Brief on the Proposed Regulation of Midwives under the Health Disciplines Act.*

Alberta Health and Wellness. 2000. Health Innovation Fund Projects Announced. Press release, Edmonton, 22 March.

Alberta Medical Association. 1998. *Position Statement on Midwifery*. April.

Alberta Premier's Commission on Future Health Care for Albertans. 1989. *The Rainbow Report: Our Vision for Health*. Volume I. Edmonton.

Alford, Robert R. 1972. The Political Economy of Health Care: Dynamics Without Change. *Politics and Society* 12 (Winter 1972): 127-64.

Barrington, Eleanor. 1985. *Midwifery is Catching*. Toronto: NC Press.

Benoit, Cecilia. 2000. *Women, Work and Social Rights. Canada in Historical and Comparative Perspective*. Scarborough, Ontario: Prentice Hall Canada.

Bourgeault, Ivy, Eugene Declercq, and Jane Sandall. 2001. Changing Birth: Interest Groups and Maternity Care Policy. In *Birth by Design: The Social and Cultural Aspects of Maternity Care in Europe and North America*. Routledge: New York.

Bourgeault, Ivy and Mary Fynes. 1996/97. Delivering Midwifery in Ontario: How and Why Midwifery Was Integrated into the Provincial Health Care System. *Health and Canadian Society/Santé et Société Canadienne* 4, no. 1: 227–60.

Briskin, Linda. 1999. Mapping Women's Organizing in Sweden and Canada: Some Thematic Considerations. In *Women's Organizing and Public Policy in Sweden and Canada*, edited by Linda Briskin and Mona Eliasson. Montreal and Kingston: McGill-Queen's University Press.

Brooymans, Hanneke. 2001. Midwives Await Minister's 'Solution.' University of Alberta Study Also at Risk. *Edmonton Journal*, 31 March.

Canada Labour News. 1999. Midwives at a Loss to Practise their Profession in Alberta: Local Women Feel They Could Be Part of the Solution to Health Care Woes. *Canada Labour News*, June.

Church, John, and Paul Barker. 1998. Regionalization of Health Services in Canada: A Critical Perspective. *International Journal of Health Services* 28: 467–86.

Conway, Margaret, David Ahern, and Gertrude Steuernagel. 1999. *Women and Public Policy: A Revolution in Progress*. Washington: CQ Press.

Cowan, Paul. 1998. Docs' Job Action Isn't Helping Us: Midwives. *Edmonton Sun*, 22 June.

Eduards, Maud. 1991. Toward a Third Way: Women's Politics and Welfare Policies in Sweden. *Social Research* 58, no. 3: 667–705.

Feldberg, Georgina, and Marianne Carlsson. 1999. Organized for Health: women's Activism in Canada and Sweden. In *Women's Organizing and Public Policy in Sweden and Canada*, edited by Linda Briskin and Mona Eliasson. Montreal and Kingston: McGill-Queen's University Press.

Folden, Rachelle. 2000. Birthing Choices Limited in Alberta. *Mt. Royal College Journal* 3, no. 3 (10 March).

Fox Piven, Frances. 1990. Ideology and the State: Women, Power and the Welfare State. In *Women, the State, and Welfare*, edited by L. Gordon. Madison: University of Wisconsin Press.

Freidson, P. 1970. *Professional Dominance: The Social Structure of Medical Care*. New York: Atherton.

Fudge, J. 1996. Fragmentation and Feminization: The Challenge of Equity for Labour-Relations Policy. In *Women and Canadian Public Policy*, edited by J. Brodie. Toronto: Harcourt Brace and Company.

Geddes, Ashley. 1999. Midwives 'Never Agreed' Not to Seek Government Funding. *Edmonton Journal*, 8 May.

Gotell, L. 1996. Policing Desire: Obscenity Law, Pornography Politics, and Feminism in Canada. In *Women and Canadian Public Policy*, edited by J. Brodie. Toronto: Harcourt Brace and Company.

Government of Alberta. 2002. Alberta Continues Grant for Midwives Insurance. *Government of Alberta News Release*, 4 May.

Jeffs, Allyson. 1998. Midwives Want Chance to Prove Proficiency. *Edmonton Journal*, 20 January.

Kingdon, John W. 1995. *Agendas, Alternatives, and Public Policies. New York: Harper Collins*.

Klein, M. 2000. "Canadian Family Physicians Shrinking from Maternity Care." The Future of Maternity Care in Canada: Crisis and Opportunity. London, 24-25 November.

Ko, Marnie. 1998. What is Unassisted Childbirth? *Nurturing Magazine Online*. http://www.nurturing.ca/ub7.htm

Marner, Paul. 1997. Letter to the editor. *Edmonton Journal*, 26 March.

McDermott, Pat. 1996. Pay and Employment Equity: Why Separate Policies? In *Women and Canadian Public Policy*, edited by J. Brodie. Toronto: Harcourt Brace and Company.

McKendry, Rebecca, and Tom Langford. 2001. Legalized, Regulated, but Unfunded: Midwifery's Laborious Professionalization in Alberta, Canada, 1975–99. *Social Science and Medicine* 53, no. 4: 531-42.

McLean, Candis. 1998. A Medical Argument Rages On. Alberta Midwives Win Accreditation While Doctors Release Alarming Contrary Statistics. *Alberta Report*, 8 June.

Midwifery Services Review Committee (MSRC). 1992. *Report of the Midwifery Services Review Committee*. Edmonton: Government of Alberta.

Molnar, Wendy. 1998. The Global Witch Hunt Reaches Alberta. *The Newsletter of the Alberta Association of Midwives*. April.

O'Brien, Ben. 1999. Evaluation of the Integration of Midwifery Services. *Birth* 14, no. 1 (summer 1999).

Olsen, Tom. 2001. Province May Rescue Midwives from Insurance Cash-crunch. *Calgary Herald*, 23 March.

Pedersen, Rick. 1998a. Deliveries Plan Catches Midwives Off Guard. *Edmonton Journal*, 26 November.

– 1998b. Midwives Offered $2,000 but Obstetricians $563 tops. *Edmonton Journal*, 2 May.

Phillips, Anne. 1995. *The Politics of Presence*. Oxford: Clarendon Press.

Rowntree, Carol, Hal Irvine, Jim Thompson, Darien Larsen, and Janet Morse. 1994. Rural Physicians' Perspective on Midwifery. http://www.srpc.ca/perspective.html

Sabatier, Paul. 1991. Toward Better Theories of the Policy Process. *Political Science and Politics* 24: 144–56.

Taft, Kevin. 1997. *Shredding the Public Interest: Ralph Klein and 25 Years of One-party Government*. Edmonton: University of Alberta Press.

Taft, Kevin, and Gillian Steward. 2000. *Clear Answers. The Economics and Politics of For-profit Medicine*. Edmonton: Parkland Institute and University of Alberta Press.

Tait, Mark. 1982. MDs to Battle Bid Allowing Midwives. *Calgary Herald*, 28 Oct.

Vlessides, Mike. 2000. Alberta Allows Midwives to Practice in Hospitals if Patients Pay. *Canadian Medical Association Journal* 163, no. 1: 74.

Walker, Noreen. 1999. Twenty Years of Midwifery. *Birth Issues* 14, no. 2. http://www.asac.ab.ca/BI_fall99/index.html

Walt, Gill. 1994. *Health Policy: An Introduction to Process and Power*. London: Zed Press

Williams, L. Sears, and J. Chris Levy. 1992. In the Absence of Medical Men. Midwife-attended Home Birth, the Charter of Rights and Antique Alberta Legislation. *Alberta Law Review* 30, no. 2: 555–96.

Wysong, Pippa. 1998. Obstetrics Crisis Looms. *Medical Post*. 7 July. http://www.cofp.com/obstetrics.htm

7

Exploring Legislated Midwifery: Texts and Rulings[1]

Mary Sharpe

On 1 January 1994, with the implementation of the Midwifery Act, Ontario midwives began to practise as autonomous, regulated health professionals. Midwifery, long considered peripheral to traditional medical practice, became legally integrated into the Ontario health care system. The act altered the status of the Ontario midwife and required the establishment of new work structures, processes, and relationships.

In this paper, I examine the role that written documents, official language, structures, and institutionalized processes (henceforth referred to as texts and/or rulings), have increasingly played in midwives' work through the integration process. To do this, I draw upon the theoretical work of sociologist Dorothy Smith (1990, 1995). I also bring my own reflections from twenty-eight years as a white, middle-class lay midwife in Toronto, as a registered midwife, and as my daughter Jenny's midwife. As well, I present relevant research (Sharpe 1995) from interviews with newly legislated midwives. I argue that the texts midwives use frame women's experiences in particular ways that can inhibit care. These texts also protect women, midwives, and the profession of midwifery.

DOROTHY SMITH

Dorothy Smith's idea is that texts not only alter, shape, and rule people's lives but over time become invisible limiting forces. What people experience and speak about in their ordinary lives, their "primary narratives," is often not captured or understood in the various texts that are created from the primary narrative. Special attention called a "bifurcated consciousness" is necessary to recover a measure of freedom to coexist with these texts. These arguments, presented in Dorothy Smith's work; resonate in my grappling with the implications of legislation.

PRE-LEGISLATIVE PRACTICE AND LAY MIDWIVES

I begin exploring my pre-theoretical life and looking at where I found knowledge. Throughout my youth, formal schooling often felt unreal. Ideas and information floated around me in a way that didn't relate to me. It wasn't until I gave birth to my daughter, Jenny, that I came in touch with intuitive knowing or, my mother would say, "the real thing." I found a knowing that was clear, meaningful, and powerful, arising from my body and the unfolding of the raw acts of birthing and breastfeeding. I lived as in a damp green forest where call and response were immediate and where feeling loomed large.

With the birth of Jenny in 1970, a natural birth with an obstetrician, I began to meet with other parents. We formed a strong subculture, exploring and sharing childbearing, breastfeeding, and parenting practices. We began to read, research, and write. I discovered that knowing from direct experience, intuition, and work with relationship has a valid place in the intellectual, academic, and professional worlds. This led me toward becoming a midwife and influenced my future birth choices: nurse-midwifery care in a U.S. birthing centre, home births with doctors in Ontario, and a midwife-attended home birth in France.

These forms of knowing become critically visible along what Dorothy Smith calls "fault lines" (1995, 13), where one can see distinctions – for instance, between the obstetrical care to which some feel subjected and the kind of birthing care they desire. It appeared that the greatest reason for having a home birth was to avoid the hospital's dictates: procedures like fetal monitoring, separation from loved ones during parts of the labour, and from the baby shortly after birth.

In the early 1970s, a small number of family physicians were attending home births, often assisted by the Victorian Order of Nurses. In 1976, when funding for this nursing service was discontinued, this need was met by some of us who aspired to become midwives. From 1976 to 1982, as a "lay" (of the people) midwife, I assisted thirteen family physicians willing to offer home births to women. In other settings, particularly in rural areas in Ontario, some lay midwives and nurses attended home births without the support of physicians or even their own colleagues. In hospital, lay midwives offered themselves as birth attendants and advocates working to protect women from interference that would unreasonably interrupt the delicate balance of labour.

The philosophy, experience, and socio-economic status of the lay midwife and the parturient women were often quite similar. We often approached this care together as friends, in the context of the woman's primary narrative. The woman told the lay midwife what she wanted and the lay midwife responded with a minimum of interpretation.

By 1979, lay midwives began to network and attend courses and midwifery schools in other jurisdictions.[2] We established study groups and informal clinics in our homes. In one setting, pregnant women, who had learned of the clinic through word of mouth, would gather one morning a week in the living room, bringing snacks to share. Herbal tea was on the stove, on a shelf, there was a donation jar to help pay expenses, and a collection of books to borrow. Children played together and women conversed while they waited to see the lay midwife of their choice in one of the bedrooms upstairs. At noon, we lay midwives would gather in the kitchen over a potluck lunch *separately* from the other women, discuss what we had learned from the morning contact, and make plans for educational activities. Out of this, we began to develop standards and forms, a statement of philosophy, and a code of ethics. Ideas and actions that originally seemed to be simply a response to a woman's requests for care became encoded in writing.

Perhaps the earliest record by lay midwives of events surrounding the birth of the baby, the gender, the date and time of birth – if not for a birth certificate, certainly for the child's astrological chart – casually written on the back of sterile glove packages or on note paper, were primarily for the woman, and sometimes for the midwife's personal diary. Gradually, we began to develop discourses and texts that influenced our practice and interpreted the woman's experiences.

In our early work, we were shielded from certain clinical details and from the large body of paper work required after legislation. Even if the home birth doctor had not been present, the signing of the birth certificate was left to her or him. A kind of parallel prenatal care occurred in those days. The woman would regularly visit the physician as well as the lay midwife. The lay midwife would dip into the clinical world for a while, leisurely checking, for example, the position of the baby, the fetal heart tones, and the blood pressure, and would often provide additional information and alternative views about testing and procedures suggested by the physician. This division of labour that existed between physicians and midwives pre-legislation reproduced elements of traditional male/female roles. The physician, with access to laboratory tests and the obligation to do the formal documentation of care, dealt with "public" matters, leaving "private" matters, such as discussing the woman's feelings and experience, to the midwife. For some midwives, this exchange facilitated their role, while for others it restricted and undermined them as primary caregivers (Van Wagner 1999).

Women increasingly requested the help of these lay midwives at home and in hospital. For some of us, this became a full-time vocation. Some recompense for care was provided: loaves of bread, childcare, gifts, and later money.

In 1981, lay midwives created the Ontario Association of Midwives (OAM), which later became the Association of Ontario Midwives (AOM). In 1982 the College of Physicians and Surgeons of Ontario, through a letter to its members, declared home birth unsafe and discouraged support for lay midwives. Hospitals threatened to withdraw privileges from physicians who attended home births, and by 1983, few doctors offered this service. In response to this lack, lay midwives became primary caregivers at home births. We formed cooperative working arrangements, meeting each other's clients and providing back-up for one another, and took on apprentices.[3]

In 1982 and 1985, inquests were called into the deaths of two babies whose births had been attended by lay midwives. We quickly learned that written accounts were key in investigations and that to protect ourselves we should keep "good" records. Experience taught us that, *if it is not written down, it did not occur.*

We created record-keeping systems and a disciplinary process for our members. Self-regulation was considered to be more palatable than possible court action and led the majority of midwives and consumers to support the lobby for registration. Thus a model of midwifery that had developed organically over many years became articulated in writing. This process helped us become clear about what we collectively wanted for women, ourselves, and midwifery.

Legalization was effected by a group[4] of midwives who worked according to a consensus model through committees in the Association of Ontario Midwives that invited participation from the membership. Working with the Health Professions Legislative Review, these midwives learned the necessary ingredients and processes of professionalism in order to prepare documentation with specific language and categories so that Ontario midwifery would fit within the requirements of a regulated health profession. The professional project implicated midwives in what Dorothy Smith would call "father-tongue language: a condition of speaking beyond what we learned from our mothers" (1990, 4). Many of the texts and documents developed were used as bases for decisions of the Interim Regulatory Council of Midwifery and its successors, the Transitional Council and ultimately the College of Midwives, and thus were key in the achievement of midwifery legislation in January 1994.

If we accept the thesis that feminist work comes out of women's efforts to effect structural changes, we see the energetic struggle to recreate midwifery as a profession and as a meaningful feminist endeavour and triumph. The Ontario midwifery model is different from and challenges current obstetrical practice – a shift from male-dominated maternity care to woman-centred care, provided principally by women caregivers.

PROFESSIONAL REGISTERED MIDWIVES

With legislation, the Ontario midwife was catapulted into a new status, role, and context. We wondered what the new legislation would mean for our lives, our practices, and our relationships with clients. Something utilitarian was coming into my midwifery practice; although I *thought* that I could care for my clients better after legislation, I *felt* as if I cared less. This mixture of ambivalence and excitement about new possibilities led me to interview midwives in 1994 for my master's thesis. Sixteen of twenty-four licensed midwives practising in Ontario for at least five years prior to and during the first year following legislation were interviewed, ten months after legislation. They were selected from eleven practices in six geographical areas, including rural and urban sites: one midwife in solo practice, the others in shared practices of from two to five midwives. Questions asked were open-ended, such as: "What changes have you noticed in your practice since legislation?" From this question, recurring themes emerged.

Midwives felt variously delighted, freed, satisfied, acknowledged, frustrated, overworked, anxious, and cautious. Common themes arose but were regarded differently. Most often mentioned were: changes in the relationship with the client with the midwife's role of primary caregiver now expanded with prenatal, intrapartum, and postpartum care, increased paperwork, responsibility in hospitals, and new interprofessional relationships; altered work arrangements with colleagues; changes in clinic settings and administration; and government remuneration.

Most midwives I interviewed felt that the legalization of midwifery protected a model of care that one would identify as feminist and that contributed in many ways to ideal care: "universal" access to midwifery care; a baccalaureate program with practising midwives as teachers and a balance of clinical and academic experience; a funding system that supports long visits with clients; assurance of continuity of caregiver; more options; and an exceptionally positive atmosphere for home births by requiring midwives to maintain confidence and competence in the home birth setting, as well as in the hospital. The least change was noted in the care of women choosing home birth. The midwives interviewed saw the home as the site where midwifery care could be most effectively expressed: "The Ontario model gives us a framework ... there is the flexibility ... the time to really play out options and choices to do a dance around so many issues. The ideal for me is to take this model and strive to give it life and reality" (Adrienne).

Concurrent with these positive statements were some concerns. For example, unregistered midwives practising outside the system, as we all once were, now were practising not simply *alegally* but *illegally*, and subject to jail sentences and fines. For some, this felt like a betrayal, the antithesis of sisterly support. Furthermore, professional midwifery developed in response to powerful consumer interest in a model of care antithetical to the medical model. Ironically, professionalism necessitates engaging in activities closely linked to the medical model. Some midwives appreciated of the new dialogue with doctors and professional procedures, and others worried about co-option and the disappearance of the unique quality of midwifery.

Formerly the woman and the lay midwife learned together throughout the pregnancy. In the evolution of the profession, along with greater experience and expertise, the midwife's education increased in "sophistication" and took place increasingly in sites separate from the woman: workshops, the assessment process for registering midwives, continuing education, and the baccalaureate midwifery education program.

CLINICAL CARE

When a pregnant woman enters into "care," she brings her "primary narratives," drawn directly from her experience. The midwife picks out certain aspects of that narrative for a written report. One could say that this narrative is operated upon by certain obstetrical schemata where parity, gravidity, blood pressure, certain measurements are extracted as data important to providing good care. The midwife engages in selecting terms and grammatical and logical connections that express the appropriate sequencing when she utilizes prenatal, intrapartum, and postpartum records. Even the items the midwife is interested in picking out of the narrative are determined by an interpretive schema (Smith 1995).

Regulated midwifery involves an intersection with the texts of other existing professional acts. Many acts already in place had to be altered to accommodate the professional midwife so that she could dispense and prescribe drugs and write requisitions for ultrasounds and laboratory testing, for example. Most notable was the change to the Ontario Hospitals Act, which legislated admitting privileges for midwives, previously held exclusively by doctors.

Midwives were clear that careful documentation was an important aspect of the business of their care. Documentation properly provided a record of the woman's clinical care and offered a measure of legal protection from the courts, the media, and even clients themselves. However, some midwives found that during visits with women, attention was given more to notes than to the mother and baby. Standardized prenatal and postpartum forms were constraining. If a place on the form was not filled out, the record was incomplete. Much of the affective care provided to the woman was lost on this record. It was alarming how readily aspects of the primary narrative that didn't easily fit could be discarded. Much of the woman's story was invisible in these records.

(In the past) there was more oral ... my visits were focused more on talking about the birth and how the woman was doing. Now there's the: "Oh, I've got to write all this down!" To me, that does change what I'm doing. It puts the focus on recording and making sure I have properly covered everything and asked people questions I might not have even asked them before. Like how often the baby is feeding when they're not expressing any concern about it and the baby ... appears to be thriving. I ask the question so I can fill the proper blank. It's a shift. I used to get a really good sense of where things are just by sitting there for a while and talking about lots of things. Now I'm more focused about filling in the blanks and writing it down. My attention is not face to face with the person, but onto the piece of paper. (Amanda)

Although the content of the clinic visits generally had changed, midwives believed women still felt well cared for. Some midwives said that they needed to pay attention to *how* they provided clinical care in order to adequately address emotional and social needs and the participation of the woman's family. Others reported that they were consciously working on balancing what they saw as good midwifery with the changes, and that they looked forward to increased adaptation to their new expanded role.

No longer were midwives primarily emphasizing the alternative view to the one generally offered by the physician, but now they were required to incorporate views that reflected the community medical standard as well. A dilemma arose for some midwives who felt that describing tests might be construed as condoning them. The requirement to offer testing shifted the focus to *verifying* rather than *assuming* that the pregnancy was normal. Assuming *normal* recreates that possibility. Midwives were concerned that they might be moving away from a wellness model towards a pathology-oriented model, relying on ultrasounds and an increased use of the system and spending less time on woman-generated discussions relating to her feelings, questions and circumstances.

I feel myself sliding more into the use of technology in the accepted medical standard. I see the changes in the trends and I am unsettled by them. (Aisha)
The list of tests grows and will continue to grow because science provides us with more ability to detect things. It's a cumulative thing and the normality of pregnancy is being lost even on the majority of women. This is us changing since legislation. (Ruth)

What is hidden here is the former reliance on doctors to engage in many of these activities. Effectively a three-way discussion (doctor – woman – midwife) around issues of care became a two-way discussion (woman – midwife). Although midwives attributed some of these changes to legislation, they have occurred within the childbirth culture in which, over the last twenty years, technology is increasingly used (Duden 1993).

Many appreciated how "[t]he ability to write orders and various lab tests and diagnostic procedures ... allow[s] us to ensure the well being of our clients is more holistically taken care of. The care is less fragmented. This truly is continuity because we have access to that piece the doctors were doing before. That's the big change for us" (Joan).

WORK IN HOSPITAL

Midwives found themselves on a steep learning curve with respect to hospital procedures, protocols, equipment and paperwork, and client admission and discharge. After their first hospital births as primary caregivers, it would take two midwives up to four hours to accomplish the postpartum care and paperwork. Hundreds of new details were included in the hospital discourse. With the exception of those whose previous nursing experience had already immersed them in charting and procedures, most midwives found this stressful at first but, with time, were able to adapt.

"The hospital is the most disturbing situation to me because I'm finding it difficult to feel like I'm fulfilling both my expected role as a health care professional in the hierarchy of the system in the hospital as well as just being with someone, which is what I feel is my primary role" (Anna). For planned hospital births, midwives usually labour with the woman at home, come into the hospital for the birth, and then return home several hours later. The journey to the hospital for the birth can be a hiatus in care. Most midwives wished to assume the three roles of primary caregiver, documenter, and labour supporter, but felt this was difficult to accomplish in hospital, where they were distracted.

The women choosing hospital births needed preparation for the challenge of administrative duties taking their midwife in and out of

the room. Some midwives brought their clients and/or the second midwife into the hospital early to provide enough people for support and
time to accomplish the admitting tasks. Experiences in hospital were
influencing how midwives worked at home births – less hands-on care:
massages, cool cloths, encouraging words. No longer were we making
meals, doing the laundry, and washing the dishes after a home birth.
Some midwives would argue that in their maturing, less action is appropriate, allowing space for the woman's friends and families to take
on the supportive work.

Now some women are hiring labour attendants, who could move the
midwife into a more impersonal role and reproduce the labour relations that existed previously between physicians and lay midwives. One
client hired an attendant who called herself a "spiritual midwife." Was
the registered midwife now the "clinical midwife"?

"It could be that midwives are going to get so busy that we're going
to be just like obstetricians and rush in catch the baby and rush out
again and the labour coach will do all the work" (Gabrielle).

Recently, I received a notice from a hospital health records department that records I made while attending a client's birth in the hospital
had not been completed. I had to complete them within a designated
time or my hospital privileges might be suspended. With fear and trem-
bling I entered that office, the great repository of hospital texts in the
bowels of the institution, to accomplish this task. The chief record
keeper's assistant directed me to my single chart. All around I saw
piles, one or two feet high, of charts with physicians' names on top. I
had been initiated into the massive world of text that links me to all
other professionals in the hospital. Paperwork is a great leveller. No
one else can do this work; you can't escape. This is one way in which
you, as midwife or physician, pay for your privilege.

Some midwives felt closely monitored and scrutinized in hospital,
and that hospital staff were testing them, waiting to assess their level of
competence. It was important to look professional in order to be accepted by the medical staff and maintain hospital privileges. Proper
documentation and the appropriate manner of making written referrals
were some of the new professional skills. In exchange for hospital privileges, some midwives felt compromised, required to comply with certain hospital rules with which they didn't agree.

Questions emerging for me liken midwives to those early home birth
doctors who supported women's choices to have their babies at home.
Their actions instigated the threat of loss of hospital privileges, and in
some cases disciplinary actions from their colleges. Will midwives be
forced to discontinue home births? Obstetrical departments in different

hospitals have various protocols that differ from each other and some-times from midwifery standards. While midwives would like their work to be research-based, it is likely that certain hospital or govern-ment requirements will come to dictate some of their practices. Perhaps midwives have been thrown, as Dorothy Smith would say, into a situa-tion that may undermine their original intentions and trap them in the very institutional web from which they endeavoured to extricate women. It seems essential that midwives continue to try to influence policy and local rulings.

These findings are echoed by other Canadian and American re-searchers. It has been argued, for example, that the Ontario midwifery legislation has changed the egalitarian feminist relationships between women and midwives; midwifery is now controlled by the professional body rather than by clients (Bourgeault 1996). Once regulated, mid-wifery no longer represents counter-cultural alternatives, community, and the emotional and spiritual aspects of life; it can no longer be seen in opposition to the dominant social order (Durish 1996). Similarly, midwives feel the tension between practising according to women's wishes and abiding by professional standards and hospital procedures (Benoit 1994). What my analysis adds to this discourse is how the texts created by or thrust upon midwives help to create these new relations of ruling.

LANGUAGE BEFORE AND AFTER LEGISLATION

Roles and ideologies are powerfully connected with words; the sound of the voice permeates everything. In an attempt to distance themselves from "patients," used in medical professional language, implying pas-sivity in a patriarchal model, Ontario midwives began to call the women they worked with "clients." Like "consumer," this appellation is problematic. While it accents the advocacy and contractual nature of the relationship, it is a shift to the language associated with law and business and a more formal working relationship.

Dorothy Smith provides illustrations of how particular language is representative of rulings, and she inspired me to look at similar occur-rences in birth language. We see how certain phrases express ideologies and represent different paradigms. Smith compares the two phrases "she committed suicide" and "she killed herself," and notes a disjunc-ture between them. They are embedded in different social relations and contexts, and as "she committed suicide" replaces "she killed herself," there takes place "an ideological move that subordinates the individual within the relations of rulings" (1990, 142–3).

The phrases "the doctor delivered the baby" and "the woman gave birth" colour our picture of the same event quite differently. In the first, it may be implied that the woman is merely a vessel, a foil or background for the occurrence, whereas the practitioner is at centre stage. Although in the phrase "the doctor delivered the baby," there appears to be some formal connection or act occurring between the doctor and the baby, the woman herself is invisible. Her name isn't even mentioned. Furthermore, this phrase may imply that the woman is subject to the rulings of the practitioner's discipline and the local setting, usually a hospital, to which the practitioner is connected. One might imagine that assistants, nurses, anaesthetists, and paediatricians were gathered around to help the doctor deliver the *baby* rather than to help the *woman* give birth. One could also say that the word "delivered" is part of the "institutional discourse" (Smith 1995) of the hospital, and a particular mode of telling what happened.

Ontario government antenatal forms require a notation of EDD, the expected date of *delivery*. Midwives have become implicated in this discourse by the required use of the antenatal forms 1 and 2 that use this term. Earlier, the acronym for this event was EDC, the expected date of *confinement*. Here the woman is suggested; it is she who is *confined* or, as my thesaurus notes, bed-ridden, incarcerated, or restricted. By saying the midwife "caught"[5] the baby rather than "delivered" the baby, we shift the concept of agency somewhat. The attendant's job is less active. It is to receive the baby already *delivered by the woman*. "Caught" was used pre-legislation and is used predominantly now, but there are pressures to move toward the mainstream use of "deliver."

In the phrase "the woman gave birth," the word "woman" is in the nominative case; the focus is on the woman and her agency, not on the practitioner or the baby. Here, the practitioner is invisible; in fact, there may not even have been one. Indeed, some women who have felt obstetrically abused dream of going to the woods to birth their subsequent babies by themselves.

Because research claims that births unattended by an experienced and equipped practitioner bear greater risk, the phrase "the woman gave birth assisted by the midwife" would be more consonant with current midwifery ideology and practice, which acknowledges the woman's central position in her own experience accompanied by trained caregivers. If we further expand this phrase to say "the woman gave birth *assisted by her supporters, (as defined by her)* and by *her* doctor/midwife" we add other important elements. Here *her* friends and family are acknowledged caregivers; *her* practitioner is personalized and is optimally someone that she knows and has chosen.

FULL CIRCLE: GRANDMOTHER/MIDWIFE

Recently, I became a grandmother. At the same time, I was acting as my daughter Jenny's midwife. I was living on the cusp of professional/public and private/familial that Smith describes. This was bifurcation! The juxtaposition of these two roles, the personal and the professional, provides a new point of departure.

Could I be both a professional midwife and my "client's" mother? Being my daughter's midwife seemed as natural as had simply putting her to my breast years earlier. However, I see how the discourse of midwifery entered into my caring activities with her at specific points along the continuum of her "lived experience" of carrying her baby, releasing him from her body, and caring for him in the days and weeks following that moment. (For a detailed description of Jenny's birthing experience see Sharpe 2001).

TEXTS AND MEDICO-LEGAL CONSIDERATIONS

A question arises for me from this experience with my daughter. Should midwives work with their own families? Why is there a convention that physicians do not treat their families? Do considerations of conflict of interest undermine the ability to perform? I would like to engage in these musings quickly, before the cement dries! I want to explore this before somebody, perhaps even the College of Midwives, tells us that we ought not attend to family members. So far, midwifery is still associated with many cultures where mothers, mothers-in-law, aunts, and grandmothers often are the midwives. It may also be associated with a postmodern feminist ethic that encourages reciprocal and open relationships in health care.

I introduced Jenny to other midwives; I asked her, "Are you sure you don't want someone else?" She was impatient. The phenomenon of choosing your mother. I had hoped that I could be Jenny's mother, midwife, and friend. Are our definitions of these roles too tight? Could we have a more holistic view of mother, as mentor, feminist, facilitator of independence, and careful practitioner?

I asked my colleagues what they thought: I might find it hard to be objective or make decisions in emergency situations because of my special caring for Jenny as her mother. Knowing how much she wanted to avoid the hospital setting for giving birth, I might sidestep or minimize indications for transporting, thereby ignoring the texts and rulings of midwifery discourse. The authority of the professional relationship might be overruled by motherly sensitivities. I might find it hard to see her in pain. If I felt I needed Jenny's cooperation in some situation, she might not respond as readily as other women, hampered by some mother/daughter dynamic or power struggle, or by habits that had evolved from our long and intimate association. Some said it would be out of the question with their own daughter, others felt it would be very comfortable and desirable. These considerations were mitigated by the Ontario requirement of having a second midwife present at every birth.

If the outcome was unfortunate, our relationship might be jeopardized. The consideration of "something going wrong" highlights a distinction between relationships with family and with other clients. There is an assumption that families will stay together forever. Although we know this is often not so, there is usually sadness associated with family disharmony and break-ups. It is assumed that the relationship with the midwife will become less central over time. In fact, a ruling makes us legally responsible for women and their babies until six weeks postpartum. Usually after this, there is little contact until a subsequent pregnancy.

When circumstances are tragic, unfortunate, or disappointing, in an agonizing search for an explanation for what happened and why, in an attempt to shift the overwhelming sense of helplessness of the present reality of the situation, in order to rationalize past or ongoing events, parents may blame the caregiver, the one whom they trusted or saw as a conduit of information and knowledge (Rosser 1999). They may be angry, hurt, and frustrated; this anger may never go away, and contact with this person may be abruptly cut off. However, this view implies that pain and difficulty lead to fractured relationships. These situations also contain possibilities for closeness and support, perhaps aided by a more intimate relationship between caregiver and client.

Midwives, though watchful for difficulties, are guardians of the normal. The orientation of "something going wrong" is more consonant with the discourse of obstetrics with its crisis management, reliance on technology and intervention, and expensive malpractice insurance.

Predicated by medico-legal considerations, I have become aware of yet another discourse, that of the insurance company to which my profession is contracted. When discussing a difficult situation recently with a client, what was profoundly disturbing was that, along with my authentic behaviour and real caring for the woman, I found myself playing a role influenced by the insurance company and prompted by my colleagues. This role was scripted to protect the insurance company, the midwifery profession, and me, and to model a way of behaving appropriately with the client under these circumstances.

What was required was a carefully mediated way of behaving, rehearsed before meeting to discuss the issue with the family. Although I found this role disturbing, it brought a heightened consciousness with it. It was the same kind of discipline that I observed while attempting to reconcile, adapt, and enter into with fullness, the roles of midwife and mother with my daughter Jenny.

Midwives bring a number of invisible partners to their relationships with women – insurers, legislators, physicians, other providers and regulators. The midwife is painfully aware of the invisible partners even when the woman has no or limited knowledge of them. A strange oppression of both the woman and midwife can result from the unspoken expectations, limitations, and rules of the invisible partners. The midwife's ideas and suggestions may remain unspoken, now considered inappropriate, too radical, too dangerous. In the midwife's silence, there is no invitation to the woman to join in discourse in these dangerous topics (James 1999).

Similarly, physician Michael Klein, in his article "Too Close for Comfort" (1997), questions whether medical professionals should be excluded from their loved ones' care. He concludes that this ethic should be re-examined. After all, the health professional has the best interests of his or her family member in mind and should, in Klein's opinion, be integrated into the loved one's care.

I conclude that in spite of medico-legal considerations, family members' requests for midwifery care are based on the choice of the woman, and midwives, where comfortable, might respond to these requests as for any other woman.

To me, family/midwifery connections feel ancient and historical. They deepen our caring for each other and link me and my daughter, Jenny, to the many midwives in the world and to earlier lay midwives in Ontario. I am now propelled toward a new family adventure. With enthusiasm, I take up these roles again as I prepare for the birthing experience of my next daughter, Lucy.

CONCLUSION

Central to the issue of texts and rulings in the context of midwifery is the interplay between public interest and self-interest. I want to conclude by exploring the concept of protection. Is protection for the public a paternalistic notion? We suspected that legislation was meant to control us midwives and protect the public. Midwives began their work to protect women from mistreatment around their births. Was this a maternalistic notion? Now the insurance company and its texts offer to protect us from the women with whom we work. The record keeping, the note taking, the indications for care are all to protect. Perhaps one could look at the continuum between public interest and self-interest. The success of a profession may be in how it locates itself practically in relation to these interests. Bad service may be the result of too much self-interest, and burnout the result of too much attention to the needs of the public and too little to the needs of the profession or the professional. The purpose of texts may be to clarify and organize behaviour so as to find the ideal balance between these interests. However, texts can never encompass all situations that will arise and can become a Procrustean bed if followed too literally. One can too radically alter the lived experience to fit the text.

With legislation, midwives are learning new texts and engaging in new rulings. Are these rulings slowing us down, fixing us gradually and inexorably into new relationships and new ways of acting and being? Or do these rulings provide structure and support and free us? Implicit in feminism is mutual respect in relationship: effective kinship. One needs to consider the needs of both the midwife, nearly always a woman, and the woman for whom she cares. In addition, one needs to consider the needs of the profession, which can offer women so much. The bottom line for midwives is: can legislation enhance creativity and expand possibilities for women and midwifery or limit them? Can midwifery text and discourse itself change and affect other institutions? Are there relationships here that are reciprocal and mutually helpful?

Through our attention to the details of our practices, we might reevaluate the degree to which the practice of midwifery in fact ultimately supports women and woman-centred care. We need continuously to hold our behaviour in question. Central to this issue for me is caring about the details of practice, being careful: full of care, midwifing the material. There is no place for complacency or resting. A tireless vigilance is required to maintain what some would say are midwifery's gains and others call our compromises. And we must continue, as Dorothy Smith would urge us, to examine our practices in order to recognize how, for better or for worse, we are implicated in the rulings of our profession.

NOTES

1 A previous version of this chapter was published in *Resources for Feminist Research*. See Mary Sharpe 2001.
2 The Maternity Centre in El Paso, which I attended for six months in 1979, and others like it in Texas have seen, from 1978 until the present, a steady

stream of lay midwives from Ontario seeking birthing experiences principally with Mexican women. See Nestel 2000.

3 See Nestel (2000) for an exploration of the forces that led to the exclusion
of foreign-trained midwives in this seed group of practising midwives.

4 According to Ivy Bourgeault (1996), who has explored the development of
other professions, the clarity of vision of this elite group of midwives and
their maintenance of power was essential to the goal of achieving legislation.

5 Dr John McCulloch, early supporter of woman's rights to home birth, used
to insist that he did not "deliver" babies but "caught" them. This phrase
was taken up by the midwifery community and later by Eleanor Barrington
in her popular book about midwifery in Ontario called *Midwifery is Catching*, published by Pandora in Toronto in 1987.

REFERENCES

Benoit, Cecilia. 1994. Paradigm Conflict in the Sociology of Professionals:
Midwifery As a Case Study. *Canadian Journal of Sociology* 19, no. 3: 303–
29.

Bourgeault, Ivy. 1996. Delivering Midwifery: An Examination of the Process
and Outcome of the Incorporation of Midwifery in Ontario. Ph.D. dissertation, Graduate Department of Community Health, University of Toronto.

Duden, Barbara. 1993. *Disembodying Women*. Cambridge: Harvard University Press.

Durish, Pat. 1996. Licensed Midwifery in Ontario: A Social Movement Transformed. Unpublished Master's thesis. Carleton University, Ottawa.

James, Susan (director of the Laurentian University Midwifery Education Program, Sudbury). 1999. Personal communication.

Klein, Michael. 1997. Too Close for Comfort. *Canadian Medical Association
Journal* 156 (1): 53–5.

Nestel, Sheryl. 2000. Delivering subjects: Race, Space and the Emergence of legalized Midwifery in Canada. *Canadian Journal of Law and Society* 15,
no. 2: 187-215.

Rosser, Jilly. 1999. Women Behaving Badly. *The Practising Midwife* 2, no. 8
(September).

Sharpe, Mary. 1995. Ontario Midwifery in Transition: an Exploration of the
Perceptions of Midwives on the Impact of Recent Legislation on Their Prac-
tices. Unpublished master's thesis, Ontario Institute for Studies in Education,
University of Toronto.

– 1997. Ontario Midwifery in Transition: an Exploration of Midwives' Per-
ceptions of the Impact of Legislation in its First Year. In *The New Midwifery:
Reflections on Renaissance and Regulation*, edited by Farah Shroff. Toronto:
The Women's Press.

– 2001. Exploring Legislated Ontario Midwifery: Texts, Ruling Relations and Ideological Practices. *Resources for Feminist Research* 28, no. 3/4: 39–63.

Smith, Dorothy. 1990. *The Conceptual Practices of Power.* Toronto: University of Toronto Press.

– 1995. *Knowledge, Experience and Ruling Relations.* Toronto: University of Toronto Press.

Van Wagner, Vicki (Ryerson Midwifery Education Program, Toronto). 1999. Personal communication.

PART THREE

Educating Midwives and Entry to Practice

INTRODUCTION

Midwifery education and training have been highlighted as critical issues in the chapters on midwifery history and legislation in the preceedings two sections. Part III delves more fully into the specific models of education for midwives and other entry-to-midwifery-practice issues. Sociologist Cecilia Benoit and anthropologist Robbie Davis-Floyd begin by describing the three basic models of midwifery education – apprenticeship, vocational, and university training – that have been adopted by midwives in altered forms in different times and places across Canada. They argue that each model has its strengths and weaknesses but at the same time needs to be contextualized within Western technocratic societies that value ever higher levels of education and ever more advanced university degrees as a means to measure "success." The authors then reflect on the range of educational choices available to Canadian midwives in various provinces today as they achieve legislation, and conclude by mentioning some of the implications this has for the evolution of midwifery in Canada.

The chapter by Benoit and Davis-Floyd provides an excellent backdrop for the description of the "pioneer" midwifery education program in Ontario presented by program director Karyn Kaufman and instructor Bobbi Soderstrom. The authors discuss the evolution of the program from its origins in the Task Force on the Implementation of Midwifery in Ontario to the Curriculum Design Committee. They highlight the special features of the program that was ultimately established, including the organization of the consortium of universities that currently house the program, structure of the curriculum, the preceptor model of clinical teaching, and a profile of students and graduates. Kaufman and Soderstrom discuss the changes that have been made to the program over the last half-decade in response to faculty, preceptors, and student concerns as well as two external reviews. They conclude with noting some of the implications the program has for the future of the profession.

The next chapter, by anthropologist Pat Kaufert and midwife Kris Robinson, focuses on a single transformative moment in the history of midwifery implementation in Manitoba: the crisis that developed around a decision made by the Midwifery Implementation Council as it set up an assessment and registration process for the first group of midwives to be licensed to practice. In the first part of the chapter, Kaufert and Robinson provide a brief description of the key players, the events that triggered the crisis, and its successful resolution. The second part of the chapter explores both the language and the cultural and ideological assumptions about the nature of midwifery as an occupation, midwifery education, and midwifery practice that contributed to the crisis. By focusing on this event from a broader cultural perspective, the authors present an important counter-narrative to the Canadian dialogue about who and, indeed, what is a midwife.

8

Becoming a Midwife in Canada: Models of Midwifery Education[1]

Cecilia Benoit and Robbie Davis-Floyd

INTRODUCTION

How should aspiring midwives be best prepared for their future service role? What types of knowledge should be transmitted, and who are the ideal teachers to transmit this knowledge? Where should such preparation take place? There were no definitive answers to these questions in the past, nor are there in the present. Each educational model that has been developed for midwifery has its strengths and weaknesses, as does the diversity of their applications in Canada and other countries.

Characteristic of Western technocratic societies in general is a marked trend toward requiring ever higher levels of education and ever more advanced university degrees for professional status and success. This trend heavily influences midwifery education. For example, in the UK, midwifery training until the late 1980s was purely vocational, but it is now based in universities and leads to either a diploma or a first degree. Midwives in the Netherlands have resisted this trend toward university education, deliberately choosing to retain their vocational style of training. In the U.S., nurse-midwives have recently moved midwifery education to the postgraduate level by effectively requiring an undergraduate degree as the prerequisite for entry into all their educational programs (Rooks 1997). Some U.S. midwives, however, have actively resisted this trend, insisting on preserving stand-alone apprenticeship as a viable educational path. Ontario midwives have recently accepted university education at the undergraduate level but stopped short of following their American nurse-midwifery colleagues into the postgraduate realm (see Kaufman and Soderstrom, this volume). Midwives in Quebec and British Columbia are following a similar path, while the midwives of Manitoba have chosen to preserve multiple routes, including apprenticeship (see Kaufert and Robinson, this volume).

In addition to this trend toward higher education, within midwifery we also see a trend toward direct-entry midwifery education and away from nursing training as a prerequisite. To some, to be trained as a nurse means to be socialized into accepting structural subordination to physicians and a concomitant lack of decision-making power. Thus, in many countries where midwifery is closely linked to nursing, we find either incipient or full-fledged movements toward dissociating midwifery and nursing and increasing autonomy and self-regulation for midwives. Nurse-midwives in the U.S., for example, have recently created a new direct-entry educational track. The new midwifery in Ontario and British Columbia resulted from an early alliance between nurse- and direct-entry midwives[2] that included agreement that nursing would not be a requirement.

Our overview of midwifery education in Canada will encompass the twin prongs of education and socialization. We use the term "education" to refer to the formal educational requirements and organization of the training program; we use "socialization" to point to the informal process or "hidden curriculum" (Illich 1973) by which a person, influenced by teachers, peers, and society, becomes a member of an occupation and acquires its values, beliefs, attitudes, behaviour patterns, and social identity – that is, the occupational group's "shared culture." The shared culture that the novice midwife eventually internalizes includes notions and patterns of appropriate practice and behaviour towards colleagues, other health professionals, and clientele, and an often unstated ideology that underlies those ideas and behaviour patterns.

Just as it can be shown that the knowledge base and the educational programs for midwives' preparation for practice vary across time and place, so too does the socialization process become transformed in response to changes in the wider socio-cultural context. Midwifery education is always embedded in and reflective of that wider context. Its evolution will reflect educational trends in the wider society, as well as medical and technological advances, gender relations, state policies, and socio-economic and cultural changes.

In this chapter we present an overview of the diverse forms that midwifery education has taken in Canada and evaluate these forms in relation to each other, demonstrating some of the complex interrelationships between these variations and wider societal evolutionary trends and trajectories. We describe three basic models of midwifery education, which serve as our analytical frame for understanding changes in Canadian midwifery over time. These include the apprenticeship, vocational, and university models. For the sake of analytical clarity, we present each model separately. In practice, however, these models rarely take the form of discrete ideal-types but rather constitute points along a fluid continuum. We first provide the reader with a window into the lived experience of that educational type through a fictional descriptive story. We then delineate the characteristics of that type, offer a brief case study of its use in a part or parts of Canada, and conclude each section by looking at the strengths and weaknesses of the model under examination.

APPRENTICESHIP

Heather (not her real name) was born in a large U.S. city but left there when she was twenty years of age to come out to Canada. As she recollects, many of her friends started talking about opting out and going back to the land. Heather says that she was very involved in this movement. She and her then partner of the time headed to western Canada, met people along the way who were homesteading there, followed a group, and ended up in B.C. Heather eventually moved to Saltspring Island, where she soon gave birth to her first child. She then moved up-island while pregnant with her second child. Her husband brought home a book from Vancouver by Raven Lang called *The Birth Book*, which was the only book out on birth at the time. As Heather recalls, he said, "You know, we should have this baby at home." Heather replied: "Well you know, who's going to help us?" Heather read the book and found it very inspiring. And only a few months later she discovered that Raven Lang was living in a nearby community and delivering babies. Heather met Raven in person soon thereafter. Heather says that as soon as she walked into Raven's office and spent that first hour with her she knew she was going to be okay delivering her baby at home. "I would never have had the courage, or maybe the naiveté to do that birth at home." Heather went on to relate that "after the second baby, I really felt I had kind of faced my demons in a very personal way and I really felt interested in helping." Heather started teaching some prenatal classes. She lived at a distance from the closest hospital and people in her community wanted to have their babies at home. Raven had moved away for a while and there wasn't anyone around to attend births. So the local women came to call on Heather. She remembers: "My daughter had been born in February, I went to my first birth in August, and I delivered the baby. And then I did a second birth. When Raven returned and I said, 'you know I need you; I can't do these by myself; I want to be trained.' And she said, 'Good, I'll train you.'" So Raven started a year of classes for a group of five, which included Heather. Heather accompanied Raven at births for nearly two years before Raven left for the U.S. for good. As Heather puts it, "Raven was an incredible teacher. I was now an apprenticed midwife."

Like many of her contemporaries in B.C., Heather eventually augmented her apprenticeship training with formal midwifery education. In 1998 she received an official license to practice. (Based on interviews conducted by Benoit, 1995.)

History and Characteristics of Apprenticeship

Midwives have traditionally learned their craft through apprenticeship. Historically, there was but one type of knowledge transmitted to neophyte midwives – "lay" knowledge or "lifeworld" knowledge that was gained by watching an experienced midwife at work, and eventually by the trainee doing more and more of the work herself (Benoit 1989a).

Apprenticeship learning is full-bodied, experiential learning that involves all the senses (Davis-Floyd 1998a, b). In apprenticeship systems, even watching is participatory; the apprentice rarely or never simply observes. Rather, she almost always uses her hands in some way, carrying water, providing clean cloths, preparing food, and massaging the mother. Ideally (but not always in practice), over time the apprentice midwife becomes an expert in lifeworld knowledge, which consists of a sustained social and intuitive knowledge of the women she serves, as well as a body of techniques acquired by "doing" midwifery work with other women who share a similar social world. This method of learning correlates well with the demands of the job: the apprentice learns in the sorts of environments in which she will practice. Traditionally, midwives were also expected to acquire a body of cultural-religious knowledge, which included how to deal with a stillbirth or a death in childbirth as well as how to dispose of the afterbirth and so forth. Still, this cultural-religious knowledge, like the embodied social knowledge and practical techniques acquired by the apprentice midwife, was gained largely through sustained observation and interaction with others within the local community, after which the midwife came to master the shared values, codes of behaviour, and common mores of those in her lifeworld (Böhme 1984).

Although pure apprenticeship training has been largely superseded in high-income countries by more didactic vocational and university-based models, apprenticeship nevertheless continues to play an important role in those models in various forms. Just as medical training, which has for centuries been university-based, has also retained a strong apprenticeship component, so midwifery training, which only became formally institutionalized in high-income countries over the last two centuries, has retained aspects of apprenticeship in the form of clinical training under preceptors, who often take on roles similar to those played by the mentor in the apprenticeship relationship. Hands-on, one-on-one interactions with preceptors reminiscent of apprenticeship characterize midwives' training in all high-income countries. Nevertheless, there are important differences between pure apprenticeship and the kinds of apprenticeship or clinical preceptorship (i.e., practicum in a clinical or home setting under the guidance of a preceptor/teacher) that form part of vocational and university-based midwifery training. In pure apprenticeship, the student-mentor relationship takes on a particularly close and intense quality and may last for years.

Canada and the U.S. are unique among high-income countries in that apprenticeship training is still extant inside their borders, in the former case notably in northern Aboriginal communities and some Native reserves (see Carroll and Benoit, this volume). The roots of this development can be traced to the rise of North American lay midwifery during the 1970s and 1980s. The pioneers of this social movement, who include such internationally known midwives as Raven Lang, Ina May Gaskin, and Elizabeth Davis, learned about birth by attending the births of friends, reading books, and apprenticing with other midwives or with nurses or an occasional willing physician where midwives did not exist (see Van Wagner and Sharpe, this volume). Over time they developed a unique body of knowledge that reflected their lived experience of home birth and sought to develop educational methods and programs that would preserve that knowledge system and help to avoid it being incorporated into universities – which they saw as medicalized and subordinated to medical control. A sophisticated system of apprenticeship was one of the methods they developed. Some of the earliest midwives were largely self-taught, but as their knowledge base grew, they began to train others.

As these lay midwives gained licensure and regulation in various U.S. states, they developed a number of formal programs, including some three-year vocational schools (see below). Eventually they dropped the appellation "lay" in favour of the more professional "independent "or "direct-entry." Yet even as they professionalized, apprenticeship remained central to their values and sense of identity as autonomous and independent out-of-hospital practitioners. In 1982 they founded the Midwives Alliance of North America (MANA), an organization that primarily represents independent (non-nurse) midwives who practise outside of hospitals and that since its beginnings has remained open to membership from midwives in both Canada and Mexico, as well as the U.S. Throughout the 1980s MANA members, including Canadian midwives, developed standards for practice and core competencies in which they believed all midwives should be trained. In the early 1990s

MANA encouraged its associate, the North American Registry of Mid-wives (NARM), to develop a new national certification, the Certified Professional Midwife (CPM). A primary motivator for the development of this credential was a desire among MANA members to legitimize apprenticeship through creating a mechanism for evaluating the knowledge, skills, and experience of the apprentice-trained midwife. This certification has recently been made part of the licensure process in Manitoba (see Kaufert and Robinson, this volume).

Most Canadian midwives learned through apprenticeship until the recent decade or so. In fact, all the original Ontario non-nurse-midwives were apprentice-trained, as were those in B.C., Quebec, Alberta, and the other provinces where non-nurse-midwives were in practice. Indeed, it is important to point out that the midwives who are creating the formal educational programs now were mostly apprentice-trained in the beginning, so apprenticeship is essential to the development of Canadian midwifery. As noted above and discussed in detail by Carroll and Benoit in this volume, apprenticeship is still currently functioning in a variety of forms in northern pockets of the country and in some Aboriginal communities and is integral to the new legislation for midwives in Manitoba.

Apprenticeship training fundamentally involves attending births with one or more practising midwives, assisting them in myriad ways, and observing the way they interact with and care for pregnant, labouring, and postpartum women. Apprentices also watch and help with emergencies, frequently discussing every detail of care. Through extensive face-to-face contact the midwife and apprentice come to develop a deeply bonded relationship that many midwives see as essential to successful midwifery education. All published descriptions of midwifery apprenticeship stress the importance of this relationship; two even contain sections on what to do when the relationship is not "working" as it should. Most of the time, mentors care deeply about the apprentices they take on, get to know them intimately, are committed to making sure they obtain the best education possible, and work to bolster the student's trust in birth and in herself as she learns. The average duration of such apprenticeships is around three years.

In the community of Puvirnituk, located on the east coast of Canada's Hudson Bay, women selected by other local indigenous women to fill the position of community midwives receive their training primarily from working side-by-side with the professional direct-entry midwives employed at the local maternity centre attached to the regional hospital (see Daviss 1997; Carroll and Benoit, this volume). Morewood-Northrop (1997) describes a similar community-based birthing project in the Northwest Territories of Canada. In other northern villages, nurse-midwives have arrived to attend births, sometimes for years, so that the Inuit women will not have to be evacuated to southern hospitals to give birth. But most of these nurse-midwives have left the north without training indigenous midwives who will remain in their communities, as has been done in Puvirnituk. In circumstances like these, the apprenticeship model remains an especially appropriate route for midwifery education.

Strengths and Limitations of Apprenticeship Training

Midwives' deep commitment to apprenticeship arises from two basic premises: (1) to fear birth is to generate complications that result from the fear; and (2) midwives who trust birth profoundly tend to help women give birth more effectively. The argument used in favour of apprenticeship training is that "to trust a woman to give birth is to help her trust herself." Birth turns out well without requiring intervention most of the time; thus, apprentice-trained midwives are mostly exposed to women working hard and successfully giving birth. Although they have opportunities to experience pathology and emergency management over the course of their apprenticeship training, these incidences form the periodic punctuation, not the defining ethos, of their clinical experience (Davis-Floyd 1998a). Their training gives them a much broader experience of the wide range "normal" birth can take when it occurs outside of hospitals and thus is not technologically controlled (Mason 1987). Apprentice midwives from B.C., for example, have often included as part of their training a stint in a high-volume midwifery service either overseas or in the U.S., where they will encounter many births with complications, but this exposure takes place against an already-established background of trust in the power of women and in the normal process of birth.

Another part of apprenticeship's strength is the continuity of care it offers to pregnant women (Mason 1988). Continuity of care constitutes part of the essence of apprenticeship training, where the student accompanies her mentor not only to the birth of a given client but also to every prenatal and postpartum visit. It is apprenticeship training that establishes the midwifery ideal for continuity of care, an ideal that other training programs can only strive to emulate. Providing that a mentor midwife is locally available, an additional benefit of apprenticeship training is that it allows women who do not have the money or the mobility to attend a university-based program or to study abroad to become competent practitioners. Apprenticeship learning is connection-based. If the apprentice attends a birth with her mentor, for example, during which the woman haemorrhages, the apprentice might spend the next day studying any literature she can find on postpartum haemorrhage and quizzing her mentor about its management. She knows, in an immediate and visceral sense, why this knowledge matters (James 1997).

Apprenticeship is often limited, however, by a small number of experienced midwives available to serve as mentors (Burtch 1994). It also depends upon the motivation of the learner, the abilities of the teacher, and the quality of their relationship (Van Wagner 1994). If they do not communicate well, if the student is unmotivated, or if the mentor is deficient in knowledge, clinical judgment, skills, or the ability to interact with clients, the student can be at risk, and therefore also the future clients she may serve. Other limitations of pure apprenticeship include the absence of in-hospital training and the fact that because birth turns out well most of the time, exposure to birth complications can be rare for midwives who learn purely through low-volume home birth practice. Apprenticeship training alone is in general not recognized in the technocracy as a valid educational route in most professions, although because of its special combination of intimacy and efficacy, there is a growing trend in adult education toward re-valuing apprenticeship (a.k.a. mentorship) as a viable educational style for the twenty-first century.

It is because of these limitations, as well as the fact that most of the recent provincial midwifery legislation does not recognize apprenticeship training as adequate unless combined with other forms of knowledge transmission, that it is increasingly rare in most parts of Canada.

VOCATIONAL TRAINING

Lou-Anne (not her real name) was born in a small outport community on the southwest coast of Newfoundland. Though now retired from midwifery practice, Lou-Anne still has vivid memories of her vocational training and subsequent practice in the local cottage hospital serving the people of her own and neighbouring communities. In the 1980s, the provincial highway connected Lou-Anne's community to the larger urban areas, and access to the new regional hospitals located there led to the demise of the cottage hospital system and eventually the vocational style of training midwives as well. However, prior to these developments of modernization, Lou-Anne and her co-workers literally "ran the show" on the cottage hospital maternity ward and were held in high esteem by the local birthing women and their families.

Lou-Anne stresses that she was a trained midwife; in her view acquisition of skills via practical experience and specialized formal knowledge achieved through a vocational program are both essential for qualified midwifery practice. Lou-Anne also stresses that her formal qualifications and practical experience gave her a government license and access to public employment, granting her a kind of occupational status and economic security not enjoyed by her predecessors. Her vocational midwifery training included formal lectures, technical training on the use of obstetrical instruments, and extensive clinical experience, both on the hospital's maternity ward and in women's homes. As Lou-Anne explains, "What I didn't learn from the midwifery training, I could learn on the cottage hospital ward because we had to do these things, emergency things as well as the practical delivery of babies."

Today Lou-Anne's workplace, the cottage hospital, is confined to the northern areas of the province and the vocational style of training midwives for practice in Canada has completely disappeared. (Adapted from Benoit 1991, 1–2.)

History and Characteristics of Vocational Training

As high-income countries began to industrialize, a process that included the gradual secularization of life, a new form of "vocational" midwifery education came to include "book learning" and the formal lecture, with midwives in some countries (especially those with national state endorsement of midwifery as an important service for the population's health, such as Sweden, Finland, and the Netherlands) receiving part of their education in a more structured manner, through the reading of textbooks on obstetrics and attending lectures given by obstetricians and senior midwives on the emerging "science" of childbearing. Typically, such lectures took place in a formal setting – a cottage hospital, a birthing centre, and later in larger hospital settings where student midwives observed women during labour and delivery and sometimes physicians. At first, these formal midwifery training programs ran for only a number of weeks; later they were extended to three to six months of theoretical instruction, and became longer still as the twentieth century unfolded (Benoit 1991; Carter and Duriez 1986). Didactic learning in the classroom was complemented with hospital observation and practical experience with birthing mothers who, at the beginning of this period, tended to be poor women who were either homeless or without adequate living conditions for home birth.

Midwives in vocational training continued to learn much of their art and science by actually *doing* midwifery. At first training sites included clients' own homes or perhaps the home or workplace of the midwife; later they encompassed publicly funded midwife clinics, small community cottage hospitals, and eventually larger maternity wards where, depending on the particular time and country, the midwife may or may not have been permitted to use all of her acquired knowledge in everyday practice.

Case Study: Vocational Training In Canada

In Canada, a short-lived vocational School of Midwifery located in Vancouver, B.C. took in two classes of midwives in 1984 and 1985. The school was loosely affiliated with Seattle Midwifery School and accredited by Washington State. Upon completing the Washington state's licensing examination and applying for a license, the successful midwife candidate gained the title "Licensed Midwife" (Rice 1997). The only other part of the country where a vocational training has been researched is in the former British colony of Newfoundland (Benoit 1989b). The program, initiated in the early 1920s, was located in the capital city of St John's. Graduate midwives found work in outlying clinics or one of the eighteen small (thirty- to fifty-bed) cottage hospitals strategically located around the island of Newfoundland, or in one of the few parallel institutions located in the even more isolated northern region of Labrador. Formal union with mainland Canada in 1949, where midwifery had all but become defunct by the time, led to a demise of vocational education for midwives in the renamed eastern province of Newfoundland and Labrador (Benoit 1991).

Strengths and Limitations of Vocational Training

Vocational programs tend to stay concretely focused on the vocation they are designed to teach, offering a balance of practical skills and theoretical knowledge oriented towards real-world application. Vocational training mixes experiential and didactic educational methods and concentrates on socializing its students into the practical requirements of their jobs, from institutional rules and regulations to training in the requisite technologies. Vocational curricula are formalized and are often evaluated for content and quality by an outside body so that an education system based on vocational training will produce midwives of a measurable and uniform minimum standard. The quality of the learning is not based solely on the quality of one or a limited number of mentors, as might be the case under an apprenticeship model. As with apprenticeship, preserving the vocational model helps to assure the preservation of midwifery; in vocational schools, there is no mixing of midwifery education with other fields, as might be the case in universities.

In countries where midwifery education is moving or has moved to universities, vocationally trained midwives may suffer from the stereotype of the "second-class citizen" and their training may seem incomplete. For example, in the UK, vocational training, while providing student midwives with a basic salary and birthing women with the care of a valuable health provider, also awarded employers with a cheap source of labour and allowed them to emphasize the needs of the organization rather than the educational and developmental needs of the student midwives. Such criticisms have been a driving force for moving midwifery education into higher education in the UK.

On the other hand, the midwives of the Netherlands have steadfastly resisted moving their education into an academic setting. After finishing five years of secondary schooling, students apply to enter one of the three midwifery schools in the country, which are part of the Dutch "HBO" system – Higher Occupational Education (Hoger Beroepsonderwijs). The demand for entry far exceeds the supply of available spots, indicating the popularity of midwifery as a future occupation among young Dutch people. The four-year midwifery educational program covers prenatal and postnatal care, normal low-risk deliveries – both at home and clinic – the identification of high-risk situations across the reproductive period, and techniques of scientific research. Some believe that the status of Dutch midwives would be enhanced and protected if midwifery education moved into the university, but research suggests that location outside the university has allowed midwives to protect their special knowledge and thus their autonomy. Dutch midwives feel strongly that their vocational model works to preserve midwifery as separate, woman-centred, and unique, and they do not want it "compromised" by being moved to the university and mixed with other health professions or sciences (Van Teijlingen 1994; Benoit et al 2001). They have, however, worked to create streamlined mechanisms for vocationally trained midwives who later want to pursue university degrees.

In the U.S., like apprenticeship training, vocational midwifery training is presently being developed and preserved only by direct-entry midwives. Some nurse-midwifery educators, stressing the value of university-affiliated programs, dismiss vocational programs as "trade schools" that represent an outdated educational model. Nevertheless, for American direct-entry midwives vocational programs are increasingly proving to be viable means of expanding their educational scope beyond the numerical limitations of one-on-one apprenticeship while still preserving their unique body of knowledge about out-of-hospital pregnancy and birth. Unlike vocational programs in the UK, these U.S. vocational schools put great emphasis on the development of a sense of autonomy and of critical thinking and decision-making skills.

UNIVERSITY EDUCATION

Nicole entered the postgraduate nurse-midwifery program offered at Memorial University's School of Nursing in the late 1960s. She says that she applied for the program because she realized that advanced university education was "the trend these days" but also because she

hoped to work "up north" for a stint helping birthing women in remote locations of the country. A midwifery credential, in her mind,
would be a great asset, especially given the fact that very few Canadian
nurses at the time had one. Nicole also mentioned that, even if she
didn't go north, the credential would give her extra "clout" in clinical
settings where she would be working alongside doctors, nurses, and
other health professionals. Despite these attractions, Nicole has mixed
feelings about what the program offered her: on the one hand, she enjoyed the opportunity to do advanced research, problem solve, and
learn to understand pregnant women as a group in a broad sense – that
is, to see the big picture. Nicole says that her university education
taught her, above all else, to "figure things out on her own," something
that she still likes to do very much today. On the other hand, she won-
ders if her clinical training was adequate for dealing with what she had
to face in the "real world of work." She wishes in particular that she
had leaned more about the practicalities of good midwifery care as well
as about the diverse home conditions of birthing women. This would
have prepared her better, she says, for the "cultural shock" she experienced when she went to northern Quebec to work as a midwife.

By the late 1980s, academic nurse-midwifery training programs
across Canada, including the one that Nicole graduated from, had become defunct. It would not be until another decade and a half before
university education for midwives was offered again in Canada.
(Adapted from Benoit 1991, 84–90.)

History and Characteristics of University Training

Mid- to late twentieth-century Europe and North America are marked
by a new style of midwifery knowledge – academic – and a new site for
imparting it – the university. Midwives, along with an assortment of
other health providers, found themselves drawn to the post-industrial
academy for the training and socialization of new recruits to their own
profession.

Canada also took this route, although comparatively late in its development. In many countries where midwifery survived the modernization process relatively intact or has recently been reintroduced as a
legitimate health profession in its own right, the neophyte's educational
preparation more or less follows this route: high school/gymnasium or
parallel graduation, application to a university-level direct-entry or
nurse-midwifery program of three to five years duration and, in some
countries, advanced/further education at the masters level. The biological and also more recently the social sciences are deemed highly important in regard to the student's knowledge acquisition.

Case Study: University Training in Canada

Until the late 1980s, three university nursing schools – located in Alberta, Nova Scotia, and Newfoundland – offered nurses additional courses in midwifery training within an Outpost Nursing program. These academic programs were focused on placing nursing students interested in providing maternity and general nursing care to residents in northern and remote communities of the respective provinces (Benoit 1991). While noteworthy because of their focus on the need for additional expertise in maternity care, these programs suffered from the fact that they were all postgraduate, necessitating a nursing degree as a prerequisite. A second shortcoming was that the curriculum tended to be taught by nursing and medical instructors and thus was medicalized in content. Further, the clinical experience of students was largely confined to medical settings, and students had little or no access to clients in community clinics and the home. This contrasts to some extent with the new university undergraduate program for midwives in Ontario discussed by Kaufman and Soderstrom later in this volume.

Strengths and Limitations of University Education

College- or university-based training is in alignment with the values, beliefs, and status consciousness of mainstream society; it is culturally thought of as the bottom line for service occupations. As a socially valued educational pathway, it carries concomitant benefits, including social recognition and prestige, easy access to government loans, and straightforward routes to advanced degrees, which bring prestige and salary raises and empower their recipients to teach, to start new programs, to effect changes in legislation, and to carry out research on client needs and various aspects of midwifery care. In short, academic credentials carry with them "cultural capital" for the new midwifery graduate, and her new-found degree can carry weight (but there is no guarantee that this will occur) when negotiating attractive work options, helping her to compete on an equal standing with other similarly credentialed health professionals, not least of all physicians.

Presence on a university campus can be a distinct advantage, with all the facilities and educational and research opportunities that entails. Moreover, academic institutions and university hospitals are often the sites of development for innovative knowledge and technologies about childbearing that, if permitted to acquire, midwives can subsequently make judicious use of in their place of work. Universities' greater resource base has facilitated, in various countries, the development of sophisticated learning technologies and the elaboration of educational theories and methods. Distance learning, for example, allows the student to remain grounded in her community, gaining clinical experience with a preceptor in her local hospital, while the case study approach allows for the reintegration of theory and method through the careful didactic study of specific birth experiences.

Students trained in the large teaching hospitals often associated with universities oriented toward the health sciences are exposed to and develop expertise in dealing with individuals of diverse socio-cultural and economic backgrounds, a wide range of birth complications and unusual health conditions, and the "latest and greatest" in medical technologies. Educators generally work with students to help them develop good risk assessment skills, competence in giving culturally sensitive care, a critical sense of which technologies have efficacy, under which circumstances, and which ones do not, and good research skills that can enable them to sift the data for themselves.

Of course, university education is not at all of one type, but rather varies in the degree of medicalization of the curriculum, distance between students and the lifeworlds of the women they will eventually serve, and whether the midwife in the long run is reduced to a technical expert possessing merely "scientized" knowledge or can maintain a more holistic approach. Yet it cannot be denied that the clinical component of academic education for the most part takes place in tertiary hospital settings removed from the life experiences of birthing women. And universities may further this divide between the lifeworld and the ivory tower by increasing the physical distance between educational facilities and practice settings (Hall 1994; Warwick 1992) and by carrying out clinical training in large university hospitals, rather than in the actual lifeworlds of clients or in smaller sites closer to their geographic communities.

In addition, there is always a risk (either real or perceived) that the education of health practitioners may become divorced from practice, that is, that teaching and learning curricula may become more academically than clinically focused. Hunt (1996, 31) found that practising midwives feel this danger strongly. Some commentators are convinced that university education has great potential to improve clinical care (Alexander 1994, 25), while others question this assumption (Jackson 1993, 275).

Training offered in large cultural institutions such as universities often comes to reflect hegemonic philosophies and practices. In the cultural realm of birth in Canada and many other high-income countries, the patriarchal medical model is hegemonic. Thus midwifery training carried out in such institutions will be pressured to incorporate many elements of a highly medicalized, patriarchal, and technocratic approach to birth (Davis-Floyd 1992), and midwives so educated may often be required to intervene in birth in ways contrary to both scientific evidence and the non-interventive principles of midwifery care in order to successfully graduate.

CONCLUSION

Midwifery students have gained their special body of knowledge in various ways. There has not been in the past nor is there today a single way to prepare midwives for practice. Instead we observe a range of different educational models, all of which have both positive and negative aspects, as we have shown. Our journey has emphasized the variability in preparation of midwives for practice through an examination of both their formal education and informal socialization into the role of midwife. We have shown that neither midwives' knowledge base nor their socialization are arbitrary; rather, each is shaped by the larger culture and structure of the society that generates it. We have also shown that the degree of professional autonomy midwives may be able to achieve is greatly affected by the educational system they have experienced, as is their social status within the complex system of medical and health professions.

It is also important to note that these three models are not mutually exclusive. As we have seen, apprenticeship programs that include didactic classes are moving toward vocational models, and some form of apprenticeship forms part of almost all vocational and university-based educational programs. As discussed in the chapter by Kaufman and Soderstrom in this volume, an altered form of preceptorship is integral to the Ontario direct-entry university education program, as well as to the Quebec and B.C. academic midwifery programs that have recently been established. University programs that are practically focused and retain the integrity of midwifery without dilution can carry over some of the benefits of vocational programs.

To some extent at least, the recent trend toward academic education has raised the status of midwives, granting them more authority vis-à-vis medicine and nursing. (This was, for example, an important consideration in choosing the university-based program in Ontario, as Kaufman and Soderstrom discuss in this volume). Academic education thus seems to enhance midwives' autonomy as long as the higher education does not merely socialize them into accepting hegemonic models and practices. This problem has not so far occurred in Canada for degree-holding midwives there, and the future appears promising in this respect, although it may be more difficult to sustain the caseload apprenticeship/continuity model when the number of students being educated increases.

There is no agreement in the scholarly literature as a whole about whether academic education in the long run will better train midwives than apprenticeship or vocational training. The philosophy of care must be woman-centred, we argue, for a move into the university to represent a genuine improvement instead of co-option. Whether a woman-centred philosophy of care can be maintained in the Canadian university setting remains to be seen. Here socialization into midwifery plays a major role. Historically and in the present, it seems clear that the kind of midwives a given program produces will have as much to do with *how* they are taught as with *what* they are taught. Midwives who are trained in a humanistic manner and in a nurturing atmosphere will find it easier to become woman-centred caregivers when they go into practice than midwives who are trained according to techno-medical norms. In other words, the application of the midwifery model of care is as important to midwifery education as it is to midwifery practice.

Of course, in the final analysis, it is how midwives *practise* that matters most. The conclusion that emerges is that in order to gain competence in the full spectrum of care, from the woman-centred holistic approach to techno-medical interventions, it can be argued that midwives need to be educated in a full spectrum of settings, from home to birth centre to hospital. They must be able to integrate the lifeworlds of the women they attend with the work world of midwifery in such a way that the client's needs are fully met. Systems that provide training environments where midwives can function fluidly in both home and hospital, like those so far developed in Canada, can be seen as more beneficial to more women than hospital-dominated systems, which in effect splits home and hospital, allocating hospital care to university-trained nurse-midwives and home care to direct-entry midwives who are apprentice- or vocationally trained.

In this new millennium, we expect to find midwives around the world working to develop philosophies of care that are evidence-based and woman-centred and that encourage midwives' independence of mind, educational programs that effectively blend theory and practice in the full spectrum of settings, and work worlds that encompass that full spectrum. Such developments will assist midwives to become fully respected as practitioners within their country's health care system and to more effectively do what they exist to do: give childbearing women the best possible care.

NOTES

1 This chapter borrows extensively from Cecilia Benoit, Robbie Davis-Floyd, Edwin Van Teijlingen, Jane Sandall, and Janneli Miller, 2001, Designing Midwives: A Comparison of Educational Models. In *Birth by Design: Pregnancy, Maternity Care and Midwifery in North America and Europe,* edited by Ray

DeVries, Cecilia Benoit, Edwin Van Teijlingen, and Sirpa Wrede, 139–65. Reproduced by permission of Routledge/Taylor & Francis Books, Inc.

2 The correspondence we point to here between nursing training as a prerequisite to midwifery training and midwives' lack of autonomy does not hold for all countries. Swedish nurse-midwives, for example, enjoy extensive autonomy.

REFERENCES

Alexander, J. 1994. Degree of Difference. *Modern Midwife* 4, no. 8: 24–6.

Benoit, Cecilia. 1989a. Traditional Midwifery Practice: The Limits of Occupational Autonomy. *The Canadian Review of Sociology and Anthropology* 26, no. 4: 663–49.

– 1989b. The Professional Socialization of Midwives: Balancing Art and Science. *Sociology of Health and Illness* 11, no. 2: 160–80.

– 1991. *Midwives in Passage: The Modernization of Maternity Care.* St John's, Nfld.: Institute of Social and Economic Research.

Benoit, Cecilia, Robbie Davis-Floyd, Edwin Van Teijlingen, Jane Sandall, and Janneli Miller. 2001. Designing Midwives: A Comparison of Educational Models. In *Birth by Design: Pregnancy, Maternity Care, and Midwifery in North America and Europe,* edited by Ray De Vries, Cecilia Benoit, Edwin Van Teijlingen, and Sirpa Wrede, 139–65. London: Routledge.

Böhme, G. 1984. Midwifery as Science: An Essay on the Relationship Between Scientific and Everyday Knowledge. In *Society and Knowledge,* edited by N. Stehr and V. Meja, 365–85. New Brunswick, NJ: Transaction Books.

Burtch, Brian. 1994. *The Trials of Labour: The Re-emergence of Midwifery.* Montreal and Kingston: McGill-Queen's University Press.

Carter, J., and T. Duriez. 1986. *With Child: Birth Through the Ages.* Edinburgh: Mainstream Publishing.

Davis-Floyd, Robbie. 1992. *Birth as an American Rite of Passage.* Berkeley: University of California Press.

– 1998a. The Ups, Downs, and Interlinkages of Nurse- and Direct-Entry Midwifery. In *Getting an Education: Paths to Becoming a Midwife,* edited by J. Tritten and J. Southern, 67–118. Eugene, OR: Midwifery Today.

– 1998b. Types of Midwifery Training: An Anthropological Overview. In *Getting an Education: Paths to Becoming a Midwife,* edited by J. Tritten and J. Southern, 119–33. Eugene, OR: Midwifery Today.

Daviss, Betty Anne. 1997. Heeding Warnings from the Canary, the Whale, and the Inuit: A Framework for Analyzing Competing Types of Authoritative Knowledge about Birth. *Childbirth and Authoritative Knowledge: Cross-Cultural Perspectives,* edited by Robbie Davis-Floyd and Carolyn Sargent, 441–72. Berkeley: University of California Press.

Hall, J. 1994. Midwifery Education: Where Is It Going? *MIDIRS Midwifery Digest* 4, no. 4: 384–6.

Hunt, S. C. 1996. Marketing Midwifery Education: Findings from a Survey. *Midwifery* 12, no.1: 31–6.

Illich, Ivan. 1973. *Deschooling Society.* Harmondsworth: Penguin.

Jackson, K. 1993. Midwifery Degree Programmes: Who Benefits? *British Journal of Midwifery* 1, no. 6: 274–5.

James, Susan. 1997. Regulation: Changing the Face of Midwifery? In *The New Midwifery: Reflections on Renaissance and Regulation,* edited by Farah Shroff, 181–200. Toronto: The Women's Press.

Mason, Jutta. 1987. A History of Midwifery in Canada. In *Report of the Task Force on the Implementation of Midwifery in Ontario,* edited by M. Eberts, A. Schwartz, R. Edney, and K. Kaufman, 195–232. Toronto: Queen's Park Printer.

– 1988. Midwifery in Canada. In *The Midwife Challenge,* edited by Sheila Kitzinger, 99–133. London: Pandora.

Morewood-Northrop, Maureen. 1997. Community Birthing Project: Northwest Territories. In *The New Midwifery: Reflections on Renaissance and Regulation,* edited by Farah Shroff, 343–56. Toronto: The Women's Press.

Rice, J. Allison. 1997. Becoming Regulated: The Re-emergence of Midwifery in British Columbia. In *The New Midwifery: Reflections on Renaissance and Regulation,* edited by Farah Shroff, 149–80. Toronto: The Women's Press.

Rooks, Judith P. 1997. *Midwifery and Childbirth in America.* Philadelphia: Temple University Press.

Van Teijlingen, Edwin R. 1994. A Social or Medical Model of Childbirth? Comparing the Arguments in Grampian (Scotland) and the Netherlands. Ph.D. dissertation. University of Aberdeen.

Van Wagner, Vicki. 1994. "Why Legislation? The Regulation of Midwifery in Ontario from a Feminist Perspective." Paper presented at the CSAA meetings, University of Calgary.

Warwick, C. 1992. Reflections on the Current Management of Midwifery Education. *MIDIRS Midwifery Digest* 2, no. 3: 251–4.

9

Midwifery Education in Ontario: Its Origins, Operation, and Impact on the Profession

Karyn Kaufman and Bobbi Soderstrom

INTRODUCTION

On 7 September 1996 the first eighteen women to graduate from the Ontario Midwifery Education Programme stood in front of their families, midwife teachers, and fellow students and read aloud their promise:

This is our promise to all of you, our way of thanking you for what you have done for us.
This is our affirmation to our community.

We Promise
To serve and attend to the women in our community;
To protect the sanctity of the birth process as a normal and profound life event;
To respond to the psychosocial, physical, emotional, and spiritual needs and choices of women;
To honour the principles of equity and accessibility;
To recognize and honour human interdependence and the cultural diversity within our communities;
To advocate for a safe world where women and children live with dignity and hope and have adequate shelter and sustenance;
To continue to work with the birthing community to develop and maintain standards of maternity care that are directed by and responsive to women's expressed needs;
To contribute to the growth of a unique body of knowledge and to pursue life-long learning;
To be accountable for our actions;

To promote and develop interprofessional collaboration and cooperation;
To broaden and support women's choices and help them recognize their own strengths and social power;
To respect and promote women's decisions, their right to informed choice, choice of birthplace, and active participation in their care;
To ensure the safe passage and well-being of the newborn child;
To support women to give birth safely, with dignity and power.

We Also Promise
To kiss our children, to nurture our partners, and to respect and honour those that came before us;
To be mentors and friends to those who will join us as midwives in the future.

To each other, members of today's graduating class:
We promise to continue to sustain and support each other in our professional roles and personal lives, and to actively nurture our own and others' sense of self-worth.

These first graduates symbolized both the realization of a decade or more of planning and preparation and the future of a newly established profession. Their commitment to the ideals that were central to the creation of the profession was an inspiration to the students to follow and a tribute to the many midwives who had contributed to their education.

The Ontario Midwifery Education Programme was Canada's first degree-granting university program in midwifery. The second and third programs to open are in Quebec (1999) and British Columbia (2002). Manitoba has proposed a program but not yet received funding.

In this chapter we will reflect on the key events in the policy-making process that led to Ontario's university program, describe the structure and curriculum of the program, and speculate about its impact on the development of midwifery education in Canada. Our perspective of developments in Ontario is first-hand, personal, and rooted in our extensive involvement in the profession. We hold faculty appointments in the program and are also practising midwives and leaders within our professional association. Our own very different backgrounds (Bobbi Soderstrom from a graduate degree in library science, an apprentice midwife, and a nursing degree; Karyn Kaufman a CNM and DrPH from the U.S. with an academic career in Canada) reflect the variety of experience not only among the faculty overall but also among the first registrants in Ontario.

ONTARIO'S DEVELOPMENT
OF MIDWIFERY EDUCATION

Provincial Task Force

In 1986–87, an independent task force appointed by the provincial government conducted an intensive investigation of how midwifery was to be established in Ontario including midwifery regulation, practice, and education.

When the Task Force on the Implementation of Midwifery in Ontario began its work, no province in Canada extended legal recognition to midwives and there were no formal preparatory programs. The closest approximations to midwifery preparation were the advanced obstetrical nursing course in Alberta and the outpost nursing programs in Newfoundland and Nova Scotia (see Benoit and Davis-Floyd, this volume). The women practising midwifery in various places across the country were graduates of formal programs outside Canada, apprentice-trained, or self-taught. Many of the so-called "lay" midwives had extensive university backgrounds and had devised intensive self-study and skill development opportunities.

The task force gathered information about these forms of preparation and turned to other countries, especially those where midwives were well established and a respected part of the health care system such as the United Kingdom, the Netherlands, and Denmark, to learn about other forms of midwifery education. Task force members examined their curricula and talked with teachers, practitioners, and government officials. The inescapable conclusion was that no universal recipe existed for midwifery education. Sometimes nursing was a prerequisite, but often it was not. Programs varied in length and were sited in hospitals, independent schools, or other educational institutions. The essential element for a successful program was the larger context of midwifery in the setting, i.e. whether midwives had an established role and whether midwifery education was financially supported as part of post-secondary education.

Even though midwifery is not available in the U.S. to the extent that it is in Europe, the proximity and potential influence of the U.S. on Ontario developments made it imperative that we investigate midwifery there. The stark contrast in legalization, organization, integration with other practitioners, site of practice, and inclusion in third-party payer arrangements between U.S. nurse-midwives and those who were not nurses was clearly evident. The education of nurse-midwives was primarily in the university sector, often at the master's degree level, while non-nurse midwives relied on a few private, independent schools, self-study, and apprenticeship training. There was considerable organizational division between the two categories of midwives that further eroded the strength of the profession and the potential impact on society that might have been realized with a unified profession. It was a lesson to be heeded by the Ontario task force.

During the public hearings held by the task force in 1986, several consumers and midwives spoke of their support for the apprenticeship model because of the close relationship fostered between teacher and student and client. The one-on-one supervision allowed for variation in teaching and learning styles so that apprentice and mentor could individually pace the learning. The task force was mindful of these benefits of apprenticeship in formulating recommendations, but was also aware that midwifery, as a newly regulated profession in the North American context and as a woman's profession, had high potential to be marginalized. Its visible presence in the post-secondary sector was, therefore, an important goal.

The final recommendations of the task force sought to blend the benefits of the apprentice model with the benefits of formal systematic study of the biological and social foundations of midwifery. The recommended place of education of midwives was the university sector, the setting consistent with that of the majority of North American health care professionals. The task force also believed that university preparation would provide for the future development of research and scholarship within the profession and provide midwives with a background suitable for advanced academic study.

The report of the task force (Eberts 1987), issued in late 1987, specifically recommended that:

1   the education of midwives be within a university program that could foster research and academic debate, and that the location be one of the health sciences centres where specialized health studies, medical disciplines, and broad university offerings would be available to midwifery, and interdisciplinary opportunities would help to cross-educate medical and nursing students about midwifery and midwifery students about them;
2   the program confer a baccalaureate degree on successful graduates since an undergraduate degree is the most common credential for health professionals and because this background provides opportunity for the academic development of scholarship and practice and the pursuit of advanced degrees;
3   there be "multiple routes of entry" to enable both those with or without nursing preparation to be educated in the same program and meet the same clinical practice requirements; and
4   modes of distance education be used to enhance access for students who would find it difficult to leave their home community for the duration of a university program.

The task force also made recommendations about the admissions process and emphasized the importance of assessing motivation to enter midwifery and interpersonal skills in addition to academic preparation. Other recommendations were directed to the importance of extended periods of clinical learning to acquire hands-on skills and having opportunities for elective placements both within and outside Canada.

RESPONSE TO TASK FORCE RECOMMENDATIONS ABOUT EDUCATION

The recommendations were submitted to the minister of health and also to the minister of colleges and universities. Within the Ministry of Health, the Women's Health Bureau was charged with the task of responding and preparing an implementation strategy. Karyn was seconded temporarily from McMaster University to the Bureau to coordinate ministry activity. The process of taking recommendations from paper to reality was not straightforward. Formulating policy is an inherently political process that is shaped by more than advice from an external panel, no matter its degree of expertise. There were conflicting opinions within the midwifery profession and its supporters about the merits of having midwifery education at a university level. Supporters of the recommendation thought that university preparation would lead to better acceptance from physicians, nurses, and hospital administrators, who were key to successful integration. Others worried that university preparation would overly medicalize the profession and distance midwives from the women who sought their services. There were also conflicting opinions within the government bureaucracy about the location of an educational program. Some of this concern was about costs, but the same arguments that divided the midwives were heard also. Even among those who supported the general recommendation of university level preparation, there was disagreement about whether a health sciences centre was the best location. The major concerns were about the relative costs, the possibility of medical dominance of the program, the difficulty of establishing a new program in a large institution, and accessibility for future students.

The Curriculum Design Committee

Without a clear consensus about the appropriate location for midwifery education, the Women's Health Bureau staff suggested a further consultation strategy. The minister of health agreed and in May 1989 a Curriculum Design Committee was appointed, chaired by a leader in the midwifery community, Holliday Tyson. The committee's twelve members included consumers, midwives, physicians, and nurses with diverse educational backgrounds including college diplomas, university degrees, and apprentice training. The committee was directed to describe in detail the essential components of midwifery education and to recommend options for the type of educational institution in which to locate a program.

In addition to reviewing the content and organization of several European, British, and American midwifery programs, the committee met with representatives of several post-secondary institutions who expressed an interest in offering a midwifery program. An independent private school was briefly considered and had the attractive feature of complete responsiveness to midwives only, but was rejected because of the enormous financial obstacles and the inability of such a school to confer a recognized credential. The two most obvious choices of site in order to secure provincial funding were a community college or a university. Community colleges were viewed as more accessible and less expensive for students and more likely to develop programs in communities across the province. Universities were viewed as better able to support the midwifery curriculum and foster midwifery science, research, and the potential for graduate study. A university degree was also deemed to be a more credible credential. Creatively, the committee suggested a collaboration of the two types of institutions in order to capture the benefits of both.

In the report of the Curriculum Design Committee (May 1990) the members reported their consensus that "a baccalaureate degree was the appropriate credential for midwifery education in Ontario" (Tyson 1990). In addition they wrote a set of guiding principles for an educational program that set forth the importance of community learning environments, the clinical competencies expected of graduates, and the desire to be responsive to learners from a variety of geographic and cultural backgrounds. They included recommendations about the didactic and clinical content of a program that were invaluable in formulating the actual curriculum.

The committee also recommended that faculty hold joint teaching and practice positions. The teacher-practitioner model was highly desirable for avoiding a split in the profession between academic and practising midwives. The committee also thought this was one method of promoting participation in research among practitioners and strengthening the commitment to evidence-based practice.

A further recommendation given substantial emphasis was that a four-year baccalaureate program be compressed into three. This format was based on values very central to midwifery. The year-round schedule would provide students with greater opportunity for continuous clinical experience and therefore greater ability to provide continuity of care for women. As well, since most students were likely to be women, many with young children, there were perceived advantages to having the program be as short as possible.

SELECTION OF A PROGRAM SITE

Upon accepting the reports of the task force and the Curriculum Design Committee, the Ministry of Health and the Ministry of Colleges and Universities approved a budget for the program based on an average enrolment of thirty-five to forty students per year. This number was considered to be the minimum for a viable program, and it was a number that could be accommodated within existing midwifery practices for clinical teaching. The Ministry of Colleges and Universities issued a request for proposals (RFP) inviting colleges and universities with health sciences programs to provide evidence of their ability to offer a program consistent with the major features described by the Curriculum Design Committee. Groups of institutions were encouraged to make a joint submission since it was clear that any single university would have difficulty meeting all the terms of the RFP.

Considerations of northern-southern, anglophone-francophone linkages as well as histories of working relationships across institutions were major driving forces in shaping the two multi-institutional proposals that were prepared in response to the RFP. McMaster, Laurentian, and Ryerson universities comprised one consortium, led by Karyn at McMaster. Lakehead, Ottawa, and Windsor universities along with the Michener Institute and Cité Collegiale of Ottawa formed the second consortium, led by Monique Begin, then dean of the Faculty of Health Sciences at the University of Ottawa.

The Ministry of Colleges and Universities appointed an external review panel to assist it in making its decision about a program site. The panel included Bobbi and a second midwife, Michelle Kryzanauskas, who later became the first president of the College of Midwives of Ontario. Physicians, nurses, a consumer, and persons with administrative, legal, and financial expertise in the university sector were appointed also. The panel was co-chaired by an expert in university programs and Mary Eberts because of her former work as chair of the task force. The panel members represented also the views and concerns of special constituencies such as First Nations, francophones, and residents of the north. In this way the ministry sought to have broad input into a potentially divisive decision.

After evaluating the written proposals and conducting site visits, the panel recommended that the McMaster consortium be awarded the program based on McMaster's experience with an interdisciplinary approach to health science education and its use of problem-based learning, Ryerson's expertise in part-time adult education, and Laurentian's ability to attract northern students and francophone students.

In December 1992, the minister of colleges and universities and the minister of health officially announced the selected consortium. The Ministry of Colleges and Universities provided a targeted operating grant for the first years of funding. Start-up funds were made available immediately, contingent upon a commitment that the first students would be admitted nine months hence in September 1993. The pace was hectic, although some observers noted wryly that midwives were used to working on nine-month time lines. The three initial directors exemplified three different routes of entry to midwifery: nurse-midwifery (Karyn at McMaster), direct-entry midwifery (Holliday Tyson at Laurentian), and apprenticeship (Vicki Van Wagner at Ryerson). Others appointed to the faculty included the then president and two former presidents of the Association of Ontario Midwives (Eileen Hutton, Rena Porteous, and Bobbi). The accumulated experience, varied backgrounds, and commitment of the entire faculty group were (and continue to be) its major assets.

The faculty set to work to prepare course materials for the fall term and conduct the assessment of the first applicants. With equal amounts of exuberance and exhaustion, we welcomed the first students on schedule and immediately began work on the courses for the following term.

FEATURES OF THE MCMASTER-LAURENTIAN-RYERSON POLYTECHNIC UNIVERSITIES PROGRAMME

Three Universities – One Program

A fundamental organizing principle of the consortium was an equal partnership among the three collaborating sites. The students and faculty all participate in and benefit from being part of a consortium. Decision-making is a shared responsibility. Therefore all committees of the Programme include representation from the three sites.

Each of the three sites has a unique role within the overall program. Laurentian University is located in northeastern Ontario and offers degrees in French and English. It serves northern and francophone students. Ryerson University offers a part-time course of study that permits students to take up to seven years to complete all requirements. McMaster University is the main administrative and financial centre and provides access to many of the teaching resources that are available within its Faculty of Health Sciences.

Each site has a small core group of faculty who work together to organize and deliver the program content. The biological and social scientists are responsible for several of the foundation courses and the midwives organize and teach the applied midwifery courses. All the faculty members have graduate degrees (required for appointment to a university faculty) but among the midwives, their preparation in midwifery has been acquired in a variety of different places and ways including apprenticeship. In addition to the core faculty, there are a large number of practising midwives who provide supervision of students during their clinical placements.

Admissions Process

Applicants to the program must apply to one of the three sites; each site then carries out its own assessment of applicants. All applications are reviewed for previous academic performance at the secondary school level or beyond. Each site requests personal letters or interviews or both as part of the final selection process. The ratio of applicants to available places has varied from 8:1 to 4:1 in recent years. The annual intake has increased from just over thirty (1993) to fifty-six in 2002.

The large majority of applicants are female and all students admitted to date have been female. About 90 per cent are from Ontario. The mean age of students at the time of application decreased from thirty-three in 1993 to twenty-nine in 1997 (the last year of complete data). The majority are married or in a stable relationship. The proportion with children has deceased from 70 per cent of the earliest admitted students to under 45 per cent more recently. On average, about 20 per cent of the entrants have prior nursing preparation and about 50 per cent have a prior degree in arts or sciences. To date, 12 per cent of all admitted students were in the French language stream at Laurentian University. Another 8 per cent of students across all sites had a language other than English as their first language (Stewart and Pong 1998).

The Centre for Rural and Northern Health Research at Laurentian University, under a contract with the Midwifery Education Programme, surveyed students at entry to the program from 1993 to 1997. Students were asked about their reasons for becoming a midwife. Most commonly they cited the promotion of women's health care, empowering women, and providing physical, emotional, and spiritual support to women and families. These reasons have remained stable over the groups surveyed. More recent cohorts have also indicated their support of the philosophy of midwifery as an added reason for their choice of the profession (Stewart and Pong 1998).

Organization of the Curriculum: What We Teach and How We Do It

Students spend six of nine academic terms in clinical placements. The other three terms have a heavy concentration of courses in sciences, social sciences, women's studies, and research fundamentals. In addition to these foundation courses, first-year students have several follow-through experiences where the objective is to be "with woman," to learn from the woman about her experience of pregnancy, birth, and the postnatal period by observation and interview. Through reflection and analysis, the student begins to consider her role as a caregiver and the nature of the midwife-client relationship.

Placement in a midwifery practice begins in the fourth term and continues, with one exception, until the end of the program. The exception includes a one-month elective opportunity of the student's choosing and placements for one month each in a hospital maternity unit and in an obstetrician's practice. Anecdotally, these placements enhance students' skills, foster interprofessional relationships, and provide students with a greater appreciation of others' roles in the health care system.

The theoretical content about midwifery care is studied throughout the placement terms, both independently as the student encounters issues in her clinical work and formally in a weekly small group tutorial with a faculty tutor. The topics of study in tutorials move from normal pregnancy and parturition to variations of normal, and then to pathologic problems including emergency situations. By the end of the clinical courses the students have studied in-depth both common and less common maternal and newborn situations.

At specified times each year, we hold intensive workshop sessions where all students in a given course are brought together in one place for a period of time, typically five to ten days. This format helps to build relationships among the students and enhances the sense of the common program. Guest experts and specialized teaching resources, such as professional patients who teach pelvic examination, can be made available for all students.

A few courses are available by distance education, i.e. the student has no requirement to attend class and submits all work by mail or by e-mail. For some in-person classes, a variety of media have been used (teleconference, videoconference, net meeting) to link two or three groups of students together with one instructor. Students much prefer personal contact with an instructor and become frustrated with the limits of the technology. When students begin their sequence of clinical placements, many are located far away from one of the university campuses. To accomplish the necessary high level of student interaction that is mandatory in their tutorial groups, groups of nine to eleven students are linked with a tutor by telephone conferencing when they cannot meet in person. Students and faculty have become skilled at conducting group discussions over the phone and using e-mail transmission for class notes and assignments. Students, therefore, experience a range of teaching-learning venues, from large to very small groups, from in-person to electronic contact, and from intensive residence with other students to being remote from all other students.

Organization of Clinical Learning Experiences

In the five academic terms of midwifery clinical learning, each student is assigned to a midwifery practice group and a designated midwife preceptor, i.e. supervisor/teacher/mentor. The preceptor is responsible for facilitating the student's entry to the practice and providing her with opportunities to acquire the necessary midwifery skills and judgments, in much the same way as an apprenticeship. The student must be available for all antenatal and postnatal visits and is on-call with the preceptor for labours. The student provides care to women under the watchful eyes and guiding hands of the preceptor. This role evolves gradually from the first placement to the last, when the student should function as the "primary" midwife with the preceptor being a consultant colleague.

As faculty, we strongly endorse the value of a student-preceptor relationship that develops over time and believe that students benefit from continuity of supervision. Their professional socialization is facilitated within a close long-term relationship. Students and preceptors spend many hours in each other's company as they travel to home visits, await the birth of a baby, and conduct visits in the clinic and at home. The student experiences first hand the rich relationships that develop between midwives and their clients. The preceptor is key in modelling the values and qualities of a midwife and in shaping the growth and development of the student. The preceptor is able to observe the student over a period of time and provide the necessary feedback. When the relationship works well, the learning is enhanced and the entire practice benefits from the presence of students. There can be strains for both preceptors and students as they struggle to accomplish the learning goals and the important work of providing individual care to women. Faculty must sometimes assist in conflict resolution between students and preceptors. Rarely are placements changed to resolve problems, since our approach is to work through the issues for mutual benefit.

While there are a number of similarities between student clinical placements and an apprenticeship, there are differences. Unlike an apprenticeship, preceptors do not choose their students, nor do students choose their preceptors. Student placements are assigned through a lottery system that takes account of but cannot guarantee personal choice of geographic location. Students who must relocate to a community that is not of their choosing find this very stressful. Practice groups contract to provide a placement for one or more students usually for two consecutive terms. In an apprenticeship, the student usually gains all of her clinical learning from the same midwife or small group of midwives, whereas our students are placed in at least two different practices in order to gain different experience, e.g. a rural and then an urban setting. If an apprenticeship flounders, the learner may find herself without a placement whereas a student in the program has recourse to a structure to obtain another placement if needed.

PREPARATION OF CLINICAL PRECEPTORS

Almost all practising midwives throughout the province who have a minimum of one to two years of experience participate in the clinical teaching of students. Of necessity, the educational program must provide preceptors with skills and information required to be teachers and evaluators of students in the clinical area. Workshops and the program's *Guide to Teaching, Learning and Assessment for Midwifery Preceptors and Student Midwives* are used for this purpose. An initial workshop orients midwives to the structure of the education program and the role of midwives as preceptors. We offer tips to new preceptors about clinical teaching and how to demonstrate to clients the value of including a student in their care.

In follow-up workshops, midwives focus on exchanging ideas for teaching effectively, especially for students having difficulties. They also problem-solve about how best to cope with the stresses of simultaneously being a midwife and a clinical teacher. Several preceptors reported that their initial anxieties about the responsibilities of being a preceptor were abated by opportunities for interaction with other preceptors in the workshops. Beyond the challenges of being a preceptor, some midwives reported that the workshops provided a valuable opportunity for the exchange of information and strategies for the inevitable problems they faced as newly regulated professionals in the health care system. Preceptors have expressed the rewards for themselves of providing student supervision. They have mentioned that they gain ideas from the students who have worked in other practices or who have heard ideas from other students during tutorial sessions. Students have enriched the clinical practice of midwives by posing challenging questions and doing literature searches about client questions or clinical problems.

The program continues to recruit new preceptors. In recent years, graduates of the program and registrants educated in other jurisdictions have been valuable additions to the preceptor group. Many of the first-recruited preceptors have expressed a desire to take time off from teaching, so the continued recruitment of new preceptors is vital. One of the challenges faced by the program is maintaining a critical mass of experienced and dedicated preceptors.

What Have We Changed?

Like many new ventures, we made excellent decisions about some aspects of the program and faced problems with others. The accelerated pace of preparing course materials existed throughout the first three years because we had such a short time to prepare for the arrival of students. We were continuing to write new courses just a few months before they were first taught. In 1996, at the end of the first three years, we organized an external review to assist us in taking stock of what had been accomplished.

Two eminent reviewers, Lesley Page from the UK and Diony Young from the U.S., familiar with issues in maternity care and midwifery education, conducted on-site assessments of course materials and interviewed students, preceptors, and faculty. Their report was laudatory and provided immensely helpful suggestions for improvements, including the need to reduce its intensity and increase the time for completion. The reviewers commented that the program was too rigorous and intensive for a three-year degree and that changes were needed to slow the pace and reduce stress, especially for full-time students and preceptors.

Students and the faculty found the pressures of year-round study to be very intense. Students were unable to pursue any outside employment, which increased their financial burdens. The hoped-for benefits of the three-year program were not realized in the day-to-day experience of that timetable. A faculty retreat was held in late 1996 and a plan emerged to reorganize the program from three calendar years to four academic years. The revised program has the same number of academic terms as the original format, but full-time students have two of three summers available for work and/or family time. For part-time students, the change allows them to plan a course sequence that can be completed in as many as seven years.

A second major change that was supported by the external review was to increase the biological science content and broaden the options in the social science and health science offerings. Student feedback strongly supported increasing pharmacology, biochemistry, and microbiology content. Two new courses have been added to address this concern. More recently students have asked that they receive instruction in business management skills. They are aware from their clinical placements that midwives must manage their practice workload, budgets, and support staff.

The external review, while pointing out areas for improvement, also provided great encouragement and support to everyone involved. The reviewers wrote that "in comparison with programmes elsewhere in the world, this one may well be the best available to midwifery students anywhere in meeting all academic and clinical practice standards" (Young and Page 1996). This strong vote of approval was important to validate the enormous time and energy that had been invested by both faculty and students.

A second external review was conducted in 2001. The panel concurred with the conclusion of the first reviewers. They also provided recommendations to assist with organizational issues, increase support to students and preceptors, and increase recruitment of applicants from diverse communities (Cooke, Kaufert, and Martin 2002).

ASSESSING THE IMPACT OF THE EDUCATIONAL PROGRAMME

Expanding the Profession

By the autumn of 2002, 153 students had completed program requirements and were eligible to apply for registration with the College of Midwives. The number of graduates has increased each year from eighteen in 1996 to thirty-three in 2002. As greater numbers of part-time students (who spend a longer time in the program) complete their studies, the number of graduates will be over forty by 2004. The graduates of the program now constitute nearly two-thirds of the number of registered midwives in Ontario. Of the graduates, only those who completed in the first years have now acquired five or more years of clinical practice experience. Concurrently, the number of original registrants, many of whom had many years of practice experience, has declined as some have retired and others have chosen a lighter workload by reducing the number of clients they attend. The experience profile of the registrant population has, therefore, shifted rapidly. Yet the demand for midwives to provide supervision for students is critical for continued growth. A challenge for the program is supporting the learning needs of "newer" midwives as they become preceptors. Workshops, mentoring of new preceptors, and faculty support when problems arise are strategies recently and commonly employed.

There is at the same time an interest in learning about the work life of graduates. The Centre for Rural and Northern Health Research at Laurentian University conducted follow-up surveys by mailed questionnaires of the graduates from 1996 to 1998 (Stewart and Pong 1999a, b). Their results show that most graduates were practising within Ontario and felt adequately prepared for the realities of midwifery clinical practice. They were satisfied with their decision to become a midwife and would make the same decision if given the choice again. A few graduates opted not to become registered midwives, citing the lifestyle problems they experienced as a student as the major reason. Graduates who were surveyed one or two years after graduation reported that time away from their families and balancing their personal and practice obligations were the most stressful aspects of their work. Several respondents planned to reduce their workload because of a decision to become pregnant themselves.

Overall, graduates rated their educational experience as highly positive. The clinical "hands on" preparation was perceived as very effective in preparing them for day-to-day work as a midwife. One graduate described it as "the heart of my work." They were able to obtain sufficient experience in both home and hospital birth to feel confident about their skills in both locations. The intensives were described by one graduate as "crucial foundation blocks for learning." The majority of respondents said the program met their expectations and many took the opportunity to offer suggestions for further changes. Most of those surveyed were either involved or planning involvement in the educational program as preceptors. Many were leaders in the midwives' professional association or the regulatory college. A small number were planning to pursue graduate education with a view toward obtaining a future faculty appointment.

There is preparation underway for a repeat graduate survey in order to develop a better understanding of their career paths and practice patterns. There is also a desire to glean useful information for the continual process of curriculum revision.

INTEGRATION INTO THE HEALTH CARE SYSTEM

The development of the educational program has contributed to greater visibility of the profession, strengthened the autonomy of the profession, and also furthered its integration into the overall health care system. Midwifery faculty members take part in interprofessional activities within their university site and in external committees related to maternity care. Midwifery students participate in department and university activities that help promote a greater understanding in the general student population of the profession and the educational program.

Midwifery students accompany midwives into hospitals and have elective placements in hospital units. Their presence across the province helps a greater number of hospital staff to become familiar with the principles of midwifery care. The students' socialization and adherence to principles of informed choice, choice of birth place, non-authoritarian client relationships, and evidence-based practice furthers the overall goal of improved health care for women. In turn, hospital staff members have an important role in assisting students to understand organizational issues in hospitals.

Future Challenges

One of the goals of establishing midwifery education in the university sector was to facilitate midwifery research and scholarship. This has been a challenge. Faculty teacher-practitioners are subject to unpredictable schedules and disrupted work activities that pose substantial barriers to conducting scholarly work. However, half of the present complement of midwifery faculty either have doctoral preparation or are engaged in doctoral studies. Four faculty members have obtained external awards for conducting research and most have published in midwifery and health journals. One faculty member has been instrumental in the development of the first Canadian peer-reviewed midwifery journal. With time, midwifery research will be able to contribute to an understanding of the way women give birth in Canada.

Recent graduates and several midwifery preceptors have expressed interest in research and in obtaining graduate preparation. Currently, there are no programs within Canada that offer a master's or doctoral level program in midwifery. Those who decide to pursue graduate work either leave the country for a period of time or enrol in a complementary discipline, e.g. education, women's studies, epidemiology. The requests for a Canadian graduate program are increasing and it looms as an important future challenge.

The Ontario Midwifery Education Programme is an important resource for the development of educational programs in other provinces. The newly established programs in Quebec and British Columbia signed formal consultation agreements with Ontario's program in order adapt course materials to their respective programs.

Over the next one to two years, the program will be participating in a comprehensive evaluation of midwifery implementation in Ontario. The outcome of the evaluation will help guide human resource planning for the next several years. It is likely that the outcomes will also influence curriculum changes as more is learned about the variations in practice activities and the needs of a growing profession.

Each phase of program development has brought new challenges. It is unlikely that demands will lessen any time soon. Energy, commitment, and creativity will continue to be necessary ingredients in meeting the challenges ahead.

REFERENCES

Cooke, Pauline, Patricia Kaufert, and Kerstin Martin. 2002. *Midwifery Education Programme, Report of the External Review.* Unpublished report.

Eberts, Mary (Chair). 1987. *Report of the Task Force on the Implementation of Midwifery in Ontario.* Ontario Ministry of Health.

Stewart, Dianne, and Raymond Pong. 1998. *Summary Report of the 1997 Midwifery Entry Survey.* Centre for Rural and Northern Health Research, Laurentian University. Unpublished report.

– 1999a. *Summary Report of the 1996 and 1997 Cohorts of Graduates of the Midwifery Education Programme.* Centre for Rural and Northern Health Research, Laurentian University. Unpublished report.

– 1999b. *Summary Report of the 1998 Cohort of Graduates of the Midwifery Education Programme.* Centre for Rural and Northern Health Research, Laurentian University. Unpublished report.

Tyson, Holliday (Chair). 1990. *Report of the Curriculum Design Committee on the Development of Midwifery Education in Ontario.* Ontario Ministry of Health.

Young, Diony, and Lesley Page. 1996. *External Review Report of the Midwifery Education Programme.* Unpublished report.

Midwifery on the Prairies: Visionaries and Realists in Manitoba

Pat Kaufert and Kris Robinson

Discussing issues of language and childbirth, Paula Treichler argues that definitions "are social, cultural and political as well as linguistic and they are constructed by specific speakers with specific aims and interests." She continues: "Thus a definition is not, as conventional wisdom assumes, the set of necessary and sufficient conditions that constitutes a fixed starting point for political, economic and ideological struggle. Rather a definition represents the outcome of such struggles – an unstable, negotiated and often quite temporary cultural prescription" (1990, 133).

This paper deals not with childbirth but with midwifery. Like Treichler, however, our concern is with issues of definition, more particularly with the emergence of a new definition of the midwife, carefully crafted to be uniquely Canadian and, more particularly, uniquely suited to the Province of Manitoba.

Rather than presenting a history of the re-establishment of midwifery in Manitoba, chronicled committee by committee and report by report, we have focused on a single transformative moment in this history, the crisis that developed around a decision made by the Midwifery Implementation Council (MIC) as it set up an assessment and registration process for the first group of midwives to be licensed to practice in Manitoba. As many other provinces have found, creating an equitable framework for enabling midwives with varied backgrounds to seek registration is a difficult task, legally and administratively, and it may aggravate existing tensions between those with different aims and interests. This is also a story, however, of the MIC, a group of indi-

viduals, midwives, and others, who worked hard and creatively to resolve differences, to compromise and reach consensus. Out of this
consensus emerged a new definition not only of the midwife but also of
the women for whom she should care. In the first part of this paper we
provide a brief description of the key players, the events that triggered
the crisis, and its successful resolution. The second part of the paper explores both the language and the cultural and ideological assumptions
about the nature of midwifery and midwifery practice that contributed
to the creation of the crisis. In the final section of the paper, we consider some of the factors that contributed to the resolution of this crisis
and their implications for midwifery practice in Manitoba.

One of us (Kris Robinson) was closely involved in these events,
whereas the other (Pat Kaufert) was an outsider, being neither a midwife nor a member of MIC or even any longer a potentially childbearing woman. She was, however, once chair of an earlier committee on
the implementation of midwifery in Manitoba and has a particular interest the role of history, politics, economics, and ideology in the creation of the Canadian midwife. We have kept our account of this
sequence of protest, negotiation, and eventual resolution deliberately
bare of detail on the individuals involved, using only material already
in the public domain. This is partly protection of confidentiality, but
also because we are concerned not with the behaviour of specific individuals but rather with exploring the broader political, social, and linguistic context within which this crisis erupted, simmered for a time,
and was resolved.

IMPLEMENTING MIDWIFERY:
A CRISIS AND ITS RESOLUTION

The Government of Manitoba appointed the MIC in 1995, shortly after
it had announced its intention to legalize the practice of midwifery and
make it an insured service. The MIC included representatives from government, members of the medical profession, nurses, educators, lawyers, and representatives of various community-based organizations
including the Winnipeg Women's Health Clinic. Most importantly, it
included both nurse-midwives and community-based midwives.

An earlier report to the provincial government had made a series of
recommendations that together outlined the essential characteristics of
a made-for-Manitoba midwife (*Report* 1993). Signatories to that report agreed that midwifery should be a regulated profession, that it
should be an insured service within the provincially funded health insurance system, that there must be multiple routes of entry into midwifery training, and that midwives should practice in many different

settings. Midwives should have hospital privileges but also the right to conduct home births. (This was the most contentious of the recommendations and the most difficult on which to reach agreement.) While not original to Manitoba, each of these recommendations had been carefully debated by the committee that wrote the report and provided the provincial government with a definition of the midwife to which all the key stakeholders had given general agreement, including the representatives of both the community and nurse-midwives.

The mandate of the MIC was to transform these recommendations into reality. This included developing some method of retraining and evaluating midwives already active in the province so that they would be ready and eligible for licensing as soon as the act was promulgated. At the time, only very incomplete information was available to the MIC on the number of midwives in Manitoba, who they were, or how many would want to be licensed. Once it started to hold information sessions for midwives, the council discovered that the midwifery community was larger and more diverse than had been anticipated, and could be divided into three relatively distinct groups of uneven size.

The smallest group is identified in MIC reports as "unregulated" or "community" midwives. A few of the community midwives had trained abroad or taken courses offered by U.S.-based midwifery education programs, but as a group they were deeply committed to a model of midwifery based on training by apprenticeship and through the experience of attending to women as they gave birth. Although limited in number, the community midwives were the most publicly visible of the three groups, having been the primary target of critics of the home birth movement and the most vociferous of the lobbyists for midwifery.

The second group was made up of nurse-midwives. A few had been educated in Europe, but the majority had been trained under the British midwifery model, either in the UK or in other Commonwealth countries. Some were Canadians who had returned home after training abroad, but others had been recruited to work in Canada by the federal government under a policy of hiring midwives to work in the Arctic and in remote northern communities. The majority of these midwives left Canada at the end of their contract, but some drifted southwards, often finding work in hospital-based departments of obstetrics where their skills and experience were highly valued. (A few of these midwives worked in programs targeting special needs populations, such as teens and women from the inner city.) As their midwifery licenses were unrecognized under provincial law and their legal status was dubious, the opportunities to practise the full range of their midwifery skills were highly dependent on the good will of a few physicians.

The largest of the three groups attending the MIC information meetings was made up of midwives who had been trained in the Philippines, China, and southeast Asia. Many worked at the peripheries of the health care system in personal care homes or as nannies. Migrant midwives were shut out entirely from being able to practise. They could not risk their immigrant status by copying the community midwives and providing midwifery care outside the law, but neither could they work as obstetric nurses. Some had been trained in direct-entry midwifery programs and did not have nursing qualifications; others had nursing qualifications not recognized in Canada. Although the largest of the three groups, they were also the group on whom the MIC had the least information.

At a practical level of conditions of work, legal status, and economic security, each group had different possibilities of gain or loss from the implementation of regulated midwifery. As independent practitioners, the community midwives were accustomed to high control over such elements of their work as the choice of client, the number of clients, the structure of the workday, and the choice of work partners. Only their clients, or occasionally their peers, had any oversight over their management of a birth. They operated, however, in legally contested space, were fiercely opposed by many physicians, and were at constant risk of criminal prosecution. Midwifery was restricted to physicians by the Manitoba Medical Act with the result that midwives could be prosecuted for practising medicine without a license. While they were economic entrepreneurs, self-employed and free to determine their own fees, the market was small and midwifery provided at best a relatively unstable income. Regulation promised legal and economic security, but also the risk of losing control over their choice of client, the site of birth, and their freedom to practise with minimal regulation or oversight.

The nurse-midwives were health professionals with incomes that were higher and more secure than those of the community midwives, but as nurses within a hospital hierarchy, their control over their work setting was low and subject to the authority of the hospital administration, senior nurses, and physicians. Regulation would gain them a greater independence and autonomy of practice, but at the risk of having to work in ways with which they are not fully comfortable. Many of their anxieties focused around the probability that doing home births would be a precondition of being able to practise. Immigrant midwives might seem to have least to lose, for whatever they had gained by coming to Canada, they had lost their professional status, and the employment opportunities that remained to them were often low paid and marginal to the health care system.

The question for the MIC was how best to transform these three very different groups of midwives into a single entity, the Manitoba midwife. The MIC did not want to discard its own vision of the midwife or jeopardise women's safety by regulating the incompetent, but it also wanted to move the assessment process forward with some speed. The time pressure was the result of a commitment to having a group of midwives in place, registered, and able to practise as soon as the Midwifery Act was proclaimed. (The act was given Royal Assent on 28 June 1997, but its proclamation was delayed at the request of the MIC until the first group of midwives had been assessed and would be ready to move into practice.) The dual challenge was to ensure not only clinical competency but a form of philosophical competency as well.

Seen from an assessment perspective, the nurse-midwives offered the advantage of having been trained and having worked in a setting in which the evaluation of clinical skills was part of the culture. They were also likely to be familiar with other expectations of a midwife's role in a formal system, such as record-keeping, reading test results, making referrals, and relating to other members of the health care team. They might need to refresh or learn the clinical skills necessary to functioning outside the security of the obstetric ward and its technology, but the MIC could be somewhat reassured on their levels of clinical competence. A different question was how best to develop and assess their capacity to work with physicians on a consultative basis (given they had been trained to a more subordinate role) while at the same time preparing them to relate to pregnant women on a more egalitarian footing than customary in the culture of the hospital.

Community midwifery was based on relationships with women that were already companionate rather than professional; however, if they were to work effectively with other health professionals, then the MIC had to ensure that they could discard an often deep-seated hostility to hospitals and physicians. A rather different problem was that having been trained by apprenticeship, many of the community midwives were less accustomed than nurses to being evaluated and having their clinical knowledge tested and measured. Complicating the need to evaluate their clinical competence was the commitment of the community midwifery movement to a philosophy of knowledge as intuitive and experiential and, therefore, not amenable to testing and evaluation. Yet the MIC had to find some method of ensuring their ability to follow clinical guidelines and work to protocols of midwifery practice.

Finally, there were the immigrant midwives, who probably posed the greatest challenge for the MIC's own philosophies. At this point in time, the MIC knew relatively little about their academic or language skills, their clinical competence or philosophy of midwifery. Clinical skills could be taught and assessed and barriers of language were potentially remediable, although not necessarily in the time available. Philosophies of midwifery care could be determined and the degree to which these diverged from those of the MIC could be explored. The more fundamental challenge, however, was to set up an assessment process that would respect the cultural diversity of the immigrant midwives without abandoning the MIC's own principles of midwifery care.

The MIC reviewed the assessment methods that other provinces had used, including the special, time-limited program that had been created in Ontario. Based in Toronto at the Michener Institute, it had been staffed by three midwives imported as tutors from the Netherlands, Sweden, and New Zealand. The choice of tutors reflected the influence of the European midwifery model on the Ontario program, whereas many MIC members had a strong commitment to the American midwifery movement, with its emphasis on home birthing, apprenticeship training, and the absolute autonomy of the midwife. Wanting to ensure that this should be the basis for the Manitoba system, the council decided to design its own program and adopt the system of examination and skills assessment set up by the North American Registry of Midwives (NARM). NARM was the creation of the Midwives Alliance of North America (MANA) and was created by the Alliance to develop and implement a national certification process for direct-entry midwives.

NARM's regulations laid out a series of conditions that had to be satisfied before a midwife could begin the assessment process. These conditions included having attended ten home births as a primary midwife with a certain percentage of these births having occurred within the previous ten years. Attendance at in-hospital births was not required. NARM also demanded evidence that the midwife had provided continuous care to women throughout pregnancy and childbirth and into the postpartum period.

When the MIC made a preliminary announcement to the midwifery community on the proposed use of the NARM process, the statement of these conditions evoked a storm of protest. As seen by the nurse-midwives, the stipulation on the number of home births would exclude all but the community midwives. Immigrant midwives could not count births attended as midwives before coming to Canada unless they had occured in the last ten years, and for both groups the requirement for continuity of care was problematic. The main resistance came from nurse-midwives who were quite comfortable with the concept of renewed professional autonomy and continuity of care but objected to having to do ten home births as a condition of assessment. Even if some nurse-midwives had delivered the required number of babies, it was rarely as the officially recognized birth attendant and never officially as a home birth. The fact that community midwives were not being asked to demonstrate their capacity to function within the hospital environment further fuelled the resentment and anger of both the immigrant midwives and nurse-midwives.

Being excluded from the assessment process was not a minor matter. The only other choice for those wanting to become licensed midwives was to wait until the proposed midwifery degree program had been set up and then hope to be accepted. The advantages of becoming licensed through the MIC included speed and lower costs. The most important factor, however, was that it might be the only route into midwifery for those who could not qualify for entrance into a degree program (a possibility for some of the immigrant midwives) or who could not afford the time or the expense of getting a degree. (The degree program would have to operate under university regulations rather than those of the MIC or NARM.)

It is unlikely that the use of the home birth as the yardstick defining who could or could not enter the assessment process was deliberately exclusionary. Nevertheless, the MIC's critics accused it of adopting a policy that not only was in contradiction to its own commitment to ensuring the existence of multiple routes of entry into the profession but would severely affect the chances of both the immigrant midwives and nurse-midwives of becoming regulated midwives. Faced with these protests and wanting to avoid splitting the midwifery community just on the verge of its success, but committed also to its own vision of the Manitoba midwife, the MIC decided to renegotiate the conditions set by NARM.

NARM was cooperative, agreeing to suspend the regulation on the number of home births and their timing within the previous ten years. NARM also agreed to two compromises that would allow Manitoba midwives to write their examination. The first allowed a midwife who had not practised in the last ten years to write the NARM exam provided they were enrolled in the Manitoba assessment and upgrade program, which they would accept as currency. Second, NARM would allow midwives without out-of-hospital births to write the NARM exam but would not grant them their certification as a Certified Professional Midwife unless they fulfilled the requirement for out-of-hospital births in the next three years. Responding to pressure from midwives who did not want to provide out-of-hospital births, the MIC agreed to allow those who registered in the first three years following proclamation of the Midwifery Act to have the option of choosing a form of registration that would entail permanently restricting their practice to their own choice of birth setting. This condition could be removed later, but only if a midwife agreed to a period of supervised practice in the setting with which she was least familiar.

The decision brought the crisis to an end and allowed the MIC to move forward into organizing the assessment process. The change may seem slight: midwives as a group would still work in both home and hospital, although not all midwives would work in both settings. Furthermore, the option of choosing a birth setting would be available only to midwives going through the assessment process, not to those who would enter practice after graduating from the degree program. The significance of this change is more in terms of its implications for the definition of the midwife. It meant that doing home births had become an option rather than an absolute requirement of being registered to practise and, therefore, was no longer the defining characteristic of the true midwife. Many saw this as critical because of the symbolic place of home birth within the long drawn out, still continuing, process of negotiating between different visions of the midwife, different philosophies of midwifery care, and conflicting claims over who is (or is not) a true midwife.

HOME BIRTHS: SACRED SYMBOL
OR SEED OF DISSENT

Language has played a key role in maintaining and reinforcing the divisions within the midwifery community. Rosalind Petchesky's statement that "Reproductive politics is in large part about language and the contestation of meanings" (1995, 387) was written with reference to women and ownership of the body but applies equally to the place of language in the politics of midwifery. The naming of midwives, for example, the ways in which names are claimed or rejected, what names mean in different contexts, who has the right to a name and who does not, all these are contested ground. An early example would be the distinction between the male and the female midwife in the seventeenth century. More recently, there has been the proliferation of names in North America for non-nurse-midwives including "lay," "independent," "unregulated," "community," and "traditional" midwives.

The title "nurse-midwife" seems self-explanatory: a nurse who is also a midwife. In most settings outside North America, it is an indication of professional education, the possession of a professional license, and legality of practice in most countries other than Canada. Yet in the context of the debates over the implementation of midwifery in Manitoba, it has also been seen as indicative of the co-optation of midwifery into the world of medicine and the absorption of the midwife into the identity of the nurse. The nurse-midwives were themselves ambivalent, changing the name of their association in 1992 from the Nurse Midwives Association of Manitoba into the Association of Manitoba

Midwives. The name change was to show their support for multiple routes of entry into midwifery, but by dropping "nurse" out of their title they were also rewriting their "narrative of origin" by asserting a claim to be recognized as midwives *tout court*. Their vision of the Manitoba midwife was close to that of the European midwife, a highly educated, highly skilled, autonomous health professional, very different from the reality of their position within the Canadian medical and nursing hierarchy.

The titles "community midwife" and "traditional midwife" were chosen to distinguish them from the nurse-midwife, but also to indicate their total independence from the world of biomedicine. Their naming also carried a message about their roots, their "narratives of origin." As defined by Yanagisako and Delaney:

Narratives of origin tell people what kind of world it is, what it consists of and where they stand in it; they make it seem natural to them. By anchoring individual lives to some kind of larger cosmic order, identities are secured ... Narratives of origin incorporate classificatory schemes that describe the order of things, as well as relations between the order of things, as well as the relations between things and between different kinds of people. For people whose origin story it is, these things take on the aura of the sacred. (1995, 2)

Narratives of origin are not histories, but rather they are statements of philosophy about the present, contained in a story about the past. They answer the questions "Who am I?" and "Where did I come from?" In this case, they reflect a very particular vision of what it is to be a midwife.

The title "community midwife" has different meanings in different contexts. The British National Health Service used it in the 1960s and 1970s to describe nurse-midwives who worked for a local health authority, running mother and baby clinics, advising on breastfeeding, and doing postpartum visits (Macfarlane and Mugford 1984). A-political and non-ideological, it was essentially an administrative label in the UK setting, distinguishing these midwives from the hospital-based midwife. "Community" in this definition is a spatial and organizational construct, a set of people living in a bounded space or, more specifically, a subset of the population comprising all the new mothers in that population. Used in Manitoba as a designation for the non-nurse-midwife, the word "community" becomes a philosophical rather than a spatial construct. Loosely based on the distinction between the community and the state, it denotes the emergence of the midwife out of the community, more particularly out of the community of women, rather than out of the institutions of biomedical science (Burtch 1994).

"Traditional," also used in Manitoba as a designation for the non-nurse-midwife, has different meanings within the discourse on midwifery depending on the speaker and the context. Anthropologists tend to use the word "traditional" in contraposition to "modern" or "colonial" or "Western" or, if medical anthropologists, to biomedicine. Gertrude Fraser (1995), for example, uses the term "traditional midwife" in her study of an African American community of Green River in the southern United States. A few of the old midwives were still alive, seen by Fraser as lingering figures in a vanishing culture, soon to disappear. Used in this sense, the word "traditional" would also describe the midwives who once cared for women living on the Canadian prairies. Like the midwives of Green River, each of these midwives will have drawn on whatever were the traditions of childbirth in their own community, whether Ojibway, Cree, French, Scottish, Mennonite, Ukrainian, or any of the other cultures represented in the history of Manitoba. Rather than one form of traditional midwifery, there must have been several varying from culture to culture, changing with time and assimilation, eventually disappearing except in the memory of the elders.

The word "traditional" in the "Traditional Midwives Collective" (the title chosen by community midwives for their association in 1985) appears to have been a generic term, an expression of spiritual kinship with all the long-dead midwives of the province's past, rather than a reference to a specific midwife in a specific culture. The idealization of past midwives as wise women, crones, close to nature, close also to natural ways of childbearing, is not unique to Manitoba. Figures of this type are part of the folklore of the midwifery and home birth movement. In her fascinating analysis of the writings on childbirth by novelists and social scientists, Tess Coslett (1994) found repeated images of the midwife as "filthy peasant crone" – a term Coslett borrows from Adrienne Rich – her ancient wisdom contrasted with the new knowledge of the physician. Other versions of this figure are to be found in the mythic mother-goddess imagery of some new age style North American writing and art. Although their resemblance to the real midwives of Green River as described by Gertrude Fraser, or to the Cree or Ukrainian midwives of turn-of-the-century Manitoba, is probably slight, these imaginary figures are powerful because they imply a direct linkage between the community midwife of today and the traditional midwife of the past (see MacDonald, this volume).

This is the vision; the reality is rather different. The Manitoba Home Birth Network was formed in 1981 and the Manitoba Traditional Midwives Collective in 1985. Their roots trace back not to the midwives who practised in the nineteenth century in rural Manitoba but to the natural childbirth and home birth movements of the 1960s and 1970s in the United States. These movements had drifted northward across the Canadian border in the late 1970s and early 1980s, winning supporters in Ontario and British Columbia and spreading into Manitoba. Close ties exist between the leadership of the home birth/midwifery movements in Manitoba and Ontario, but also between the Canadian movements and the midwifery movement in the United States. Canadian midwives took U.S.-based courses, read the U.S. literature, attended meetings and workshops in the U.S. Along with the more formal transmission of information and training came a strong commitment to a particular vision of woman in childbirth, the midwife and setting of birth within the home rather than the hospital.

For Robbie Davis-Floyd in her study of pregnancy and childbirth among middle-class women in the southwestern U.S., women having home births are radicals against medical orthodoxy, people leading at the edge of a new paradigm. She writes:

The home birthers in my study who espouse the holistic model do so in direct and very conscious opposition to the dominant technocratic model. They represent the one percent of American women who choose to give birth at home. I suggest that the importance to American society of this tiny percentage of alternative model women is tremendous, for they are holding open a giant conceptual space in which mothers and babies can find room to be jointly embodied and spiritually linked ... They speak of mothers and babies as unified energy fields, co-participants in the creative mysteries, entrained and joyous dancers in the rhythms and harmonies of life. (1992, 154)

This passage captures the beauty and the excitement of this particular vision of childbirth, as well as the fervour that drove the home birth movement in Manitoba, as elsewhere. As a vision, it also had an extremely powerful impact on members of the women's health movement for whom home birth became the ultimate acting out of the beliefs and values of feminism. In Yanagisako and Delaney's telling phrase, home birth had taken on "the aura of the sacred" for both midwives and their clients.

Yet, there are other views of the home birth/midwifery movement and other explanations of the reasons why home birth became so important to its identity. Barbara Katz Rothman described the women attracted to the home birth movement in the U.S. as follows:

Some of the women came from the feminist health movement, women who have been fighting for abortion rights and see birth as another issue in reproductive freedom. A very different group sees the husband/father as having a right to be with his wife and birth belonging in his territory. And still others, such as a home-birth group in Kansas see birth as bringing genuine fulfillment to husband and wife, concluding that birth belongs in the bedroom. Feminists, traditionalists, spiritualist, and sensualists: a puzzlement. (1982, 32)

Margaret Reid (1989) places both movements within the broader counter-culture of the late 1960s, whereas Gertrude Fraser sees home birth as an outgrowth of a "consumerist choice-oriented social move-ment influenced in large part by middle class (white) feminist theory and praxis" (1995, 55). Emily Martin (1987) locates the origin of the home birth movement firmly within the middle classes, seeing the rejec-tion of biomedicine and the demand for personal control in childbirth as an expression of middle-class values. In her view, middle-class women hoped to shift the balance of power between themselves and their caregivers by moving birth into their own homes and "growing" their own midwives (midwives were often self-recruited from among women who had home births).

The middle-class roots of the home birth/midwifery movement had a number of very pragmatic consequences; for example, it meant that the community midwife model of care evolved out of their experience with a relatively narrow, very select segment of the society of childbearing women. Many assumptions in this model – such as the health of the pregnant body and the quality of the home – were based on this popu-lation. The class nature of their client-base limited the experience of most community midwives to women who were not only healthy but health conscious, living in homes that usually had adequate light, wa-ter, heat, hygiene, and bed linen. Seen from this rather different angle, the "good" birth, the home birth, birth as a spiritual or sensual experi-ence, is also a birth dependent on access to the accoutrements of the middle-class income, lifestyle, and home, but also middle-class culture. Some years ago, Margaret Nelson (1983) pointed out that middle-class notions of the desirable birth were not shared across class lines; work-ing-class women, for example, wanting more rather than less pain kill-ers. Carol McClain (1983) found that the views on Caesarean birth of working-class women were not only different but reflected the very dif-ferent realities of the lives of working women.

The social and political implications of the narrowness of the class base were largely invisible so long as the backgrounds of both midwife and cli-ent were essentially the same. Each enjoyed the advantages of working with someone who was bright, articulate, highly involved in what was happening to the pregnant body, and totally convinced of the rightness of what they were doing. The result was a form of intellectual and ideologi-cal symbiosis, which contributed immensely to the cohesiveness of the two movements, strengthening their sense of common purpose. Yet, the criticisms of Emily Martin or Gertrude Fraser are also to be taken seriously and can be read as a special case of Audre Lorde's (1980) wider criticism of the assumption of sisterhood made by the early women's movement. "There is a pretense to a homogeneity of experience covered by the word *sisterhood* that does not in fact exist." The sincerity of the midwifery/home birth movement is not in question, but the naiveté of some of its assumptions about women and childbirth had potentially serious implications for the ways in which midwives might be educated, assessed, paid, regulated, and used, and in which they take their own values and experience as the norm.

VISIONS AND REALITY: A PRAIRIE SOLUTION

The middle-class basis of the community midwifery/home birth movement was largely irrelevant so long as community midwifery remained the minority choice of a few, deeply committed women in Canada and the United States. It became problematic once midwifery became a matter of public policy. A number of different options were open to provincial governments. One was to do nothing, and leave community midwives operating outside the law, albeit unlikely to be successfully prosecuted once legalized midwifery has been introduced elsewhere in Canada. This still remains the choice of some provinces. Another was simply to legalize the position of the community midwife, imposing minimal regulation but also providing minimal funding and making her payment the ongoing responsibility of her client. (The community midwifery movement in the U.S. took payment between midwife and client for granted.) A third option, slightly more attuned to Canadian values, was to allow the community midwife to continue doing home births for clients of her choosing, but with her fee paid by the government.

This third option would have preserved intact the bonding between midwife and client that was the mark of the community midwifery movement, as well as protecting that sense of birth as a deeply spiritual experience celebrated in the earlier passage from Robbie Davis-Floyd. The risk was that it would also preserve the middle-class nature of the client base. (This seems to be the case in British Columbia.) For as long as midwives could set up their own practice and select their own clients, it would be natural for them to work primarily with women who shared their vision and philosophies of birthing. These women would be largely white, largely urban, and largely highly educated.

There are many reasons why the MIC did not choose any of these options, but the most important was their vision of midwifery care for

Manitoba. There was also the presence of the immigrant midwives and lessons learned from the example of Ontario. While immigrant mid-wives was probably far more numerous in Ontario than in Manitoba, they had also been largely invisible within the debates over the imple-mentation of midwifery in that province. Preoccupied with the deep di-visions between community and nurse-midwives, no one paid much attention to this third presence or to the implications of the rules gov-erning assessment on their access to registration. It is the work of Sheryl Nestel (1996/97; this volume) that made the immigrant visible, just as Audre Lorde once made the African American woman visible to the women's movement. Once made visible, they could not be ignored. More correctly, they could not be ignored by the MIC, given the very strong commitment of its supporters within the women's community to issues of equity and diversity.

The implications and consequences for the immigrant midwives themselves is a story that must ultimately be told from their perspective. The immediate consequences for the MIC included a re-examination not only of the rules of the assessment process but also of the dichot-omy drawn between hospital and home birth. The MIC was deeply committed to ensuring equity and access for all the many different com-munities of women in Manitoba, not just the relatively small group of middle-class women already members of the home birth movement or likely to want home births. The council consulted widely, believing that the communities of women likely to benefit from midwifery care also included women living in northern, rural, and remote areas, First Na-tions women, immigrant and refugee women, the emotionally and so-cially dysfunctional, the physically or socially isolate, and women without homes suitable for childbirth, and women who wanted to birth in hospital but attended by a midwife. Midwives had to be able to work with all these different communities and meet their different needs. It was at this point that many of the assumptions of the community mid-wifery movement that had made sense when the majority of clients were highly educated and middle class became problematic.

The MIC decided to discard the dichotomy that assigned birth either to the home with the assistance of a midwife or to the hospital and oversight by a physician. Needing a practical way of deciding whether or not to define a birth as in- or out-of-hospital, the MIC adopted a pragmatic approach and agreed that the availability of back-up was the key element of difference between the hospital birth and the home birth. Midwives who had worked in rural and northern communities supported this new definition, maintaining that small community hos-pitals and nursing stations were very similar to the home in terms of levels of available technology. Using the lens of "safety" as a guiding principle and acknowledging the realities of the Manitoba climate and environments, these small hospitals and stations often offered practical advantages, such as being more accessible than a remote farm house or better provided with basic services (such as water) than houses in many First Nations communities.

This renegotiated definition of out-of-hospital birth was not embraced by all midwives, as some argued that this dilute definition undermined the philosophical concept of home birth. Others saw the MIC's decision to allow a transformation of the definition of the "home birth" into the "out-of-hospital" birth as a creative solution to a dilemma that was part practical and part philosophical. By slightly adjusting the NARM criteria and the careful wording of Manitoba's own regulations, MIC created a system in which the community midwife and nurse-midwife could coexist, while also providing an opportunity for midwives from the immigrant community to join them, regaining their legal status and ability to practice.

The history of midwifery in Manitoba is an act still in process. It is impossible to predict exactly how it will evolve once established and as other models of education take a larger role in training the midwife and shaping both her skills and her philosophy of practice. The passage from Paula Treichler quoted at the beginning of this chapter implies that it is unlikely that any one definition of the midwife will achieve stability or permanence, but the events we have described suggest that this is not necessarily a bad thing. The outcome of this particular struggle was a solution that was a better fit with the political, social, and ethical realities of the province than could have been achieved had the system been left untouched or modified to allow only one form of midwifery.

CONCLUSION

The conclusion to this paper has to be the announcement on 12 June 2000 that the first group of twelve midwives were in place and ready to start legalized practice. Some may interpret this ending as the co-optation and routinization of community midwifery and the disappearance of the midwife as romantic radical. Yet, she was a figure belonging as much to a particular time and place as the traditional midwives of Green River. Perhaps it is time that she also vanishes, if the exchange is to be the free and easy access to midwifery care of any woman in Manitoba who wants or needs that care and support, regardless of where she lives, her age, her education, her ethnicity, her social class, or her philosophy of childbirth.

Acknowledgment: We want to thank Dr Carol Scurfied for her invaluable advice and assistance.

REFERENCES

Burtch, Brian. 1994. *The Trials of Labour: The Re-emergence of Midwifery*. Montreal and Kingston: McGill-Queen's University Press.

Coslett, Tess. 1994. *Women Writing Childbirth*. Manchester: Manchester University Press.

Davis-Floyd, Robbie. 1992. *Birth as an American Rite of Passage*. Berkeley: University of California Press.

Fraser, Gertrude. 1995. Modern Bodies, Modern Minds: Midwifery and Reproductive Change in an African American Community. In *Conceiving the New World: The Global Politics of Reproduction*, edited by Faye Ginsburg and Rayna Rapp, 42–59. Berkeley: University of California Press.

Lorde, Audre. 1980. *The Cancer Journals*. San Francisco: Spinsters/aunt lute.

Macfarlane, Alison, and Miranda Mugford. 1984. *Birth Counts: Statistics of Pregnancy and Childbirth*. London: Her Majesty's Stationary Office.

Martin, Emily. 1987. *The Woman in the Body*. Boston: Beacon Press.

McClain, Carol. 1983. Perceived Risk and Choice of Childbirth Service. *Social Science and Medicine* 17, no. 23: 1857–65.

Nelson, Margaret. 1983. Working Class Women, Middle Class Women and Model of Childbirth. *Social Problems* 30, no. 3: 284–91.

Nestel, Sheryl. 1996/97. 'A New Profession to the White Population in Canada': Ontario Midwifery and the Politics of Race. *Health and Canadian Society/Santé et Société Canadienne* 4, no. 2: 315-41.

Petchesky, Rosalind. 1995. The Body as Property: a Feminist Re-Vision. In *Conceiving the New World: The Global Politics of Reproduction*, edited by Faye Ginsburg and Rayna Rapp, 387–406. Berkeley: University of California Press.

Reid, Margaret. 1989. Sisterhood and Professionalization: A Case Study of the American Lay Midwife. In *Women as Healers*, edited by Carol Shephard McClain, 219–38. New Brunswick, NJ: Rutgers University Press.

Report and Recommendations of the Working Group on the Implementation of Midwifery to the Minister of Health. 1993. February. Manitoba: Manitoba Health.

Rothman, Barbara Katz. 1982. *Giving Birth: Alternatives in Childbirth*. London: Penguin Books.

Treichler, Paula. 1990. Feminism, Medicine, and the Meaning of Childbirth. In *Body/Politics Women and the Discourses of Childbirth*, edited by Mary Jacobus, Evelyn Fox Keller, and Sally Shuttleworth, 113–38. New York: Routledge.

Yanagisako, Sylvia, and Carol Delaney. 1995. *Naturalizing Power: Essays in Feminist Cultural Analysis*. New York: Routledge.

PART FOUR

Equity and Accessibility: Confronting Some Unresolved Issues

INTRODUCTION

As Pat Kaufert and Kris Robinson's paper in the last section describes, equity and accessibility are important issues for both midwives and birthing women that have yet to be fully resolved. We take aim at these two issues more fully in this section. Concerns with equity and accessibility are particularly salient in the description of the experiences of women with unregulated midwifery care in Nova Scotia from 1975 to mid-1998 by Denise Marion. In this chapter, Marion documents 169 cases of experiences with midwifery care in a retrospective, descriptive study that involved mailed questionnaires to former midwifery clients and selected individual interviews. The socio-demographic attributes of the women, their expectations, experiences, and motivations for choosing midwifery care, and reasons why some women seek home birth care are presented. Marion shows that in the unregulated environment in Nova Scotia those women who choose midwifery care have to pay for it themselves, so that midwifery is not an option for those who cannot afford it. Some Nova Scotian women also "pay" for their care on an emotional level as a result of having to deal with the scepticism of mainstream society and contention from the medical community for choosing to rely upon lay/independent midwives working outside of the formal system. Marion concludes by expressing hope that her province will follow others in encouraging the option of regulated midwifery and making it a public service, thereby removing the economic barrier to accessing midwifery services that currently exists.

The issue of access to midwifery care comes up again in chapter 12 by Anne Ford and Vicki Van Wagner in their reflections on their experience on the Ontario Equity Committee. They describe how between 1988 and 1992, as Ontario worked on crafting the legislation that would guide the introduction of midwifery in the province, a small committee of women (including the authors) travelled around the province to meet with groups representing a variety of different constellations. Focusing on ensuring that the legislation and education for Ontario's midwifery profession reflected the history and needs of marginalized groups, the Equity Committee chronicled the histories and concerns of Aboriginal women, immigrant and refugee women, women with disabilities, teenage mothers, lesbians, incarcerated women, and women from the Mennonite community. Ford and Van Wagner recount these experiences and note how this work influenced specific elements of the 1993 legislation and the Midwifery Education Programme for Ontario.

Following this description of the Equity Committee process in Ontario, Dena Carroll and Cecilia Benoit present an alternative narrative of midwifery in Canada, with a particular focus on how traditional midwifery practices in British Columbia and in other parts of Canada have resurfaced and become recognized as a positive link to improving the health of Aboriginal people in urban and rural communities. For many centuries, Aboriginal people across the country have faced social and cultural changes that have negatively impacted their overall health, cultural identity, and traditional values. The authors argue that the revitalization of Aboriginal midwifery has resulted in a deeper understanding of the interface between medical science, traditional practices, and gender. They highlight the critical role that traditional Aboriginal midwives and birthing families have played historically within various geo-cultural communities in the province of British Columbia and across the country. They also discuss some contemporary examples of the revitalization of public interest in Aboriginal ways of birthing, traditional medicine, and midwifery across Canada in light of – and partly in contrast to – emerging Canadian models found in non-Aboriginal communities.

We conclude Part IV with Sheryl Nestel's critical analysis of the midwifery integration process in Ontario entitled "The Boundaries of Professional Belonging: How Race has Shaped the Re-emergence of Midwifery in Ontario." She describes how, despite the lengthy lapse of time post-regulation to make changes, and the fact that Ontario is Canada's most multicultural and multiracial province, midwifery in the province remains dominated by white women. Given the presence in the province of thousands of women, many who are new immigrants, who possess formal midwifery training, Nestel exposes the paradox represented by the absence of women of colour from Ontario midwifery. She argues that the current normatively white racial character of midwifery is linked both to structural inequities related to race and to the midwifery movement's many complex and problematic interactions with groups popularly understood as "racially" different.

Unregulated Midwifery: Experiences of Women in Nova Scotia

Denise Marion

INTRODUCTION

The case of midwifery in Nova Scotia offers an interesting contrast to many of the provinces discussed in this volume in terms of access and regulation. Although there has been a slow surge of interest in midwifery care since the late 1970s similar to other jurisdictions, midwifery in Nova Scotia is not (at the time of writing) a regulated health profession. Therefore when women in Nova Scotia choose midwifery care, they usually pay for the service out of pocket, according to a sliding scale determined by their financial means or by negotiating barter agreements with their midwives. Some women also "pay" for their care on an emotional level as a result of having to deal with scepticism from mainstream society and contention from the medical community.

According to anecdotal sources, a small number of women have sought out the services of midwives for maternity care and childbirth. Little information exists, however, about the reasons behind these choices or about midwifery practice in general in the province.

Midwife-assisted home births and hospital births attended by midwives in conjunction with physicians are not registered as "home births" or "midwife-assisted" by the provincial Department of Vital Statistics. The births are recorded as hospital or non-hospital birth. There is no information reported on where specifically the birth occurs outside the hospital. Deaths are reported as hospital, home, other, and other health care facility (Billard 2003).

In spite of the absence of documented information, I embarked on a study combining a quantitative and qualitative research approach to learn about these women's stories and to obtain some background demographic information about them. In this chapter I describe experiences of women choosing midwifery care in Nova Scotia from 1975 to 1998. I focus primarily on their motivations, expectations, and experiences of midwifery care and their reasons for choosing home births. I begin with a bit of detail about the context of maternity care in the province.

NOVA SCOTIA IN CONTEXT – SOME CONSIDERATIONS

Jutting out into the Atlantic Ocean, the easternmost province of mainland Canada was, in 1605, home to the first permanent European settlement north of Florida (Towler 1999). Its landmass forms Canada's second smallest province. The history of its people and the relatively sparse population density has been shaped by its natural resources – rich agricultural land amidst forests and rock and miles of shoreline.

Little is known, sadly, about the tradition of midwifery from the First Nations' people of Nova Scotia. It is recorded that midwives contributed to local health care from 1755 to 1764, when British midwives settling in Nova Scotia had their wages paid by the British government (Mason 1988). At that time, midwifery care was viewed as "one of many reciprocal activities that was part of daily life in these infant communities" (Kusisto 1980, 17).

Ambivalence toward the profession crept in as medical obstetrics came into favour. Midwives were ostracized from professionalized medicine and at the same time were criticized by physicians for their lack of lengthy apprenticeships (Kusisto 1980). Although compulsory certification of midwives was instituted in Halifax in 1872 (Hackett 1998), by the end of the nineteenth century "midwifery as an occupation for, or service to women was no longer acceptable" in Nova Scotia (Kusisto 1980, 2). Still, midwives were utilized when disaster struck: they were requested to "report to duty" to provide health care after the devastating 1917 Halifax explosion, which killed two thousand and injured many more (Maritime Museum 1999). Later in the twentieth century, midwifery certification and legislation in Nova Scotia was dissolved, leaving its practice in an "alegal" limbo.

During the mid-1980s, the provincial government attempted to address problems of rising health care costs in relation to its population. More than a third of Nova Scotia's population lived in the central eastern portion of the province. Forty per cent of the population, or 360,000 people, lived in the Halifax Regional Municipality (HRM 1997). Maternity care services outside the Halifax Regional Municipality were reduced through the restructuring of the province's health care system from 1988 to 1995: during this period, twelve community hospitals stopped providing maternal-newborn services (Reproductive Care Program 1997). Almost half of the province's births each year occur at the major women's hospital in Halifax. Consequently, funded birthing options and choices for maternity care are limited.

Not surprisingly, support for midwifery care resurfaced. The Midwifery Coalition of Nova Scotia formed in 1984 and lobbying for a self-regulating midwifery profession ensued. In 1997, the provincial Department of Health conducted a year-long review to examine the potential for regulated midwifery. Gaps in the provision of optimal maternity care were documented (Reproductive Care Program 1997). The report also revealed that many Nova Scotians were not familiar with the concept, philosophy, and modern practice of midwifery.

In June 1999, the Interdisciplinary Working Group on Midwifery Regulation delivered *Recommendations for the Regulation and Implementation of Midwifery in Nova Scotia* to the provincial minister of health. The minister agreed to strike an Implementation Committee to draft a framework for midwifery legislation and review the recommendations. Shortly thereafter, a different political party was elected and the newly elected minister of health deferred proceeding with the working group's recommendations.

The justification for this decision presumably was that a professional body could not sustain its college with a small membership of practising midwives. Such rationale dismisses the fact that many out-of-province or out-of-country certified midwives living in Nova Scotia might return to midwifery practice in a regulated environment. It also overlooks individuals who might choose a career in midwifery once an educational program is established.

One can also question why tracking of home births or midwife-assisted births in hospital has not been updated by the Department of Vital Statistics or the Reproductive Care Program of Nova Scotia. Is it lack of insight into the trend of alternate birthing options? Lack of funding? Lack of political will? Given the fact that the present and recent premiers of Nova Scotia have been medical doctors, does it hint of medical hegemony?

METHODS

My first contact with midwifery in Nova Scotia was at an annual Midwifery Coalition conference in 1995. I attended this meeting, as a midwifery supporter, to learn about the state of midwifery practice in Nova Scotia. In a series of meetings in 1997 I met with the only three practising midwives in the province at the time, as a potential researcher. They supported my proposed study to explore women's experiences with mid-wifery and provided me with the names and addresses of all their former clients. Given the province's population and the small number of women receiving midwifery care, the task of attempting to contact all previous midwife clients was feasible. I mailed retrospective anonymous question-naires to women who had chosen midwifery care for one of their preg-nancies, births, or postpartum periods in Nova Scotia. I also placed a two-day ad in the province-wide *Chronicle Herald* newspaper in May 1998, and a notice in the summer edition of the Coalition of Nova Scotia Midwives' quarterly newsletter. In this way, I tried to recruit and account for as complete a population of these women as possible.

Along with thesis advisers, colleagues, and midwives, I devised a questionnaire with eighty-three close-ended and twenty-four open-ended questions. Relevant literature informed the development of my questions. In addition to the main questionnaire, I sent supplementary questionnaires to women who had more than one midwifery experi-ence in Nova Scotia. The questionnaires primarily requested demo-graphic information and, to a lesser extent, some descriptive data. It required approximately one hour to complete. The questionnaires were deemed to have face-validity – that is, the midwives and my thesis ad-visers felt the questionnaire was a reasonable tool to try to measure the concepts of interest. I did not test-pilot the questionnaires with a sam-ple of midwifery consumers because the target population was small: approximately 200 women. I sent consent forms and, later, postcard re-minders to all potential participants. Replacement questionnaires were mailed to participants who had agreed to participate but had not re-turned questionnaires some weeks after the initial mailing.

To follow up and provide context on key qualitative themes from the questionnaires, I conducted in-depth, face-to-face interviews with a subgroup of these women. Of the many women who signed consents to also take part in interviews, four were selected through purposive sam-pling for in-depth discussions. They were chosen to represent a diverse range of experience with differing ages and family sizes from urban and rural communities. Qualitative data – derived from their oral stories and all the responses to the open-ended questions in the questionnaire – enriched the quantitative data collected in the questionnaires.

EXCLUSIONS AND RESPONSE RATE

A physician in the rural Pictou area of Nova Scotia attended some home births alone from the mid-1970s until the mid-1980s. Later he attended home births with one or two assistants. Also, a few foreign-trained midwives assisted some home births in the Halifax area during the 1970s (MacLellan 1997). Between 1980 and 1988, a midwife and her assistant began to regularly offer midwifery care. The assistant midwife provided individual labour support to a small number of women from 1980 to 1983 (Wheeler 1999). I did not obtain the names of these clients for possible inclusion in the study; nor did I locate the women who birthed at home with the physician. The currently practising midwives confirmed that, to the best of their knowledge, there had been no other practising midwives in the province since 1980.

The search for former Nova Scotia midwifery clients turned up the names of 200 women. No additional women were found through the newspaper or newsletter notice. Names came entirely from the midwives' list except for two, which were given to me through chance discussions. The current addresses of former clients came from all the Canadian provinces, the U.S., Japan, France, and the Netherlands. I could not locate thirty-four women despite address checks and phone searches. Four women declined to participate and three women were excluded because they received all their midwifery care and gave birth outside Nova Scotia. Of 159 eligible respondents, 130 women completed and returned questionnaires for an 82 per cent response rate.

FINDINGS

Descriptive statistics were applied to the quantitative data using Stata 4.0 (StataCorp 1995). The qualitative data were obtained on a broad scale from written responses in the questionnaires and on an individualized level from the interviews. The primary questionnaire was completed by 130 women and accounted for 129 births[1] with midwifery care in Nova Scotia. Of these women, 25 per cent completed a supplementary questionnaire for additional midwifery experiences in the province. The survey therefore reported on 169 midwifery experiences and 168 births that occurred from 1975 to mid-1998 in Nova Scotia. The yearly occurrence of midwifery care in Nova Scotia is shown in table 1.

Demographic data particular to women choosing midwifery care in Nova Scotia can be found in table 2. The majority of women were Canadian by birth (76 per cent) while just under a quarter listed other countries as their place of birth. At the time of their first midwifery experience in Nova Scotia, women's ages ranged from nineteen to forty-one years, with a mean age of 30.4 years. Over half of the women (55 per cent) were multiparous (had given birth to one child already); 45 per cent were primiparous (about to give birth for the first time). Interestingly, two women each gave birth to their sixth child during their first midwifery experience in Nova Scotia. Nearly three-quarters of the respondents had some university education.

Table 1
Occurrence of midwifery care in Nova Scotia from 1975
to mid-1998* (n=169)

Years	Number of births	% of total **
1975–79	2	1
1980–84	8	5
1985–89	33	20
1990–94	52	31
1995–98	74	44

* Based on survey responses
** Decimals rounded off; totals may not equal 100.

With respect to lifestyle factors, most reported not smoking (96 per cent) or drinking alcohol (64 per cent) during pregnancy. Many also participated in regular physical activity (82 per cent). Most women (96 per cent) breastfed their infants, and three-quarters continued breastfeeding for more than eleven months.

With respect to social support, the majority of women (86 per cent) believed their partners were supportive towards midwifery. Fewer women (75 per cent) felt their partners were supportive of birthing at home. Most women (62 per cent) lived in an area with a population of 10,000 or less. Just less than half of the women (48 per cent) stated they had no religious affiliation.

Including both first and subsequent midwifery experiences, 71 per cent of births were at home and 29 per cent occurred in hospital. Of the births at home, there were one set of twins and four vaginal births after a previous Caesarean birth (VBAC). There were eight instances when births occurred at home without a midwife. These instances involved seven multiparous women and one primiparous woman and were related to rapid labours, poor weather conditions, and one intentional delivery by the woman's partner. Thirteen per cent of women planning home births were transferred to the hospital prior to birthing. Of the hospital births, there was one VBAC, nine births assisted by forceps or vacuum extraction, and six Caesarean births. There was one neonatal death at two days of age, one Caesarean birth of a premature stillborn twin, and one vaginal birth of a premature stillborn infant. There were no maternal deaths.

Compared with other women of childbearing age in the province, there are some striking differences with women choosing midwifery care in Nova Scotia. By examining provincial data from the Nova Scotia Atlee Perinatal Database[2] in 1988 and 1995 respectively, 6.5 per cent

Table 2
Demographic data at first midwifery experience in Nova Scotia (n=130)

	Number of women	% *
EDUCATION (MATERNAL)		
High school graduate or less	16	13
Some college/trade school	8	6
College/trade school grad	11	9
Some university	18	14
University graduate	51	40
Postgraduate studies	25	19
WORK STATUS **	53	41
Paid employment outside home		
Self-employed	36	28
Full-time homemaker	44	34
Student	12	9
Unemployed	11	9
TOTAL HOUSEHOLD INCOME		
< $20,000	46	36
$20,000 - 29,000	26	20
$30,000 - 50,000	33	26
> $50,000	23	18
MARITAL STATUS		
Married	98	76
Common-law	29	22
Single	2	2
RELIGIOUS AFFILIATION		
Christian	31	25
Jewish	1	1
Buddhist	6	5
Hindu	1	1
Bahai	2	2
Other	26	20
No religious affiliation	61	48

* Corrected for missing information. Decimals rounded off.

and 9.4 per cent of Nova Scotia mothers were thirty-five years of age or older at the time of delivery. This contrasts with 18.7 per cent of the study respondents who were thirty-five years of age or older when they gave birth between 1975 to mid-1998. In regards to infant feeding, 96 per cent of the study respondents breastfed during their first experience with midwifery in Nova Scotia from 1975 to mid-1998, including 74 per cent who breastfed for more than eleven months. This is markedly higher than the 50 per cent and 60 per cent of women in the general population in Nova Scotia who were breastfeeding at the time of discharge from hospital in 1988 and 1995 respectively. In regards to smoking, 4 per cent of midwifery clients in the period from 1975 to mid-1998 smoked during pregnancy. This is much lower than the nearly 34 per cent of Nova Scotia women in the general population who smoked during pregnancy in 1988 and the nearly 30 per cent of Nova Scotia women in the general population who smoked during pregnancy in 1995.

REASONS FOR CHOOSING MIDWIFERY CARE

"Birth is such a miracle, shouldn't it be a celebration?"

Many women gave more than one reason for choosing midwifery care, but desire for a home birth ranked first. In fact, 86 per cent of women wanted a home birth while 14 per cent wanted a hospital birth with a midwife. As events unfolded, 70 per cent of women gave birth at home and just under a third gave birth in hospital.

Women stated that they valued the midwifery philosophy of minimal interventions during pregnancy and birth, and the focus on birth as a natural as opposed to a medical event. An interviewee described: "I wanted a very positive birth experience, I wanted people who believed in my body's ability to work. I wanted to have as natural a birth as possible, I wanted to include my other children in the birthing process, and I wanted to be with people who knew me ... I knew I would be more tense in the hospital and when a woman is more tense, things can happen. And a respondent said: "a lot of the medical intervention that is considered necessary ... puts expedience ahead of the well-being of the mother and child. This type of medicine leaves out the spiritual side of the birth experience."

Women described looking for a connection with their caregiver. Some felt it was important to receive care from another woman, preferably one who had given birth herself. An interviewee explained:

It's the ... continuity of care, the compassion and I'm quite convinced that a lot of it has to do with ... the fact that all my midwives were women who had had babies ... and there's something about ... what comes along with motherhood that makes ... real compassion, real heart connection, real sacrifice a possibility ... I'm always absolutely flabbergasted when women tell me they're going to male obstetricians for their babies. How could they possibly ... trust somebody who's never had a baby? It's the most absurd thing imaginable. Like you know, taking tennis lessons from someone who's never held a tennis racket.

Midwifery provided an emotional connection of shared values with their caregiver for some women. The care reflected their family's beliefs: "Midwifery care was the fit for me and my family's values and lifestyles."

Women wanted to labour and birth in comfortable, familiar surroundings where they felt they had more control and could relax. Women saw the midwife as a specialist for normal pregnancy and birth and felt that the quality of care would be better, more meaningful, and a healthier choice for themselves and their babies: "I felt like I had the best care that I ever had and I felt like my newborn had the best care than any of my other children. I really felt that ... just the follow-up, checking on him ... how every step the new baby is blending in with the family and all these kinds of things. It was more like a, I suppose in a sense, more like a holistic care that you're getting than ... just being at the hospital."

Another interviewee said:

To me, midwives are more educated than MDs because they have to make sure that if something happens, they're on top of it and know what it's about because of people being against home births. So even more so do they make sure they're educated about the situation and possible problems. So I felt that I was in better hands than I would have been in the hospital with the machinery and the nurse who is ticking off the things on her chart, you know. I felt that I was being well looked after ... and that my baby and I were never in any jeopardy of any sort.

Some women wanted an advocate for pregnancy and birth: "I wanted someone to protect me when I was in a vulnerable state."

Women believed that their wishes would be respected: one woman felt her wishes would not only be respected – they would be "celebrated"! Women believed they would be empowered to feel strong and to birth in their own way. Throughout pregnancy, birth, and postpartum, midwifery care offered holistic care for the entire family. As one interviewee said: "... we'd go see the midwife for an hour and a half at a time, and [my husband] would get a lot of information and after speaking to his friends ... they weren't getting the information that he had. It's not the same thing; usually it's only the woman who goes to see the doctor for ten or fifteen minutes at a time and the guy doesn't really have (laughter) much to do with it."

Many women viewed pregnancy and birth as a natural event that affected self-esteem, confidence, and bonding with one's baby. They often wanted to be the main decision maker in their childbirth care: "[The midwives] always asked permission for everything … the eye drops, 'Do you want us to do that … the vitamin K, did you want that by injection, or did you want that orally, did you want it at all?' Everything – even when I had the heart rate checked during the labour or any dilation checks, anything – it was either at my asking to, or they asked if it was ok. You know … I found was the nicest difference of all. I was very much treated like a person, as opposed to just a woman with a baby stuck in her."

Women wanted a holistic alternative to traditional medicine, one where the spiritual aspect of pregnancy and birth could be affirmed. Birthing, as one respondent described, was "a direct connection with the life force."

EXPECTATIONS OF MIDWIFERY CARE

Previous hospital birth experiences played a significant factor in choosing midwifery care for most women. The majority of multiparous women (92 per cent) said feelings about a previous birth experience influenced them. Nearly one-fifth of the multiparous women had previously experienced midwifery care elsewhere, including nine births at home. In addition, there were five instances of previous home births, some attended by either a doctor, a doctor and nurse, or without any birth attendant.

Women whose previous birth experiences were uncomplicated and joyful events felt that subsequent births would be enhanced with midwifery care and/or a birth at home. Other women based their expectations on experiences at their friends' midwife-assisted births. Some women had read about births attended by midwives and had considered midwifery care for years. They felt midwifery made sense. Midwifery care was seen as a way to have more support and make birth more family oriented with children present or nearby. Some women knew a particular midwife personally. Others found prenatal care from their midwives more convenient. One woman wanted to labour longer at home with a skilled caregiver; another sought out midwifery care specifically for the practice of perineal massage; and a few others wanted to avoid defensive hospital medicine. Three women mentioned not knowing a doctor or being unable to get a doctor and turning to a midwife instead. In other cases the maternity wards in nearby hospitals, which some women were accustomed to, had closed. Some women disliked hospitals, believing they harboured germs, and believed doctors were for people suffering with illness. Midwifery care was recommended to two women by their doctors.

Women who previously had negative experiences and unpleasant memories with the medical system most commonly felt their wishes would not respected or their birth plan would be disregarded. As one interviewee described: "I had more fear going to the hospital than I had of ... staying at home ... I knew if I went to the hospital, I would have my previous birth history hung over my head and would not have this birth seen as an individual thing ... It was going to be ... 'Ok if the baby's breech again, you're going to have to have an epidural.' Well, have to have an epidural? Well, why? You know, who says?" Another woman said: "I know that if I had been in hospital that they would have performed a C-section. For sure. At home you keep your own confidence and are driven by nature and not by technology."

Some women felt that conventional care was impersonal and often accompanied by unnecessary interventions. One woman described her previous hospital birth as "traumatic" and felt she was treated like "an idiot" with staff rebuffing some of her requests with "Don't you want a healthy baby, a safe baby?" Another woman recalled the "nightmares" of a previous experience when her baby was discovered in labour to be breech, and her labour turned into a "circus" with "multitudes of viewers." Two women felt a lack of sensitivity and caring by hospital staff during previous miscarriages.

Most women (92 per cent) felt that their expectations of their midwifery experience were met and sometimes exceeded. Less than a fifth of women felt that their expectations had not been met. Unmet expectations were frequently related to the difficulties women had accessing midwifery services fully. Some women were disappointed that their midwives were not allowed to provide care or "catch the baby" in the hospital. A few women expected midwifery to be supported within the medical system or expected the midwife to have either more midwifery knowledge or more medical knowledge. Six women were not sure what to expect with midwifery care.

There were a few incidents based on unsatisfactory events. Concerns pertained to individual circumstances: some women wanted better communication; more postpartum care; more breastfeeding support. One woman said that she would use drugs if she had to do it again; another regretted going to hospital after a long labour; another felt that her tear was not well sutured; and another found the secondary midwife not very supportive of her husband. One respondent regretted relying so heavily on her midwife's judgment; another questioned whether she should have had more high-risk care because her premature labour in hospital resulted in a child with cerebral palsy; another said that although she was supportive of midwifery care in general, she wouldn't choose midwifery again in Nova Scotia until there was "some regulation to ensure a standard of care." One woman whose two-day-old baby died after a hospital birth said that, although she and her partner received the best prenatal care, in retrospect they questioned their choice to have midwifery care for the labour and birth because of their infant's death. Regrets and misgivings, however, were the exception.

CHALLENGES

Overall, 69 per cent of women faced challenges in receiving midwifery care. Accessibility was a big issue, both financially and logistically (see also Van Wagner, this volume). The financial burden of accessing non-funded midwifery care prevented midwifery services from being a viable option for all women in Nova Scotia (see also James and Bourgeault, this volume). It is not surprising that financial concerns were mentioned by nearly all the women who had challenges receiving midwifery care, given the fact that 36 per cent of them had annual household incomes of less than $20,000. Some women expressed regret that they could not pay their midwives more. It is interesting to note that half the respondents also received alternative therapies from other health providers, particularly chiropractic and massage therapy. Apparently these women place a high priority on their maternal health concerns, and that includes alternate health services that they likely also paid for out-of-pocket.

Accessibility was hampered by the small number of practising midwives in the province and the distance between midwife and client. Nearly three-quarters of women were forty-six minutes or more travelling distance away from their midwife. This presumably contributed to the fact that, overall, eight planned home births were not attended by their midwives.

Another challenge encountered by many women was the lack of emotional support and the sense of ostracism or "feeling apart" they experienced. Because midwifery care and home births in Nova Scotia were considered non-conventional, women often had to justify their decisions and defend their choices to families, friends, and health practitioners. As one interviewee recalled: "... a lot of our friends, we scared them at first ... They'd say ... 'You're crazy to have a home birth'". Women discovered that their choice of birth place was often detrimental to their relationship with their physicians. One woman, planning a home birth, had to change doctors four times until she found one who would agree to provide care for her. An interviewee said:

... at one point I just said "Let's just stop this. We're not going to talk about it anymore. We're not going to talk about where I'm giving birth – we're just going to have a prenatal visit." I did even say to my doctor at one point, "You know if I walked in here and you said: 'Okay, ... you're pregnant,' and I said: 'Well, I don't wish to continue this pregnancy,' that would have been my choice, and you would have, as a doctor you know, supported me in that whether you agreed or disagreed." And I said: "Why should I not have the choice of where I give birth?"

PERCEIVED OUTCOMES FROM MIDWIFERY CARE

Over three-quarters of the women believed that midwifery care changed them or their family in some way. Empowerment was a particularly important theme. Women felt empowered when they gained knowledge about birth and maternity options and a sense of mastery over themselves and their decisions. Many believed that they and their partners learned more about parenting. One respondent stated: "It [midwifery care] has empowered us to think carefully about, and question, all aspects of raising children. It has helped to make me the kind of mother I want to be ... It has nurtured and encouraged my taking responsibility for my own health and my family's health." Another respondent said: "Perhaps most significantly, it [midwifery care] was very important in helping us enter parenthood and birthing with confidence. I believe that initial experience helps us even now to trust our instincts and make informed decisions."

In turn, many women wanted to empower others: they felt other women should have the right to know about midwifery care and home births and make informed decisions. Another interviewee said: "I think a lot more women will make that choice [midwifery] too once they are confident in themselves and aware of the facts ... I think more people have to know more about it ..." Another respondent said: "... experiencing the beauty of our daughter's birth gave us both an enormous amount of self confidence as new parents. It deepened our spirituality and increased the strength of our convictions whether accepted or not in the mainstream."

Women learned to listen to their bodies and believe in their own strengths and potentials. Midwifery care increased their awareness of the naturalness of pregnancy, birthing, and mothering. One respondent said: "I was just going along for the ride. It was an expression of complete trust in my body's capacity to give birth." This confidence eased fears, and helped some see the value of self-responsibility for their and their family's health and well-being. They gained a sense of control and saw themselves affirmed as competent individuals making important, informed decisions. Some women questioned the medicalization of maternity care, and many found conventional medical care inadequate compared to midwifery.

The special, trusted relationship between the woman and her midwife was repeatedly mentioned. Most women felt supported and that their individuality was respected. As two respondents stated: "We will always have a strong tie with our midwives who gave us love and guidance ... Personally I felt that never before – from any other caregiver – have I ever received such tender and loving care"; "Midwifery care allowed us a special opportunity to experience pregnancy and birth with rapture." A number of women mentioned that they were saddened when the midwife's visits stopped at the end of the postpartum care. Indeed, it was not uncommon for some former clients to bring their children to midwifery gatherings in future years. Other women described their midwives as friends.

Some women believed their birthing experiences would eventually empower their children. Others gained insight into the potential of a healthy community through the midwifery process. One woman's description echoed that of others: "We have three daughters who will grow up aware of choices in health care that they will have control over. Midwifery care's emphasis on natural remedies and healthy living has permeated our entire family's outlook on healthcare – the result: an extremely healthy family." Another respondent said: "We feel even more strongly that a good midwifery system would reduce a great deal of birth trauma, ensure mothers and babies got off to a good breastfeeding relationship (more than a few weeks or months), have partners more deeply involved with their children and put a confident power back into taking responsibility for the health and well-being of the family."

Some women felt they were unchanged by the experience of midwifery care but acknowledged its influence. One respondent explained: "I think the 'change' begins before choosing the actual midwife. I realized that my body was made to birth a child ... midwives helped us accomplish that within our medically oriented society, in a way to honour an organic process, emotionally and physically. It hasn't changed us, it has enhanced our lives, our ability to express our humanness."

For almost everyone, midwifery care and the intimate occasion of birth brought forth positive memories, although one woman stated that midwifery care had a negative impact on her. Her first experience with midwifery resulted in a Caesarean birth and the death of her baby two days later. Her following pregnancies and births were attended by obstetricians, and she had no further midwifery care.

PERCEIVED OUTCOMES FROM BIRTHING AT HOME

With respect to their views of birthing at home, 75 per cent of women who gave birth at home felt that the birth at home had changed them in some tangible or intangible way. A home birth was seen as a "wonderful way to welcome [a] baby into a loving environment." Birthing at home was an empowering experience for many women and their families, even when the birth had taken place years earlier. As one respondent said: "It [the birth at home] brought us closer together emotionally and spiritually. It was an incredibly enriching, empowering event in our lives."

Birthing at home was frequently described as spiritual and linked with nature: "We all are changed as a result of this sacred experience. It reinforced our belief in the Universe ... it allowed me to come in contact with my spiritual self fully for the first time. Although the other two births were also spiritual, constant interruption broke that sense of wholeness." Some women also felt that their midwives connected with the spiritual aspect of birth: "It's wonderful that a midwife would come to your home and be involved with the whole family ... they see birth as such a spiritual experience too, not just some sort of mechanical thing that's happening to your body ... they seem to have a lot of faith in that event that you know for the most part, things will progress along ..." Another respondent said: "I think [her daughter's] birth at home was a spiritual experience that I find hard to put into words. There is something special about the care ... a calmness/quietness that I remember settling into the house when [the midwife] arrived ..."

Some women felt that birthing naturally gave them inner strength and mental stamina for future trying times:

When a woman is able to persevere through the hardest part of her labour and do it on her own, it does give her strength in the rest of her life ... even in my dealings with my children, it makes me understand patience and the different parts of life ... it seems to branch out into so many different areas of my life ... if a birth experience is taken from a woman – taken over – that can be really disappointing, and it can really affect how she interacts, you know, in everyday living.

Another said: "Having a home birth made me understand and work with, rather than against, the incredible forces within my body. I hope my own daughters will choose midwives to assist and guide them in their childbirth experiences. I feel honoured and proud to have known what having a baby is really about."

Other women felt their home births strengthened their convictions of self-responsibility in making major decisions in life. One interviewee said that the careful, considered decision-making process she and her husband worked through choosing home birth provided an educational opportunity for their older daughters:

... with my daughters, I think it's been wonderful for them that we can talk about these things and they see that you have to do what's right for your own family, and that doesn't matter whether that's the norm, or whether that's going with the crowd or whatever. And that's one thing that I think that children that are home ... come away with. It's not like you make a point of doing things different but it's just when that feels right for your family that you can make a choice like that – once you have the facts.

Some women discovered the value of balance: "Our family has learned about nurturing and finding a balance between letting nature take its course and the prudent use of medical intervention through our home birth experience."

Women felt that family bonds – immediate and extended – were strengthened at home. An interviewee explained:

I would have liked to have had all my babies at home ... it was really wonderful to be home. I think it was wonderful, not just for me, I think it was wonderful for the whole family that the baby arrived at home. I remember my oldest daughter saying "It just seems so different, it's just like [the baby] was always here" because of course, [the baby] was always here ... that was special for her ... my husband grew up here at the farm and all his aunts, like they're elderly. So after the baby was born, they could come down and see the new little baby, so that was wonderful for them as well.

The majority of all questionnaire respondents (96 per cent) saw advantages in giving birth at home. Home was seen as a comfortable, relaxed, calm, and safe place, where women could be in their own familiar spaces and crawl into their own beds when they wanted, with their partners and children. They had choice over birth companions and visitors, more control over events, no disruption by hospital routines, or need to travel during labour. The continuity of being in a familiar place with a known caregiver helped to sustain a focused state of mind: women could "own the process" of labour and birth. As one respondent said: "I had a wonderful primitive feeling to prowl around until I found just the right spot."

Others felt there was less risk of infection with their own germs at home and that recovery after the birth was easier, in part because of the availability of better food.

There were a few instances where women were not pleased with their home birth experiences. Two women recalled difficult births at home. This strengthened one woman's views about hospital birth. Another said that she wouldn't want the trauma of a difficult birth – "screaming all over the neighbourhood" – associated with her bedroom or home. However, one respondent stated that her difficult home birth might not have been better in hospital: "It was a very difficult labour – 14 hours – and had I been at hospital it could have been shortened perhaps with drugs but it most likely would have been equally traumatic, and more disempowering."

DISCUSSION

"Once you've had the Cadillac of care ... why would you do anything else
if you have the option?"

The characteristics of women choosing midwifery care in Nova Scotia are, in many instances, consistent with findings from earlier national and international studies (Kleiverda et al. 1990; Bastian 1993; Cunningham 1993; Ackermann-Liebrich et al. 1996; Waldenström and Nilsson 1993; Declerq, Paine, and Winter 1995; Chamberlain et al. 1991; Frank 1995). Women speak of being empowered to make appropriate choices for themselves and their families, respected in their decision-making processes, and inspired by the personal growth midwifery care creates. Damsma (1994) also reported the sense of self-confidence that women attributed to experiences with midwifery care. Almost all of the women in this study believed one's birth experience affects self-esteem and confidence. The significance of the birthing event and the importance of positive birth memories are documented in Simkin's landmark study of long-term memories associated with women's first childbirths (1992).

This study suggests that the relationship between a midwife and client is highly valued by the select group of women choosing midwifery care. They value the continuity of care and caregiver. They often experience a sense of loss at the end of their official maternity care; some women wished to be remembered by their midwives years after their birthing experiences. The study also demonstrates that midwifery care has provided many women with positive birth experiences and enhanced the well-being of many families even in its unregulated state. Women chose midwifery care because their legitimate needs and concerns were not adequately addressed by the predominant system of maternity care. Despite their seemingly small numbers, by challenging the status quo, these women have sustained the midwifery movement in Nova Scotia. They have advocated greater accessibility of midwifery care through its legalization.

Midwifery supports women's abilities to give birth through cost-effective, evidence-based birth practices. There are few other instances in health care settings where a group of people feels so strongly about a form of "care." It is this group's fervent belief that the eventual regulation of midwifery services in Nova Scotia will accommodate more women's needs equitably. Hopefully, there will soon be the political will in the province to implement the recommendations of the Working Group on Midwifery Regulation to ensure greater public access to midwifery care in Nova Scotia.

NOTES

1 One woman was having her first experience with midwifery care in Nova Scotia and had not given birth at the time of the survey.
2 The Nova Scotia Atlee Perinatal Database collects and tabulates various quantitative data about reproductive care in Nova Scotia for the provincial Department of Health.

REFERENCES

Ackermann-Liebrich, Ursula, Thomas Voegeli, Kathrin Günter-Witt, Isabelle Kuntz, Maja Züllig, Christian Schindler, and Margrit Maurer. 1996. Home versus Hospital Deliveries: Follow up Study of Matched Pairs for Procedures and Outcome. *British Medical Journal* 313: 1313–18.

Bastian, Hilda. 1993. Personal Beliefs and Alternate Childbirth Choices: A Survey of 552 Women who Planned to Give Birth at Home. *Birth* 20, no. 4: 186–92.

Billard, B.A. 2003. Personal communications, 2 September.

Chamberlain, Marie, Bobbi Soderstrom, Christabel Kaitell, and Paula J. Stewart. 1991. Consumer Interest in Alternatives to Physician-centred Hospital Births in Ottawa. *Midwifery* 7: 74–81.

Cunningham, John D. 1993. Experiences of Australian Mothers who Gave Birth at Home, at a Birth Centre, or in Hospital Wards. *Social Sciences and Medicine* 36, no. 4: 475–83.

Damsma, Annita Joy. 1994. The Experience of Choosing a Midwife. Unpublished master's thesis. University of Alberta.

Declerq, Eugene R., Lisa L. Paine, and Michael R. Winter. 1995. Home Birth in the United States, 1989-1992. A Longitudinal Descriptive Report of National Birth Certificate Data. *Journal of Nurse-Midwifery* 40, no. 6: 474–82.

Frank, Lesley Anne. 1995. Beyond Biology: Pregnancy and Childbirth as a Lived Experience of Management. Unpublished master's thesis. Acadia University, Wolfville, Nova Scotia.

Hackett, Lise L. 1998. *Midwifery in Canada, 1980 – 1997: A Brief History and Selected Annotated Bibliography of Publications in English*. Halifax: School of Library and Information Services.

Halifax Regional Municipality (HRM). 1997. *District 11 News*. Summer.

Kleiverda, Gunilla, A.M. Steen, Ingerlise Andersen, P.E. Treffers, and W. Everaerd. 1990. Place of Delivery in The Netherlands: Maternal Motives and Background Variables Related to Preferences for Home or Hospital Confinement. *European Journal of Obstetrics & Gynecology and Reproductive Biology* 36: 1–9.

Kuusisto, Kathy Moggridge. 1980. Midwives, Medical Men and Obstetrical Care in Nineteenth-century Nova Scotia. Unpublished master's thesis. University of Essex, UK.

MacLellan, Charlene. 1997. Midwifery in Atlantic Canada. In *The New Midwifery: Reflections on Renaissance and Regulation,* edited by Farah Shroff, 331–342. Toronto: The Women's Press.

Maritime Museum of the Atlantic. 1999. Ongoing display. Halifax, Nova Scotia.

Mason, Jutta. 1988. Midwifery in Canada. In *The Midwife Challenge*, edited by Sheila Kitzinger, 99-129. London: Pandora.

Nova Scotia Atlee Perinatal Database. 1997. Halifax.

Reproductive Care Program of Nova Scotia. 1997. *The Potential for Midwifery in Nova Scotia*. A review by the Reproductive Care Program of Nova Scotia on behalf of the Nova Scotia Department of Health. Principal author: Sue Daniels, MN. Halifax: Author.

Simkin, Penny. 1992. Just Another Day in a Woman's Life? *Birth* 2: 64–81.

StataCorp. 1995. *Stata Statistical Software*. College Station: Stata Corporation.

Towler, David S. 1999. *Nova Scotia*. Halifax: Excel Publishing.

Waldenström, Ulla, and Carl-Axel Nilsson. 1993. Characteristics of Women Choosing Birth Centre Care. *Acta Obstet Gynecol Scand* 72: 181–8.

Wheeler, Linda. 1999. Personal communication, 2 July.

Access to Midwifery: Reflections on the Ontario Equity Committee Experience

Anne Rochon Ford and Vicki Van Wagner

INTRODUCTION

Access to health care services is viewed as a universal right in Canada. However, it appears that some groups have better access than others. Over the past two decades, many members of marginalized communities have taken issue with federal and provincial governments and with specific health services about inequality of access to basic services and about unfair treatment within those services.

In the late 1980s and early 1990s, we were fortunate to be part of a process where we were able to hear first hand what lack of access looks like for a number of population groups in the Canadian province of Ontario. When work toward officially regulating the profession of midwifery began, an interim body responsible for crafting legislation (the Interim Regulatory Council on Midwifery, or IRCM) was established. With one exception – Jesse Russell, a Métis woman from northern Ontario – the council was composed of white women (and one man) in our thirties and forties, all able-bodied and university-educated. With a few exceptions we came from urban centres and English was our mother tongue. In a nutshell, we were not particularly representative of the full face of Ontario.

Jesse Russell found this environment uncomfortable and asked us how we were ever going to address the needs of all the women of Ontario who were not represented at the table: Aboriginal women with a long tradition of midwifery rapidly being eroded, women with disabilities who may not think midwifery services are appropriate for them, women of colour who have experienced systemic racism within the health system, refugee women with no health insurance coverage and living in fear and hyper-vigilance, francophone women who cannot find French-speaking caregivers for childbirth, lesbian women who feel left out of the mainstream heterosexual world of childbirth services, and others whose specific needs are not usually considered in the development of a new health service in this country.

As a result of this discussion, an Equity Committee was formed at one of the IRCM's first meetings. Jesse Russell agreed to sit on the committee, along with Pat Legault, a nurse educator from southwestern Ontario, Anne Rochon Ford, a writer and midwifery client from Toronto, and Vicki Van Wagner, a practising midwife also from Toronto. As members of this committee, we were given the task of speaking with a wide range of groups in the province about ways to ensure that their needs were taken into account in the creation of legislation and regulations and in the education of future midwives.

Between 1989 and 1992 members of the IRCM Equity Committee travelled to many parts of the province in an attempt to gather information about barriers to health care and the needs of groups traditionally not heard in the process of creating change in health care. We met with Aboriginal, Mennonite, immigrant, and refugee women, francophones, lesbians, teen mothers, incarcerated women, women with disabilities, and women in northern communities.

In presenting the following highlights from our consultations with these different communities, we hasten to point out that the list of those we consulted was not exhaustive. In particular, we did not speak with homeless women or low-income women except as represented in the other groups consulted, nor did we speak with women with developmental disabilities. We were uncomfortable with the notion of a "shopping list" of groups who needed to be consulted, as such lists are necessarily incomplete and can reinforce assumptions about uniformity within groups. In hindsight, we realize our work may have been richer had there been more of a focus on the commonalities and differences between and within equity groups.

We must also acknowledge that with ten years of hindsight, we may now view some of the issues differently. Along with many others in the women's movement, we have been influenced by the explosion of academic work on the intersection of race, class, gender, and sexuality that has occurred over the last decade. Other examinations of equity issues in midwifery since that time have influenced the lens through which we now view the work of the Equity Committee (see Nestel, this volume; Shroff 1997). We are currently writing at a very different moment in history than the time of the Equity Committee in the late 1980s. At the time the Equity

Committee was functioning, we were buoyed by what we perceived to be an opportunity to do things differently. We hoped to learn from some of the problems other professions were struggling with. Our work was done in a spirit of optimism that came in part from the climate of relative political and financial support for equity issues and also from the successes of the midwifery movement in gaining public and political support. The currently prevailing climate of conservatism and fiscal restraint has threatened many gains relating to equity and women's health issues across Canada.

Reviewing our past work for this chapter has given us an opportunity to reflect from a different time and perspective. In this chapter we review the work of the Equity Committee and examine how this work influenced legislation and midwifery practice in Ontario. We also explore how equity concerns have influenced midwifery across Canada. The chapter ends with our reflections on what some of the ongoing challenges are for the profession.

ABORIGINAL COMMUNITIES

"I was born in the bush and that made me strong."

A significant percentage of Equity Committee work was devoted to speaking with Aboriginal communities around the province. In total we visited ten Aboriginal communities, mostly on reserves, some urban. Aboriginal women in northern Ontario, as in other parts of northern Canada, were giving birth in conditions unheard of in the rest of the country. A federal government policy initiated in the early 1970s mandated evacuation of all pregnant women from remote communities so that they could give birth in a hospital. Aboriginal communities in the north spoke to us of how evacuation was linked with problems such as substance abuse, sexual abuse, and family violence. Historically, the period of the late 1980s and early 1990s was a critical turning point with respect to the transfer of Aboriginal health from the federal government back to Aboriginal communities, a time when key decisions about self-governance were being made in Ontario and elsewhere. The revision of the health professions legislation raised questions about how it would affect Aboriginal healers and midwives.

Although there were marked distinctions between the north and the south and on-and off-reserve, a common experience of most who spoke to us was that of overt racism and anti-Native discrimination. Experiences of those who had delivered their babies in the north were frequently characterized by well-intentioned but often harmful attitudes by health care providers who felt they knew what was best for them. This usually involved strong discouragement, if not prohibition, of Aboriginal customs relating to traditional foods and childbirth practices.

Women from remote communities in northern Ontario are flown out to Sioux Lookout or to Moose Factory, or, if they are classified as high risk, to more southern tertiary care centres. Under the policy of evacuation, women are away from their community and families for several weeks and sometimes months. We heard stories about how women would not reveal accurate information to determine due dates or deliberately "miss the plane" to avoid evacuation.

People we met with spoke of the tremendous rupture the evacuation policy has caused in many First Nations families and communities. Traditionally birth was an important part of the life of the community. Babies were delivered "in the bush" by traditional midwives or fathers. When nursing stations were set up on reserves in the 1960s they were staffed by midwives hired by the federal government to provide perinatal care. The removal of childbirth from the community in the 1970s was seen by those we interviewed as undermining both women's self-esteem and relationships between men and women. Aboriginal women told us of the loss of common knowledge about pregnancy and childbirth that would traditionally be shared among women. Also lost is the transferring of birthing skills from one Aboriginal midwife to the next.

Although the picture in the southern part of the province did not include the problem of evacuation, the experience of overt anti-Native discrimination still coloured the stories of many with whom we spoke. We heard about the revival of interest in traditional midwifery on a few southern reserves.

In all of the Aboriginal communities we visited, there was strong support for midwifery services, a desire to preserve Aboriginal traditions in midwifery, as well as a desire to have services that combine access to and knowledge of "white" medicine with respect for Aboriginal traditions. This, in fact, reflected a strong concurrence with the model Ontario was adopting – one that considered paramount the principles of continuity of care and choice of birth place (see, for example, Carroll and Benoit, this volume).

IMMIGRANT AND REFUGEE WOMEN

"Because we do not speak English, we are forced to be silent – to accept the rules; to accept the methods doctors use during birth; to be without power. Because of the language barrier, we can't say no or ask questions. Because of the environment, we are afraid to challenge what the doctors are saying and doing to us. We become the objects of medical intervention."

We met with immigrant and refugee women, and those who work in health and social services designed for them, in three Ontario metropolitan centres – Toronto, Ottawa, and Kingston. Opinions on midwifery and childbirth were as varied as their countries of origin. Some women we met with expressed the opinion that it was important to adapt to Canadian customs of birth while others felt there needed to be more openness amongst Canadian health care providers to cultural differences.

When the immigrant women were also women of colour, they felt this had a distinct impact on their experiences in Canada. Other factors that influenced a woman's experience of the health care system included whether she had her immigration papers and was covered by health insurance, whether English was her first language, whether she came from a country where female circumcision was practised, and the status of women in her country of origin. Those we interviewed strongly suggested including anti-racist education and education about culturally appropriate care in the training of midwives.

The particular history of midwifery in a woman's country of origin often had an impact on how she viewed the impending regulation of midwifery. The more midwifery was integrated into her country's health care system (e.g. in the West Indies), the more likely a woman was to feel positive about midwifery. By contrast, women from countries where midwifery was seen as second-class care or where custom was moving away from midwifery toward high interventionist birth practices (e.g. some eastern European countries) tended to view the introduction of midwifery in Ontario as a move backward.

Again, as with the Aboriginal communities visited, there was considerable congruity with the Ontario model of midwifery care. However, we were told over and over again that language was the most important issue for many of them and that many would choose a caregiver who spoke their language over one who provides their preferred style of care.

Invariably, women who had previously practised midwifery in their home countries and could not practise legally within the health care system in Canada were eager to seek out the ear of the Equity Committee. However, the focus of our consultations was on the *users* of midwifery services and not on practitioners. We had been mandated to make recommendations regarding the needs of users of midwifery services, and the IRCM's Registration Committee was to look at issues for foreign-trained midwives. In hindsight, there may have been more wisdom in combining the work of the two committees earlier on, as the process of establishing a system for the registration of midwives with education and experience from other countries proved to be a lengthy and complex one.

WOMEN WITH DISABILITIES

"Growing up disabled, you get used to being treated like a guinea pig, particularly if your disability is rare. You become 'condition X,' someone for interns and residents to observe and to learn on, like you're not a person."

We met with two groups of women with disabilities in Toronto, who shared with each other many common negative experiences with the health care system. Some had been through pregnancy and childbirth, and all had had experiences of their disability being misunderstood and their choices about sexuality and reproduction restricted. From being paraded around in front of doctors and interns in childhood to being told they could not or should not have children, their stories were chilling reminders of the insensitivity of many toward people with disabilities. And yet for some, the treatment necessitated by their disability means that their everyday lives are intricately intertwined with the health care system and health care providers.

Since midwifery has been identified as being for "normal" pregnancy and delivery, and because women with disabilities have often absorbed the cultural belief that they are not "normal," many disabled women have automatically excluded themselves from midwifery care. This group asked us to convey to midwives that the language of birth as a "normal healthy process" needs to be used with a consciousness of the impact of those words on women with disabilities.

Women with disabilities felt they would benefit greatly from midwifery services. They stressed the need for continuity of care (as women with disabilities often have to educate each caregiver about their condition), for an advocate in childbirth who could focus on the normal aspects of their experience, and for someone to help with adapting in the postpartum period.

TEENS

"Teens in the obstetrical care system are always told, never asked. They are often treated badly as if they are being punished for being pregnant ... They are afraid of the system and the system is afraid of them."

Our meetings with teenage mothers – and with caregivers working in this field – took place in Toronto. As noted in the comment above, made by a physician working with teen mothers in Toronto, they are often seen by society as being irresponsible for having become pregnant. The teens we spoke to reported feeling like there was no place for them in the world of slightly older women's pregnancy chit-chat, in prenatal classes, and on obstetrics wards. Similarly, teen culture does not provide a lot of support for young women who are pregnant, particularly if they are trying to carry on with their schooling. They reported fear that their baby might be taken from them in hospital, or that if they didn't do things "just right" after the baby was born, they would risk losing their child. It has been demonstrated in midwifery practices that work with a large population of teen mothers that this group benefits tremendously from having a consistent relationship with a known caregiver, a non-authoritarian approach, and an emphasis on individual education and counselling (Rooks 1997, 50–7).

Teens, and those with experience in caring for teen mothers, felt pregnancy, birth, and parenting were important opportunities for the teen mother to learn and to make active choices about their lives and that the midwifery approach to informed choice and personalized care could assist teens to have positive experiences with childbirth.

LESBIANS

"It was in prenatal classes where I had my first real taste of how invisible you feel as a pregnant lesbian."

Interviews with lesbian clients of midwives in the Toronto area revealed that negative experiences with the health care system had lead many of them, when pregnant, to seek out the care of midwives. We were told that the unexamined assumption of heterosexuality that lesbians often face is even more entrenched when dealing with pregnancy and parenting, both in the population generally and among many health care providers. The assumption of heterosexuality means many lesbians live the experience of feeling "invisible" when they are pregnant. Revealing their sexual orientation and family arrangements may be even more problematic than usual during pregnancy, as discrimination against lesbians and gay men can be more acute when issues of parenting are involved.

Some of the women we interviewed spoke of non-midwifery-assisted births where they felt their partner was not welcome in the labour and delivery rooms and where their ability to parent seemed called into question because of their sexual orientation. Lesbians may also feel uncomfortable about involvement in prenatal education that is almost exclusively oriented to heterosexual couples. Some of the women in the group we interviewed appreciated the efforts of some midwives to make classes more inclusive or to offer classes for lesbian women. All felt that the midwifery model could help overcome barriers, allowing a trust to develop on both sides. Some lesbian mothers reported choosing home birth in order to avoid encountering strangers and hostility and prejudice at a vulnerable time like labour. The group emphasized the importance of education of midwives about issues of particular concern to lesbians, such as methods of conception, legal issues in relation to donors, and parenting arrangements with partners and/or other co-parents.

NORTHERN AND REMOTE COMMUNITIES

"When you're driving back into town tonight from this meeting, imagine you are in labour, that you are in the middle of a snowstorm, it's −40 degrees, and you hit a moose on the highway."

Ontario's geography is such that the northern part of the province is far less densely populated than the south, with fewer large urban centres and greater distances between those there are. Combined with a harsher climate, conditions for a pregnant and labouring woman can be quite rigorous. In conjunction with some of our trips to Aboriginal communities in the north, we met with non-Native consumers in Nipigon, Sioux Lookout, Thunder Bay, and Timmins. Childbearing women and those who worked with them described a serious problem of lack of facilities, the long distances they often must travel to get to childbirth services, and lack of control over their birth experiences. They spoke of people from the north who leave and go south to train in the health professions but rarely come back; they felt there needed to be incentives to change this – grants, special funding, more programs in northern colleges and universities, distance education programs, and other alternative teaching methods.

Because of the long distances childbearing women must travel for services, many consumers we met with were highly receptive to home births and to having midwives who were trained to handle them in isolated conditions. Receptivity to midwifery by physicians and nurses working in northern and remote areas, however, was more varied. Some viewed the introduction of midwifery positively while others (mainly physicians providing obstetric care) felt that it would take away from the already very limited number of births they must assist at to maintain their skills and hospital privileges.

MENNONITE COMMUNITIES

"Birth is very private and we keep it quiet. Talking about it would detract from its sacredness. That's just the way we are."

The Equity Committee visited the heart of Mennonite country in Ontario, where we met with community leaders, visited with the clients of a Mennonite midwife at a prenatal clinic, and visited the home of an

Old Order Mennonite family who had recently had a home birth attended by midwives. Mennonites generally have an innate respect for letting nature take its course and a disdain for things technological. Particularly in the case of Old Order Mennonites, being a very private people, the link between midwifery and the Mennonites has been a logical one. Traditionally, most babies in Mennonite families were born at home with either the help of a midwife or a doctor. When doctors stopped delivering babies at home, many pregnant mothers reluctantly followed their doctors to hospitals. The resurgence of midwifery in this area in the past twenty years and the involvement and efforts of Mennonite midwives was strongly supported by the community. Our visits also emphasized the importance of educating future midwives about the significant cultural and religious differences that can have an impact on care in childbirth with groups such as the Mennonites.

INCARCERATED WOMEN

"It's not so much what they do to your body; it's what they do to your soul, your spirit, your mind."

One of the Equity Committee's final visits was to the Prison for Women in Kingston, Ontario. Although incarcerated women do not represent a large proportion of Ontario women who may use midwifery services, the committee had heard enough accounts of women pregnant in prison to warrant this visit. We met with a group of inmates and nursing staff. Although all prenatal care is provided within the prison, when a woman is due to deliver her baby, she is taken off-site to a downtown Kingston hospital. Women are routinely brought to the hospital in shackles and handcuffs with armed guards. At the time of our meeting, women in labour were expected to keep the handcuffs on and the guards remained present, but the shackles would be removed. Women inmates at that time were also forced to give up their babies at three to five days old.

The inmates we met with were intrigued with the midwifery model, where the possibility of giving birth in the prison without having to go to the hospital in shackles, and having a caregiver she knew and could trust, seemed infinitely more humane.

FRANCOPHONES

"In the hospital that serves our community – a community with a high percentage of francophones – you have about as much chance getting a French-speaking nurse when you're in labour as you have winning the lottery."

At the time the IRCM was created, Ontario was in the process of enacting legislation – the French Language Services Act – that would ensure the provision of health and social services to francophones in their mother tongue in geographical areas that would be designated as bilingual. Although compliance with the act is voluntary, the IRCM adopted a policy in favour of compliance.

From our interviews in the cities of Ottawa and Sudbury, the main concern of francophones regarding midwifery was of the need for more francophone midwives. Many voiced the need to be able to deal with someone who speaks their mother tongue while they are pregnant and throughout the entire perinatal process. Even those who could speak English with fluency emphasized that with an experience as personal and potentially emotional as childbirth, a woman needs to be able to speak her own language. At the time of the Equity Committee visits, there were no first-language francophone midwives practising in any of the predominantly francophone areas of the province. This has since changed.

EQUITY AND THE REGULATORY PROCESS

There was ongoing discussion about the results of the Equity Committee's meetings, and our findings and recommendations were infused in a number of key regulatory documents. The regulations and standards of the College of Midwives of Ontario reflect a concern for equity in a number of ways. The College's "Philosophy of Midwifery Care," which establishes a foundation through which other standards and regulations will be interpreted, attempts to ensure that a respect for diversity is integral to a midwife's approach to care: "Midwifery care respects the diversity of women's needs and the variety of personal and cultural meanings which women, families and communities bring to the pregnancy, birth and early parenting experience."

The College's "Code of Ethics" also notes that midwives must "Provide care with respect to individuals' needs, values and dignity, and [which] does not discriminate on the basis of language, culture, age, economic status, health status, sexual orientation, marital status, gender, geographic location, institutionalization, ability, race or religion."

The attempt to address issues of equity and diversity in these documents evolved out of discussion and debate with the IRCM about diversity and difference, stimulated by the experiences and perspectives of the women and communities with whom we spoke. There were lively discussions about whether midwifery care should be described as family-centred or woman-centred and about who is excluded and included by these kinds of definitions. We discussed the kinds of assumptions that were often made about women and families within the maternity care system and the childbirth and midwifery movements. These debates challenged traditionally held ideas about women, pregnancy, birth, families, and parenting and shifted the emphasis to the exploration of, and respect for, differences in women's experiences, needs, and values.

MODEL OF PRACTICE

The Equity Committee found support from all of the groups we consulted for Ontario's proposed model of midwifery care. The committee's input to the IRCM reinforced the need for continuity of care, home and hospital births, and an approach that would support women to make choices. Aspects of the model such as having a consistent small group of caregivers and choice of birth place were identified as central to working in diverse communities and meeting the needs of women from marginalized groups. Informed choice was seen as a critical element, too often lacking in the care of women who are seen as different.

STANDARDS OF PRACTICE

In the current health care system, social, economic, and demographic issues can often be "medicalized." Women with backgrounds and situations different than white, middle-class norms are often labelled as "high risk" (Rooks 1997). The CMO's "Indications for Mandatory Discussion, Consultation and Transfer of Care" were written to avoid making a woman's social and economic status, age, and the number of babies that she has had an automatic indicator of risk. The standard requires the midwife to consider and discuss these factors with the other midwives involved in the woman's care and with the woman herself. The midwife will consult with a physician if necessary, but the standard does not assume that medical care is needed.

There was also a conscious attempt in the development of regulations to try to avoid assuming urban or southern Ontario norms as the standard for the whole province. Standards and regulations were written with the hope that they would be applicable in rural and remote areas. Two standards – "When the Client Requests Care Outside Midwifery Standards of Practice" and "Temporary Alternate Practice Arrangements" – refer explicitly to isolated or remote regions and provide specific guidance for midwives in these situations. Alternate practice arrangements, which allow midwives to work with a second birth attendant other than a midwife, were devised to assist midwifery practice to grow in areas where there may not be a second midwife or the population to support the practice of more than one midwife. These standards also allow midwives to work with a second birth attendant to address needs relating to language, ability, or culture. The guidelines to the "Designated Drugs Regulation" also make allowance for the special situations that midwives may face in working in the remote north and allow a wider scope for midwives to use drugs on the order of a physician.

EXEMPTION FOR ABORIGINAL MIDWIVES

During the development of the new health professions legislation, Aboriginal organizations proposed an exemption to the draft Regulated Health Professions Act and the Midwifery Act for Aboriginal healers and midwives. The Equity Committee had found that the Aboriginal peoples we spoke to wanted both the right to establish their own systems of midwifery and to have access to education and practice as midwives within the system established under the RHPA. The exemption, which the IRCM supported, was based on the principle of Aboriginal right to self-governance, allowing Aboriginal midwives and healers to practise and learn in ways determined by their own communities without fear of prosecution.

ENTRY TO PRACTICE

As with most professions, one of the most controversial areas of midwifery regulation is the area of entry to practice. The registration process of the CMO has been critiqued as creating barriers to midwives from other countries (Nestel, this volume). In some ways, this critique is similar to that levelled at many of the other professions and trades (Cumming et al. 1989). However, the decision to create a registration process based on a specific assessment of a candidate's individual educational background, level of experience, and competence, rather than on a general assessment of the equivalency of educational programs and registration requirements in other jurisdictions, was clearly based on concerns for equity. The CMO's Prior Learning and Experience Assessment (PLEA) allows those wanting to practice as midwives in Ontario the opportunity to prove their competence through a series of written and practical assessments.

A controversial issue related to access to practice comes out of the decision to establish midwifery education at a baccalaureate level. In order to establish equivalency with this standard, the CMO asks midwives with education from other countries or with experience gained in unregulated settings (including traditional birth attendants)[1] to fulfill requirements for a minimum number of university level courses, in addition to proving midwifery knowledge and skills. This policy was adopted, after consultation with groups representing immigrant women and immigrant professionals and health care workers, in order to avoid the creation of two different classes of midwives, i.e. those with university education and those without. The goal of the policy was to avoid, as much as possible, a hierarchy in which midwives trained in Ontario universities would be seen as better educated than midwives with credentials from other countries. How successful this policy has been and whether it creates significant barriers is an important area for research.

MIDWIFERY EDUCATION

All applicants to the Ontario Midwifery Education Programme (OMEP) are asked to address their willingness and ability to work with diverse populations both in writing and during an interview in the admissions process. OMEP curriculum also reflects a belief that understanding of diversity and of racism and other forms of discrimination are a fundamental part of learning to be a midwife. The core first-year course "Social and Cultural Dimensions of Health Care" deals both with theoretical issues of social difference and social analysis and with the practical realities of working as a midwife with a diverse population. The core readings for the applied component of the course were based on the reports of the Equity Committee.[2] The program sees its attempt to balance social sciences with biological sciences in the academic component of the program as a clear statement about the need for midwives to develop the knowledge and skills required both for work with clients from diverse backgrounds and for the development of standards and policy for the profession that are grounded in an understanding of equity issues.

As was mandated by the provincial government, the program provides access to Aboriginal, northern, and francophone women. The diversity of the student population is greater than the pre-regulation midwifery community, however aspects of the program – such as the expense of participating in clinical placements, which may require relocation; the on-call nature of midwifery; and the newness of the profession – may continue to act as barriers (see Kaufman and Soderstrom, this volume).

FUNDING OF MIDWIFERY SERVICES

The development of the funding of midwifery services was also informed by the need to support diversity. Provincial funding of midwifery services has been fundamental to attempts to increase equity in access to midwifery. Without government funding in provinces such as Alberta and Saskatchewan, midwifery is in danger of remaining available only to those who can afford it or those who are extremely committed to midwifery as an "alternative" model of care (see James and Bourgeault, this volume). Without government funding, outreach to diverse communities is hampered not only by cost but also by the perception that midwifery is not an integral part of the health care system. The Ontario funding structure has supported midwives to work in communities that may require increased time for education, outreach, and actual client care. It has also paid for the use of second attendants to allow midwifery to grow in underserved areas and to function in remote areas. Devolution to local transfer payment agencies for midwifery services has been seen by Ministry of Health officials and by midwives as an opportunity to increase outreach to underserved or marginalized communities.

SURVEY OF ONTARIO MIDWIVES

In order to reflect on our past work on the Equity Committee and improve our understanding of equity issues in current practice in Ontario we surveyed all midwifery practices in Ontario in the spring of 1999 (Ford and Van Wagner 2001). We asked midwives about their perceptions of changes in their client population and changes in the community of midwives.[3] Overall, we found a majority of practices that provided care prior to legislation (88 per cent) reported that their client populations were more diverse since regulation and funding of midwifery. New practices reported serving populations that had little or no access to midwifery care prior to regulation.

Groups that were identified by practices as being better served included low-income women (reported by 94 per cent of practices); ethnic, cultural, or religious minorities (88 per cent); immigrant women (82 per cent); and visible minority women (65 per cent). About half of the practices reported an increase in teens and refugee women. A majority of practices said there has been no change in the number of Aboriginal women, disabled women, francophone women, lesbian women, or women in prison. In the case of Aboriginal women and women in prison, a small number of practices indicated a significant increase in serving these groups of women.

Practices identified funding of care as the most critical factor in increasing diversity. Hospital privileges, outreach activities, the increased credibility of midwifery since regulation, and increased diversity of midwives within the practice were all seen as important factors. A wide variety of outreach activities were reported, such as liaising with community health centres and community groups, establishing projects such as prenatal classes targeted to a specific group, and taking services into communities such as First Nations or into prisons.

Practices that reported no change or less diversity cited lack of time for outreach in a small busy practice and the fact that the practice was often full. Overwhelming workloads resulting from the transition to regulated practice, the demands of integrating into the hospital system, and a significant increase in demand for midwifery services have meant that time to undertake outreach activities has been minimal for some. Many identify outreach as one of the priorities of the next phase of midwifery as the profession grows and can begin to reach out to new and underserved communities. Most felt that outreach should be conducted by the Ministry of Health and the Association of Ontario Midwives.

Our survey also asked midwives about their perceptions of diversity in the midwifery population. Of the group registered since regulation, over twice as many midwives identified themselves as belonging to an "equity group" as compared to those who practised prior to 1994. Fifteen per cent of the group registered since regulation identified as immigrants, 11 per cent as visible minority, and 8 per cent as belonging to an ethnic, religious, or cultural minority in contrast to 3 per cent, 1 per cent, and 4 per cent respectively of the group registered prior to regulation.

REFLECTIONS AND CHALLENGES

Looking back at the work that we began a decade ago and the developments in midwifery in Ontario and across Canada since that time, we found cause both for encouragement and for concern about equity in access to midwifery care and to the profession. After eight years of regulated and funded practice in Ontario, we have seen some particular developments that highlight the potential for outreach and for serving diverse communities. For example, there are now midwifery services provided in six northern communities that did not have them prior to legislation. Rural women in some communities currently have greater access to midwifery care than urban women, as midwives in rural practices serve a greater percentage of the population in rural areas than those in large cities. The "Prison Project," a cooperative effort developed by four Toronto practices, provides midwifery care in the West-End Detention Centre.

Although most midwifery practices indicated that the increase in diversity of clients was among low income, ethnic, and cultural minorities and immigrant women, there are several indications that services for Aboriginal women are increasing as well. A practice on Manitoulin Island reports providing care to four Aboriginal communities. A birth centre that provides midwifery care and education for traditional Aboriginal midwives, under the Aboriginal healers exemption to the Midwifery Act, has been established on the Six Nations First Nation reserve near Brantford, Ontario. One Toronto practice that includes two Aboriginal registered midwives reports an increase in Aboriginal clients.

When we spoke to midwives from across Canada about how equity concerns have influenced regulation in provinces other than Ontario, they report very different degrees of success in putting equity issues on the government's agenda regarding midwifery and in the impact legislation has had on access to midwifery (Ford and Van Wagner 2001). Despite obstacles, in all of the provinces with funded care, the representatives we spoke to believed that midwifery practice has expanded to serve a much more diverse group of women and families. All expressed concerns about the barriers that remain. Regulation is recent or still pending in other provinces and it is therefore difficult to assess its impact on access. However, provinces that have regulated midwifery (or are committed to regulation) without the support of government funding may in fact be contributing to a decrease in access to midwifery care and to the decline of the profession (see James and Bourgeault, this volume). When practice in other provinces is funded, it becomes tempting for midwives to move to a more supportive environment. In this kind of context issues about equitable access become secondary to the survival of midwifery practice.

There are other disappointments. The Equity Committee identified remote Aboriginal communities as one of the areas where midwifery could make a key contribution. Although there has been discussion and planning in several northern Ontario communities about bringing birth back home, regulated, funded midwifery has yet to make a difference here. Despite the highly successful midwifery services established in northern Quebec, where Quallanat (Inuktitut for "foreign," used for non-Inuit) midwives and Inuit midwives have worked together for over ten years to integrate modern and traditional approaches to care, and the more recently opened service in Rankin Inlet in Nunavut, no such services have been developed in other provinces or territories as midwifery has become established.

Activists in the disabled women's community had hoped that midwifery would be more widely available to disabled women after regulation and funding was in place (Israel 1997). Without greater dialogue with women with disabilities many may be discouraged from seeking midwifery care due to the implications of the language used to describe the midwifery scope of practice as "normal" pregnancy and birth.

In terms of access to the profession of midwifery, it is worth noting that some of the controversy about midwifery registration has roots in previous debates that are also taking place in other countries. Some of the most heated issues pre-legislation were about (1) whether nursing should be a prerequisite to midwifery education and registration; (2) the integration of lay midwives and home birth practitioners into the health care system; and (3) the model of midwifery care that included choice of birth place and continuity of care and practice organized in autonomous groups with hospital privileges. The decision to establish midwifery separately from nursing, to include midwives who had practised outside the system pre-regulation, and to establish a community as opposed to a salaried-based model of care was met with both support and resistance from within the nursing and medical professions and from midwives who had trained in other countries.

The requirement that midwives work in all settings, including the home, and the demand for midwives to provide continuity of care created different responsibilities and working conditions than those expected by some midwives trained in other countries and by some nurses who hoped to become midwives. Some indicated that they were unhappy with the fact that midwifery would not be established in a nursing model, with practice in hospital only and organized in a shift work system as employees of the institution. Some did not see midwifery and nursing as separate professions and hoped that currently held nursing jobs could be rolled over into midwifery positions as hospital employees. These debates can be seen in the context of an international movement in similar directions that has also generated controversy among practioners in other countries.

Has midwifery begun to fulfill the promise the Equity Committee hoped for? Sheryl Nestel worries that the committee's report may have had a "vaccination effect," making the ongoing task of working to eliminate structures of racism and other discrimination seem somehow finished. As she points out, "eradicating structural racism is a full time job – it can't be done with documents and intentions." This is a worry that we share. It is a relatively easy task to write reports and to develop equity policies. It is a much more complex and challenging task to implement these policies. This is the step that Canadian midwives are currently undertaking.

Nestel also comments that the Equity Committee's reports set up the "problem" of diverse groups with midwifery posed as the "fix." This kind of approach is consistent with the role that midwifery has played in North America. The profession evolved outside the health care system as an approach to childbirth care that would not only act to "save" women from overly medicalized and technologic care but empower women in the process. This history is linked with an activist women's health movement that saw a similar role for access to safe contraception and abortion. This is very different than the British and European context, in which midwifery is seen as part of a system that itself needs to be fixed in order to meet women's needs. Although we would not want the growing profession to lose touch with its activist history and its potential to empower women, Nestel's caution about seeing midwifery as a kind of "cure" is important to reflect upon, particularly in the communities where midwifery increasingly serves more diverse populations. The roots of the midwifery movement in North America has also been in "alternative lifestyle" ideology that can be exclusionary and offensive to many outside of a small counter-culture. An equity focus on "women-centred" care pushes midwives and advocates for midwifery to be cautious about making assumptions about who that woman is and what she needs.

Midwifery in Canada is not alone in its need to learn about recognizing and respecting social difference or in its need to struggle with the structures of oppression that we all participate in. As diversity increases, the midwifery community faces challenges similar to others within the women's movement, and those working on diversity education of many kinds. As is well documented in the literature about feminism and other social justice movements, even the most well-intentioned and careful social movement will inevitably reproduce and even invent structures of oppression that must be examined and critiqued. Alternative movements such as midwifery, with strong commitments to and rhetoric about empowerment, can have particular problems examining the ways in which their actions have been problematic and even counterproductive. At the same time, an over-emphasis on critique and on getting everything just right before acting is not only impossible but can be counterproductive as well. In our discussions with midwives across the country, both those from diversity groups and those from more mainstream backgrounds worried about making mistakes, about causing offence, about the complexity of the issues, and about inevitable critique. These fears can lead to hesitation to get involved and to inaction.

The midwifery community in Canada could be seen to have set some lofty and perhaps unreachable goals. In moving from setting our goals and philosophies on paper to grappling with the realities of providing care and regulating a profession, we are concerned that midwives and their supporters may decide to shy away from confronting and "muddling through" the messy problems and challenges of diversity. We would encourage midwives and their supporters to see these challenges as an opportunity to participate in the attempts, critiques, and reassessments involved in learning to respect and work with social difference.

NOTES

1 This provision also allows a traditional Aboriginal midwife from Ontario to apply for registration with the CMO if she wishes.

2 See *An Equity Reader for Midwifery Students*, written by Anne Rochon Ford and edited by Farah Shroff (Toronto: Ryerson Polytechnic University, 1993). The course is highlighted in "All the Petals of the Flower: Celebrating the Diversity of Ontario's Birthing Women within the First Year Midwifery Curriculum" (in Shroff 1997), which also relies heavily on the Equity Committee reports.

3 It is important to note that responses to our survey were not based on actual demographic data, as practices reported that they do not have a comprehensive system for collecting data about the diversity of client population. The response rate was 56 per cent, representing 64 per cent of the midwives who practised and 71 per cent of practices that existed prior to legislation.

REFERENCES

Cumming, Peter A., Lee, Enid L. D. Lee, Dimitrios G. Oreopoulos. *Access! Task Force on Access to Professions and Trades in Ontario*. Ontario Ministry of Citizenship, Toronto, 1989.

Ford, Anne Rochon and Vicki Van Wagner. 2001. Access to Midwifery: Midwives' Perceptions of Change Post-Legislation. *Association of Ontario Midwives Journal* 7, no. 2 (Summer).

Israel, Pat. 1997. Experiences of Mothers with Disabilities and Implication for the Practice of Midwifery. In *The New Midwifery: Reflections on Renaissance and Regulation*, edited by Farah Shroff. Toronto: The Women's Press.

Rooks, Judith Pence. 1997. *Midwifery and Childbirth in America*. Philadelphia: Temple Hill University Press.

Shroff, Farah, ed. 1997. *The New Midwifery: Reflections on Renaissance and Regulation*. Toronto: The Women's Press.

13

Aboriginal Midwifery in Canada: Merging Traditional Practices and Modern Science

Dena Carroll and Cecilia Benoit

INTRODUCTION

In this chapter we present an alternative narrative of Canadian midwifery, with a particular focus on how government legislation is being applied to help revitalize Aboriginal midwifery practices in Canada. For many centuries, Aboriginal women have faced social and cultural changes that have negatively impacted their health, cultural identity, social structures, and traditional values. Several studies have examined the damaging effects of government policies, including the denigration of early healing practices and the removal of pregnant women from their communities and evacuation to southern hospitals (O'Neil and Kaufert 1990; Linehan 1992; Kaufert and O'Neil 1993; Lowell 1995). More recently, government policy makers have come full circle, recognizing the vital role that Aboriginal midwives have historically held in their communities across Canada and formally acknowledging the positive influence these traditional practitioners once had on the health outcomes of Aboriginal birthing women and their infants (Ford and Van Wagner, this volume).

While colonialism and modern medical care significantly altered many (though not all: see Chrystos 1988) early midwifery practices and maternity care services for Aboriginal[1] women, recent developments indicate that women are once again taking fiscal and political control of these services. We argue that the recognition and revitalization of Aboriginal midwifery in pockets across the country have provided Aboriginal women with greater choice and control over the design and quality of maternity care and health services at the community level. The re-emergence of traditional midwifery practices has also resulted in a deeper understanding of the relationship between medical science, ancient healing practices, and gender. Although legislation relating to Aboriginal midwifery still varies across the country, Aboriginal women are working diligently in some communities to ensure that traditional practices are merged with existing midwifery practices in order to create an alternative model of midwifery care that meets their unique needs.

OVERVIEW ON THE RE-EMERGENCE OF ABORIGINAL MIDWIFERY

Reputable studies in other parts of the world have long shown that traditional midwifery practices are instrumental to the health and well-being of birthing women and their newborns (Jordan 1992; Hird and Burtch 1997). Yet until recently, early Aboriginal midwifery practices were virtually undocumented in North America. This is despite a range of studies chronicling the pivotal role midwives play in caring for non-Aboriginal women and their newborns (Donnison 1977; Rothman 1982; Sullivan and Weitz 1988; Kitzinger 1988; Oakley and Houd 1990; Benoit 1991; Burtch 1994; Davis-Floyd 1992). While the Royal Commission on Aboriginal Peoples made reference in 1993 to the fact that midwives and herbalists within different societies were informally recognized within their local communities (O'Neil 1993, 38) as the regrettable decline of many earlier forms of Aboriginal midwifery progressed, little concrete research on the topic of Aboriginal midwifery was reported (Royal Commission 1993, 27). Complicating the matter further, Aboriginal women themselves have been reluctant to enter into public debate about mainstream midwifery and often had to lobby hard to ensure special recognition or exemption from current legislation as a means of preserving the traditional knowledge base.

Much of today's Canadian research on midwifery tends to ignore cultural and language differences and instead focuses attention on issues related to reduction in the use of sophisticated technology, medical intervention, and pharmaceuticals during childbirth; increased consumer choice of practitioners and place of birth; quality birth experiences for clients; and legitimizing childbirth as a natural event in women's lives (Bourgeault 1996; Benoit 2000; Smulders and Limburg 1988; DeVries 1996; DeVries et al. 2001; Rothman 2001).

Yet despite passage of innovative midwifery legislation over the last decade, beginning in the province of Ontario and subsequently spreading to British Columbia, Alberta, Quebec, Manitoba, and Saskatchewan, the dominant Canadian model of midwifery endorsed is still to a large extent ill-suited for counterparts in Aboriginal communities in remote or rural areas or for Aboriginal women living in inner cities of Canada (Benoit et al., 2003).

The purpose of this chapter is to attempt to unravel the threads of this largely untold history of early forms of Aboriginal midwifery, highlighting those obstacles that have impeded Aboriginal women's participation in the emerging Canadian models of midwifery care as either consumers of midwifery care or midwifery practitioners in their own right. It also provides an overview of key success stories and lessons learned from Aboriginal communities attempting to rejuvenate their traditional birthing practices.

DATA SOURCES

Primary data for this chapter were gathered during two focus groups sponsored by the B.C. Ministry of Health with Aboriginal elders and community health representatives in Kamloops and Vancouver in 1993. One of the authors, Dena Carroll, was extensively involved in the ministry's consultation and development of Aboriginal midwifery legislation in B.C.[2] The first focus group addressed issues relating to past and contemporary childbirth experiences of Aboriginal families in the province, cultural practices surrounding reproduction, education, and training of Aboriginal healers in general and midwives in particular, and alternative ways of regulating health professionals. The second focus group sought direction from the participants concerning the proposed provincial legislation to legalize midwifery in B.C.[3]

In addition to our focus group data, secondary data was gathered from consultations with Aboriginal and non-Aboriginal midwives across the country about current developments in Aboriginal midwifery in their respective provinces and territories.

A NARRATIVE ON EARLY ABORIGINAL MIDWIFERY

Aboriginal midwives traditionally played a fundamental role in the childbirth process and were largely responsible for passing down the moral and ethical values systems from one generation to the next. According to the participants from our focus groups, Aboriginal peoples of Canada from the earliest times viewed childbirth as integral to other natural and creative life processes. Like death, birth was seen as part of a cycle of life that existed within the sacred realm, governed by a ubiquitous spirituality that originated with the Creator. The arrival of a new baby reminded everyone of the delicate balance that existed between the spiritual and physical worlds.

There is limited research documenting the historical and cultural perspectives of Aboriginal midwifery, and most of these have been focused on the Canadian north (O'Neil and Kaufert 1990). In fact consultations with Aboriginal groups across Canada reveal that the term "midwife" was problematic for many different linguistic groups. Often tribal organizations used different words to describe this traditional role. Along the Northwest Coast in B.C., "midwife" was not a recognizable term among the different linguistic groups. Instead, like other parts of Canada, the linguistic translations focus on the role and responsibility. The Nuu-chah-nulth people, located on the west coast of British Columbia, translate the term into "she can do everything," the Coast Salish describe the role as "to watch/to care," the Chilcotin people define it as "women's helper," and today many people identify women elders as "keepers of the culture," due to their rich personal experience related to childbirth and other aspects of female life (Jeffries 1992, 91). This diversity and heterogeneity among the various societies is similar to the variation that existed within medicine societies of the Kwakwaka'waka and Anishina'beg and the family-based *angatquq* of the Inuit (O'Neil 1993, 38).

In all cases, the role of women's helper/midwife was assumed to be the Creator's work and viewed as a calling to a particular profession. However, midwifery practices were not limited to women; both men and women were found to be capable of providing childbirth care. Generally, the midwife was usually, but not always, the primary attendant during pregnancy and childbirth and this role was highly esteemed. Indeed, many midwives held positions of authority, decision-making, and prestige in their families, within tribal governments, and in the spiritual realm.

Focus group participants also related that Aboriginal midwives were expected to undertake a long apprenticeship with a female elder relative prior to being acknowledged by the community as a competent caregiver: youths usually started at an early age to gradually acquire the local knowledge and technical skills needed from seasoned senior midwives. Children were instructed at very young ages to respect what were commonly known as "laws of nature," including understanding the mysteries of conception and birth. The midwife apprentice was likewise tutored about human anatomy and physiology, how to prepare and administer herbal medicines and, depending on tradition and circumstance, how to perform other midwifery functions ranging from dietician and teacher to birth attendant. It was also common custom for young girls to attend the births of other women belonging to their lifeworld in order to build a solid basis of "local knowledge" (Geertz

1983) about pregnancy and childbirth, in preparation for their own personal experience of the life event.

Elders participating in our focus groups recalled that some midwives faced difficult experiences and had to be trained in recognizing the "birth energy" – the special communication between the labouring woman and her baby about to be born in order to avoid trauma. Knowing when to use natural medicines and herbs was critical for avoiding potential complications. Experienced practitioners had to be adept at dealing with protracted labour, malpositioned foetuses, and expulsion of the placenta. Infrequent haemorrhage necessitated spiritual intervention by a shaman or medicine person (who could be male or female). Not all outcomes were successful and there were times when the mother died from loss of blood or an infant suffocated in the birth canal. The arrival of a stillborn baby caused much grief, an anguish that was not limited to the family but shared generally by the entire community. Yet, despite the limited capacity of traditional Aboriginal midwives to solve obstetrical emergencies, recent evidence suggests that rates of mortality and morbidity for mothers and infants (including perinatal rates) in early Aboriginal societies were probably lower than after colonial impact (Dobyns 1983).

According to the focus group participants, Aboriginal midwives followed a continuous and holistic approach to childbirth and gave considerable time and attention to each client throughout pregnancy, birth, and the postpartum period. Their role was to counsel and instruct women on how to care for themselves while pregnant and as new mothers. Oral accounts suggest that Aboriginal midwives were often very strict with expecting mothers, as obstetrical complications were believed to be the result of failure to correctly observe such rituals. Maintaining a healthy and vigorous lifestyle, together with careful attention to diet during pregnancy, was important. In many cases, pregnant women were instructed to avoid certain foods and to remove themselves from certain social networks to avoid endangering their baby.

The act of helping another woman in childbirth required no sanction from any outside medical, legal, or political authority but instead was seen as the Creator's work. The midwife was considered the local "expert" in lifeworld knowledge about the woman's readiness to give birth. Aboriginal women were permitted – indeed expected – to show courage and to take individual responsibility for their own birthing process and a restrictive supine position was not recommended. Recovery from childbirth was usually a four-week "lying-in period" in which the midwife had considerable involvement with the newborn's family circle. In fact, the attendance of a community midwife at birth usually signified the establishment of a special, often lifelong relationship. Successful helpers/midwives also carried out significant community obligations, including leading special prayers and religious ceremonies related to childbirth. There was strong cultural symbolism and special meaning generally associated with the afterbirth and placenta. Even body parts were associated with precise beliefs and accompanying normative codes of behaviour, usually taught to the birthing woman by the attending helper/midwife or maternal or paternal grandmother. According to one elder,

The afterbirth was commonly placed in a clean, white cloth and tied in a tree in order for it to dry naturally. Such a practice symbolized keeping the stomach clean. This is why it was not burned. A boy's cord was cut and dried and put under deer or moose tracks. If [the cord] was a girl's, it was put under a berry tree. Sometimes cords were clamped on newborns' backs so that others would never lose sight of them. Still other families kept the dried cord in a drawer in a white cloth, or hid it under the house so that the infant when it got older would never run away (quoted in Benoit and Carroll 1995).

Other related cultural practices included refraining from intervening in the natural process of growth by not cutting the baby's hair.

In brief, focus group participants held strongly to the belief that traditional childbirth was viewed as an extended family/community process rather than a "medical event" or "woman's experience." Helping other women during parturition was a source of pride for female (and sometimes male) midwives, a public sign of virtue or doing good work. Available reproductive knowledge was disseminated throughout the community, usually passing from one generation to the next through oral traditions. This is unlike the present situation, where physicians claim monopoly over obstetric knowledge or, in parallel fashion, feminists claim control over female ways of knowing. Rather, participation in cultural activities surrounding pregnancy and childbirth in pre-contact Aboriginal communities took place within a closely knit nexus linking the midwife to the birthing woman, to the infant, and to the husband/partner, to the family, to the extended kin group, and to the community. According to Fiske, among pre-contact Carrier peoples of B.C.: "Reproductive roles were central to women's claims to social prominence. Carrier women who successfully raised their families and provided care and nurture to the needy became influential as family spokespersons. The wisdom of old women was and remains proclaimed in legend and song and institutionalized in the valued role of the grandmothers of the tribe" (1992, 201).

HISTORICAL DEMISE OF EARLY MIDWIFERY FORMS

The imposition of colonialism in the Aboriginal communities of B.C. and other parts of Canada resulted in significant social, economic, political, and cultural change. Among other things, the language, culture, and traditional ways/healing practices of Aboriginal peoples were called into question by the colonizers (Dickason 1992). Aboriginal peoples became increasingly dependent upon "white man's medicine," yet traders lacked the medical skills or knowledge to provide effective treatment for most who sought help (Waldrum, Herring, and Young 1994). In addition, adulterated whisky introduced by the colonial elite negatively impacted female-male relationships and altered the social, moral, and economic order of society (Shkilnyk 1985). Finally, a series of "virgin soil epidemic" diseases – including smallpox, measles, and influenza – spread like wildfire through Aboriginal populations that were without a history of exposure to these contagious diseases. This was later compounded by paternalistic government policy, all of which contributed to the weakening of Aboriginal peoples' health and well-being, not least of all that of Aboriginal women and their children. Several studies have documented how the 1867 British North America Act, in defining the legal status of registered Indians (Ponting 1998; Waldram, Herring, and Young 1995), resulted in loss of control over their organization of governance and health and social structures. Many Aboriginal healers found themselves threatened, punished, and ignored by both missionaries and non-Aboriginal government officials (Wells 1994). In relation to health matters, a government-appointed "Indian Agent," who was often without formal medical training, assumed authority over local healers. The latter had to consult the agent before admitting patients to hospital, medical emergencies excepted (Dickason 1992).

   The impact of residential school, combined with other colonial processes, furthered the negative impact on Aboriginal communities by denying access to many traditional knowledge systems, original languages, and traditional cultural practices. Between 1892 and 1957, the Roman Catholic Church set up a number of boarding and industrial schools in B.C. In 1920, governments had mandated that every Native child between the ages of seven and fifteen years attend an Indian Residential School, where widespread physical, sexual, and mental abuse often occurred. In addition, strict gendered sexual norms and religious indoctrination had a profound impact on the health and well-being of Aboriginal people. As Fiske points out, "Catholicism challenged [the Carrier peoples'] indigenous concepts of the supernatural and female fecundity. Women's curing practices, perceptions of menstrual powers, and birth rituals were scorned by the priests" (1992, 205).

Aboriginal youth "successfully" graduating from the residential school program often faced a different set of concerns. Their newly acquired foreign academic knowledge had impacted their ability to forge intimate relationships with Aboriginal people from their home communities, including their elders. As Theresa Jeffries of the Sechelt peoples explains, "The threads that bind us to our past – our language, laws, culture, and traditions – have over time become tenuous. This is the result of government intervention and the breakdown of the family unit through residential schools" (1992, 92).

The gender inequality underpinning the colonial takeover of Canada's Aboriginal peoples up until 1985 also challenged the survival of Aboriginal midwifery and seriously threatened access to local community resources. Prior to 1985, under the patriarchal provisions of the 1874 Indian Act, a status Indian woman who married a non-Aboriginal man automatically lost her official designation as status Indian, including band membership, as did her children. Consequently, these women no longer had access to the resources of their community but were required to move off-reserve and adopt Western ways. By contrast, status Indian men who married non-Aboriginal women not only retained their Indian status but were also able to gain status for their wives. It was not until 1985, in fact, that the federal government passed Bill C-31 to revise the Indian Act to allow Indian women their official access to Indian status, irrespective of marital status. This history of discrimination by race and gender continues to negatively affect Aboriginal women across Canada, placing them in an uncertain position on reserves (lands "reserved" by treaty for status Indians), as well as in urban areas of the country, where most of them live today. A Stoney Creek Band elder sums up the combined impact of these outside forces on their once intact culture: "Between 1920 and 1993 we have seen a big change in our population. Years ago there were no drugs and we used herbs. The traditional art of midwifery was learned from mother and grandmother. Today, modern medicine and doctors have taken over. In our way of life we depended on traditional medicine, and we helped ourselves."

Traditional midwifery in B.C. was officially banned (though it was not necessarily informally eliminated; see Chrystos 1988) in 1949, when the medical establishment finally succeeded in having legislation passed that classified midwifery practice as a medical act. Aboriginal midwives, along with midwives serving other communities, were henceforth liable to prosecution for "practising medicine without a license." Long before this date, however, government medical personnel had labelled Aboriginal midwives as charlatans and dismissed their original birthing practices as outdated and harmful. By the 1970s, virtually all "planned" births took place in hospitals located in the larger southern towns and cities of the province, although some reports indicate that a few midwives continued to provide assistance, especially in more rural and remote communities.

REVIVAL OF ABORIGINAL MIDWIFERY

It was not until the late 1980s that Aboriginal women began asserting their right to regain control over childbirth and health care within their own communities. A number of factors contributed to the change: revisions to the Indian Act, movement towards self-government and devolution of federal health programs, establishment of Aboriginal women's organizations and community activism. The end result over the past two decades has been the gradual transfer of control and decision-making back to Aboriginal communities. In an attempt to improve the health status, economic conditions, and education of Aboriginal people, governments have also provided resources to support community-based, Aboriginal-controlled, and culturally appropriate services. More recently, there has been recognition that health professionals such as Aboriginal midwives and traditional healers are also critical to the revitalization of Aboriginal societies.

For Aboriginal women, the revitalization of midwifery and the "recapturing" of birth and pregnancy has an added dimension related directly to regaining control after colonization and subsequent imposition of European culture. The struggle of Aboriginal women to gain back a *helper* role in the reproductive process is part of a wider community and political struggle against external oppression, including the imposition of Western, science-based medicine and political status. Survival and revival rest in the recognition that Aboriginal people (including women) must have control over their lives and their social, economic, and political futures. In health matters, this means supporting Aboriginal people in taking responsibility for decision-making on the design, delivery, and management and allocation of funds for health services in their communities. Due to the high birth rates in most Aboriginal communities, this also means having "choice" and access to appropriate maternity care services. Yet, it should not be thought that the revival of Aboriginal midwifery or other cultural practices is viewed as an alternative to mainstream childbirth practices; instead there is recognition that the two can complement and indeed cultivate each other. An examination of some of the emerging forms of Aboriginal midwifery indicates that this interface process is now on its way, and that community priorities are beginning to be addressed.

Consequently, the struggle to rejuvenate Aboriginal midwifery is less about midwives' desire for occupational autonomy and professional status, themes central to the groups trying to professionalize in mainstream society (Abbott 1988), and more about a different worldview based on long-standing cultural beliefs that embrace the physical, emotional, and spiritual factors of a woman's life and are not restricted just to the birthing process. The revitalization of community healers, including midwives, is about returning to Aboriginal women (and sometimes men) their position of honour as someone uniquely "called" to this line of work, and this revitalization therefore relies heavily on community and elder support. It is about ensuring that midwives have a legitimate place of respect in Aboriginal communities, and that they are allowed to view themselves as legitimate professionals within their communities, and that they are allowed to pass down their sacred practices or have access to resources. It is also about assurance that they give birth in their traditional lands, and that their language continues to play a critical role in this transmission of culture and in future education. In addition, midwives want their work to be viewed as integral to a much broader vision related to restoring and rebuilding those positive traditions that grant Aboriginal women and men, albeit in different ways, active roles in reproducing and socialising the next generation (Castellano 1982).

REGIONAL ABORIGINAL MIDWIFERY INITIATIVES IN CANADA

The following examples, drawn from different parts of the country, highlight current community-based midwifery services and strategies aimed at revitalizing Aboriginal midwifery. While in no sense a complete picture, we present the reader with a snapshot of what we consider to be impressive accomplishments, given the formidable challenges.

Quebec

The Inuulitsivik Health Centre   Quebec and the Northwest Territories have been the most successful in integrating the new Canadian model of midwifery, due to the implementation of pilot projects. The Quebec initiative also illustrates how midwifery training can be provided at the local level. Located in Puvirnituk in northern Quebec, the Inuulitsivik Health Centre is one of the oldest and most renowned Aboriginal midwifery initiatives in Canada.[4] The centre is an Inuit midwifery-based project that has been involved in training Inuit midwives and providing care to birthing women in the surrounding districts since 1982. The training program for Inuit "trainees" evolves with the progression of skills and knowledge, and trainees must pass a clinical assessment and written examination. Since 1990, the Inuulitsivik Health Centre has been considered a pilot project (designed to study the feasibility of midwifery as a legitimate profession) by the Quebec government (see Vadeboncoeur, this volume). Inuit women at the centre are allowed to give birth as they choose, and can communicate in Inuktitut with their birth attendant. The Inuit of Puvirnituk pride themselves on preserving the Inuit culture while also providing emergency medical backup. In 1999, the provincial government legalized midwifery as an autonomous profession and established a university training program. According to Inuit women, designated pilot projects can create obstacles for Aboriginal midwives since they delay decision-making and prevent formal recognition of traditional birthing practices.

While a breakthrough for non-Aboriginal midwives, the post-legislation situation for Aboriginal midwives in the province is far from secure (George 1999). The new Quebec Midwifery Law contains two clauses that are relevant to Aboriginal midwives. One clause recognizes the five midwives working at the Inuulitsivik Maternity in Puvirnituk. These midwives have been awarded membership to the Quebec Order of Midwives, but their licenses to practice remain restricted to the Nunavik territories. The other clause states that band/community councils are able to negotiate with the provincial Ministry of Health specific arrangements for the practice of "traditional midwives." According to Quebec midwife Jennifer Stonier:

The spirit of the law as it was intended and the current interpretation of that law by the Ministry are not the same. The intent was that communities could choose how to define and educate their midwives. However, the Ministry says the law refers only to *traditional midwives* (whatever that means) and provides the grand opportunity for the continuation of their practice provided the Ministry agrees. [Yet] these midwives cannot call themselves midwives, cannot be members of the Order of Midwives, and cannot practice in any public institution. (Stonier 2001)

The main problem is that the new Quebec law recognizes only one academic program – the one recently established at University of Québec at Trois-Rivières. Despite the fact that the birth statistics from Inuulitsivik are among the best anywhere in Quebec, including those of non-Aboriginal midwives working in southern regions of the province, no Aboriginal midwife currently in training at Inuulitsivik is able to apply for a midwifery license. In fact, she is considered to be working illegally under the strict order of the law.

On a more positive note, it has recently been announced by the federal government that the Nunavut region has the right to negotiate its own midwifery law under self-government. The existing provincial legislation is again being examined. Recent reports indicate that the government of Nunavut is starting to become involved in coordinating midwifery information and may be planning a major initiative on the midwifery issue. The major concerns under discussion are how to protect the apprenticeship model of care and ensure access to culturally relevant programs. The Inuulitsivik community and Inuulitsivik midwives have joined with the Nunavik Regional Health Board to form the Nunavik Midwifery Working Group. The group's mandate is to explore how the current provincial law might be reinterpreted or amended to finally give due recognition to the apprenticeship model of educating midwives in northern areas of the province.

The Iewirokwas Midwifery Program Located in Akwesasne, a Mohawk reserve that straddles Quebec, Ontario, and New York State, the Iewirokwas Midwifery Program is currently being set up to educate and train Aboriginal midwives, free of constraints imposed by both Quebec and Ontario provincial laws (the latter has an exemption clause for Aboriginal midwives: see Ford and Van Wagner, this volume). The General Assembly of First Nations of Quebec and Labrador have unanimously supported the initiative. The program, intended to help Aboriginal midwives to best "serve their community," is partially funded by Running Strong for American Indian Youth, a U.S. Indian-rights group that supports community initiatives. The new program aims to empower Mohawk women during pregnancy and childbirth and to build on the existing knowledge base about Aboriginal midwifery and indigenous healing (Cornacchia 1999; http://www.nativemidwifery.com/). Iewirokwas is also playing a lead role in the campaign to obtain an exemption for Aboriginal midwives in the Quebec Midwifery Law.

Ontario

Ontario undertook extensive consultations with Aboriginal midwives and Aboriginal women's groups, and in 1991 under the Midwifery Act, Aboriginal midwives in Ontario were exempted from provincial legislation.[5] The Aboriginal exemption in the Regulated Health Professions Act 1991, section 35, states that the act does not apply to Aboriginal healers or midwives providing services "to Aboriginal persons or members of an Aboriginal community." This wording has been interpreted by legal experts in Ontario to have a broader scope than "on reserve" to the extent that it covers Aboriginal persons outside of Aboriginal communities and non-Aboriginal persons inside an Aboriginal community. This exemption has provided the opportunity to rejuvenate traditional healing and midwifery practices and enables Aboriginal women to "assume their right to give birth in traditional areas without having to travel to other larger centres for care" (Aboriginal Healing 2001). Many of the Aboriginal midwives in Ontario work in conjunction with the Nurse Practitioner Association of Ontario. Since 1994, various provincial ministries in Ontario have resourced and supported the Aboriginal Healing and Wellness Strategy, which has enabled the Six Nations reserve in Ontario to gain funding to establish the Six Nations Maternal and Child Centre, or Tsi Non:we Ionnakeratstha ("the place they will be born") Ona:grahsta' (Cayuga word for "a Birthing Place"), which incorporates traditional midwifery practices. The centre, established in 1996, is located at the Six Nations of the Grand River Reserve (Brantford) and services southern Ontario. It is partly funded by the Ontario Ministry of Health and offers training for Aboriginal midwives and choice of home or centre birth to Aboriginal women. In this way, the centre is a part of the return to the pre-1924 days, when women stayed home to have their children (Gamble 2000).

Aboriginal midwives are not required to be part of either the Ontario College of Midwives or the Ontario Midwives' Association, but this may change in the future. The centre currently has two full-fledged community midwives on staff and two Aboriginal midwife apprentices. These trained community midwives graduated from the Maternidad La Luz in El Paso, Texas, and are well known on the reserve. They are involved in the care of women during all stages of their pregnancy and birth and also teach local women about sexuality and safe sex during the all-season ceremonies.

According to supervisor midwife Ruby Miller, the Aboriginal midwifery program plays a key role in community revitalization, helping to rediscover traditions and return responsibility for health care maintenance back to the local women and their families and community. Aboriginal men are also increasingly involved in the birthing process, thereby enhancing family cohesion and partnership. The focus has shifted to wellness, celebration, community revival, and bringing back traditions and teachings. While there are only a few practising traditional midwives at the centre, a concerted effort is underway to engage elders as speakers in midwifery workshops and community ceremonies. The Six Nations Aboriginal midwives would also like to expand their outreach on the reserve, as well as educate other Aboriginal communities on how to get similar initiatives underway (Wilson 2001).

A recent conference on Aboriginal midwifery, the National Aboriginal Midwifery Gathering, held in December 2002 at the Six Nations in Brantford, supported by the Society of Obstetricians and Gynecologists of Canada and the National Aboriginal Health Organization (NAHO) provided an excellent opportunity to bring Aboriginal midwives together for the first time. It focused on professional development, traditional healing practices, emergency skills offered by obstetricians, licensing, and group strategizing. This gathering was the first step toward a national organization of Aboriginal midwives and provided a venue to share practices and address emerging concerns. It also gave a rare opportunity for collaborating on a national agenda for Aboriginal midwifery and helped ensure linkage to the larger issues of Aboriginal health, maternal health, and the Aboriginal children's agenda.

British Columbia

British Columbia has taken a somewhat different path than Ontario, Quebec, and the northern regions of the country, by seeking to work *within* the current legislative framework and establishing a Committee on Aboriginal Midwifery under the umbrella of the provincial College of Midwives (Rice 1997). This committee is responsible for identifying the requirements needed for traditional Aboriginal midwives to qualify to practise, including the use of cultural and spiritual values. The committee is currently working on defining terms to "grandmother" existing traditional midwives within the legislation. At the time of writing, the College of Midwives representatives indicated that they were not aware of any Aboriginal midwives practising in B.C. Aboriginal communities (Richardson 2003). However, it is not uncommon to hear different elders or community members speak of the key role of specific women who helped deliver babies within their communities.

The Arctic

Another well-known community-based birthing centre arrangement is available to Aboriginal women residing in the central Arctic region of Rankin Inlet, Nunavut – the Rankin Inlet Birth Centre. Beginning in 1993, a pilot birthing project located in the Keewatin Regional Health Centre was developed for low risk pregnancies in collaboration with the Manitoba Department of Health, the government of the Northwest Territories, and the Keewatin Regional Health Board. Prior to this, women from the central Arctic were flown out of their communities to southern hospitals to give birth (Halifax 2000).

In 1995, the centre went from being a pilot project to a full program with a staff comprised of a small number of certified midwives, Inuit maternity care workers, and a clerk interpreter. Between seventy and eighty Aboriginal birthing women are currently cared for each year

(Canton 2000). The centre aims to have its Inuit maternity care workers progress to the point where they can take their exams to become certified midwives, although none had attained certification at the time of writing (Greer 2000). Maternity workers speak to birthing women in their own native tongue, a major step forward for central Arctic women, who have for decades received their maternity care from English-speaking attendants. While the Rankin Inlet Birth Centre is currently functioning outside provincial legislation, its long-term survival appears promising. The centre also reaches out to women in the outskirts of Rankin proper. Birthing women from out of town keep in touch via conference calls and use the centre when they are ready to give birth. There have even been some preliminary discussions about establishing another birthing centre in Pond Inlet. The opportunity to access culturally appropriate maternity services at the local level is a significant step forward for Inuit women of the central Arctic, who were just a short while ago actively discouraged from giving birth in their own communities and threatened with legal action if they used local midwives. Yet the struggle for autonomy for Inuit midwives is in no way over, and they have reason to be concerned as acceptance and regulation is moving at a slow pace. As of yet, Nunavut midwives are not funded or legalized, although Nunavut is developing a report on midwifery (Midwives Association of NWT and Nunavut).[6]

Northwest Territories

Despite strong demand from Aboriginal women and public support for community-based birthing, midwifery in the NWT remains unregulated and lacks public funding. In the NWT, the Department of Health is taking the lead to introduce a legislative framework. Aboriginal women living in this region are still required to fly out of their communities to give birth. Recent reports indicate that two community midwives provide midwifery in Fort Smith and are working on a proposal to develop a free-standing birthing centre. Their goal is to increase public awareness and education relating to traditional midwifery and traditional birthing practices.[7]

Manitoba

In Manitoba, midwifery has been funded by Manitoba Health and regulated by the College of Midwives since 2000. The focus of midwifery in Manitoba is an employer model – midwives must either work for the Health Authority or become an independent. Being an independent is not viewed as an attractive business opportunity due to the high costs

of insurance and College membership. The current midwifery legislation refers to a six-member Aboriginal committee, Kagike Daniko-
bidan, which advises the College on issues relating to Aboriginal
midwifery. The committee consists of representatives from the north,
Island Lake, and central and south areas of the province. Recent reports
indicate there are approximately four practising First Nation midwives
in Manitoba (some midwives have been trained in Ontario or are Métis), and two of these women currently sit on the committee. The committee has been struggling due to a lack of provincial funding and the
high cost of bringing northern members to meetings (most of the members are northern reps except for one). The lack of Aboriginal midwife
representation on regulatory bodies within the College has negatively
impacted its ability to engage the important people in the Aboriginal
community at critical decision-making points. In addition, there are
presently no formal midwifery education programs in Manitoba, although plans are underway at the time of writing to create an educational program to train local midwives. On the positive side, the
government of Manitoba in 2000 passed legislation that grants midwives the option of attaining accreditation through multiple routes, including apprenticeship (see Kaufert and Robinson, this volume). The
committee has determined that education at the community level is the
most important consideration and has recently approached the Chiefs
of Manitoba, who passed a resolution supporting Aboriginal midwifery. The committee has requested funding from a number of sources
to help support further meetings and a community-based mentorship
training for First Nations in the north. It is also trying to secure funding
from the Provincial Health Care Transfer Fund for a four-year project
(not pilot). Due to few options available in the north, most Aboriginal
birthing women in rural and remote communities of Manitoba are still
required to evacuate to larger cities such as Winnipeg and Thompson.
The chair of the committee, Sheila Sanderson, states there are still a
number of barriers for First Nations communities, especially those in
the north, not least of all remoteness and harsh weather conditions.

In June 2002, the Manitoba Committee of Aboriginal Midwives attended the third Society of Gynecologists World Conference in Winnipeg. Also, in the northern regions, doula training has been available for
a short period but ongoing funding has been an issue. (Lepine 2002).

Other areas of Canada

The situation of Aboriginal midwifery in the other Canadian provinces is
in flux. The fact that, to date, two provinces – Alberta and Saskatchewan

– have chosen to legalize but not publicly fund midwifery services is worrisome. The authors were unable to find any information on developments in Aboriginal midwifery in these two provinces. Nor is recent information available on initiatives targeted to Aboriginal midwives in Nova Scotia, New Brunswick, Newfoundland and Labrador, or PEI.

CONCLUSION

As evidenced above, the ability to merge traditional Aboriginal ways of knowing and modern science can be directly attributed to community-based involvement, but the challenging task is still how to overcome the results of many years of acculturation and assimilation, which caused a significant decline in traditional knowledge, values, and belief systems. One of the struggles facing community-based Aboriginal midwives is how to standardize the ways of providing midwifery services to meet community needs while at the same time allowing full autonomy and control. Equally challenging are the educational requirements for mainstream midwifery training, which is based on a bio-medical model and often limited to those with an college or university background. Recent information indicates that only a small number of Aboriginal students have entered formal midwifery training programs and still fewer have successfully graduated. According to the Equy Wuk Women's Group and the Nishawbe-Aski Nation, Aboriginal women want to be "involved in the process of accreditation, education and training of First Nations midwives in the remote north." Additional concerns have been raised about the degree of public education required to overcome Aboriginal peoples' dependency on Western medicine and consumer culture, how to rekindle the benefits of community-based approaches that include traditional and modern science, the amount of resourcing required to build a viable infrastructure, and the need for viable research to look at what the community needs to help build this capacity. As Marlene Castellano states:

Substantive Indian participation in all phases will require a radical revision of the structural relationships, which have prevailed in a colonial environment. Both Indians and government personnel will need to engage in a re-education process to facilitate the absorption of new knowledge about the other's ways, attitudinal change and the development of organizational structures to translate the promise of consultation into the reality of social change. (1982, 127)

Equally challenging are the entrenched views of the medical profession and professional colleges on standards, competencies, and barriers to professional education for Aboriginal people. The struggle remains of how to increase awareness among the medical profession and at the same time increase levels of funding to support alternate models of midwifery care.

This chapter has shown that significant strides have been made in the last decade in many provinces and territories in addressing the above concerns. There is also greater sensitivity on the part of mainstream society to the vital role of Aboriginal healers and cultural practices for individual, family, and community health. Yet the number of qualified midwives practising in Aboriginal communities has not been able to keep pace with the growing demand. The absence of services in rural and remote communities is critical, few Aboriginal women have seen shifts in "compulsory hospitalizations" and "evacuations" in their communities, and only in rare instances are these women guaranteed culturally relevant care in southern and urban hospitals. Also, time is of the essence: fewer elders of either gender are familiar with old healing practices and rituals and can transmit the embedded local knowledge crucial to the revival desired, and yet the Aboriginal population is younger and has a overall higher birth rate than the non-Aboriginal population.

Provincial health legislation has afforded modest opportunities for Aboriginal communities to revitalize their midwifery traditions, and limited funding has been forthcoming in most provinces, except Ontario. The continued revitalization of midwifery has been largely driven by Aboriginal women themselves, those who are willing to gain Western credentials as a means to support change and bring new opportunities for choice to women at the community level. The birthing centre at Six Nations Reserve in Ontario illustrates that Aboriginal communities can use the traditional knowledge and expertise of their mothers and grandmothers, and combine this with the educational aspects of modern medicine to play an important role in their communities.

We have learned from Aboriginal midwifery in B.C. and other areas of Canada that we cannot impose a foreign system on Aboriginal people: Aboriginal people must be included in the development, delivery, and decision making of services to ensure their needs are met. We have learned that Aboriginal people also want choice, access, community ownership, resources to ensure cultural and spiritual rebirthing, involvement of elders, the local community (both men and women), and information on self-care for women's health that is culturally appropriate and sensitive to the needs of women in rural and remote communities. For Aboriginal groups, the rejuvenation of Aboriginal midwifery is about restoring respect for the sacred gift of life, respecting women's status and honour, and recognizing Aboriginal sovereignty and treaty-based rights, which include land base, religious, food production, and reproductive and maternity care issues. It is also about ensuring that Aboriginal professionals are part of a system that allows access to preventative health care, appropriate use of technology, and ensures safe birthing practices for women. As illustrated above, there is no one size that fits all. The formal recognition and certification of traditional Aboriginal midwives and their unique styles of caring for birthing women and newborns is already showing great promise and deserves great celebration in communities, as mothers and grandmothers are restored to their rightful place as *keepers of the culture* and communities and families are once again given a central role in the birthing process.

ACKNOWLEDGMENTS

We would like to recognize those midwives and their supporters across the country who told us about their projects and the challenges they face to train and socialize traditional Aboriginal midwives. Without the strong commitment and hard work of Aboriginal midwives, community leaders, and elders, Aboriginal midwifery would not be on the rise across the country. We regret that due to space limitations, we are unable to explore these projects in greater depth and hope that this chapter will be a stepping stone to building a more comprehensive review of developments and perhaps contribute toward a common research agenda.

NOTES

1 According to the 1982 Constitution Act, Aboriginal peoples include status and non-status Indians, Métis, and Inuit.

2 Dena Carroll worked as an Aboriginal health consultant for the B.C. Ministry of Health and was actively involved in the Aboriginal midwifery focus groups discussed in this chapter. Dena is a member of the Chippewa of Nawash First Nations in Ontario.

3 Some of the information reported below appeared in an earlier article by the authors (see Benoit and Carroll 1995).

4 Puvurnituk and Puvurnituq are the more recent (or older as the case may be) names for Povungnituk. The change in names is the result of the re-Inuitization of place names in Nunavik, the Inuit region of Quebec.

5 The provincial legislation can be found on http://www.e-laws.gov.on.ca/home_E.asp?lang=en

6 Nunavut Statutes current to 1 April, 1999 are available on http://www.nunavutcourtofjustice.ca/library/consolacts.htm.

7 More information can be found on http://members.rogers.com/canadianmidwives/canada/nwt.html

REFERENCES

Abbott, Andrew. 1998. *System of Professions*. Chicago: University of Chicago Press.

Aboriginal Healing and Wellness Strategy. 2001. Joint Management Committee. February 16. http://www.ahwsontario.ca/policies/pdf/ IndigenousKnowledgePolicy.pdf

Alberta Midwifery Legislation: http://www.qp.gov.ab.ca/display_acts.cfm; http: //www.canlii.org/ab/sta/index.html; http: //www.qp.gov.ab.ca/display_regs.cfm

Barman, Jean. 1991. *West Beyond the West: A History of British Columbia*. Toronto: University of Toronto Press.

Benoit, Cecilia. 1991. *Midwives in Passage*. Memorial University, Nfdl.: Institute of Social and Economic Research.

– 2000. *Women, Work and Social Rights: Canada in Historical and Comparative Perspective*. Scarborough, Ontario: Prentice Hall Canada.

Benoit, C. and Dena Carroll. 1995. Aboriginal Midwifery in British Columbia: A Narrative Still Untold. *Western Geographic Series* 30: 221–46.

Benoit, C., D. Carroll, and Munaza Chaudhry. 2003. "In Search of a Healing Place: Aboriginal Women in Vancouver's Downtown Eastside." *Social Science and Medicine* 56: 821-33.

British Columbia Legislation: http: //www.qp.gov.bc.ca/stratreg/

British Columbia Royal Commission on Health Care and Costs. 1991. *Closer to Home: The Report of the British Columbia Royal Commission on Health Care and Costs*. Vols. 1 and 2.

British Columbia: British Columbia Royal Commission on Health Care and Costs.

B.C. Task Force. 1990. Issue 5 (December).

B.C. College of Midwives and Sub-Committee on Aboriginal Midwifery: conversation with Luba Lyons Richardson. June 2003.

Bourgeault, Ivy. 1996. Delivering Midwifery: An Examination of the Incorporation of Midwifery in Ontario. Ph.D. dissertation, Department of Behavioural Sciences, University of Toronto.

Bourgeault, I., and Mary Fynes. 1996/97. Delivering Midwifery in Ontario: How and Why Midwifery was Integrated into the Provincial Health Care System. *Health and Canadian Society/Santé et Société Canadienne* 4, no. 2: 227–62.

– 1997. The Integration of Nurse- and Lay Midwives in the U.S. and Canada. *Social Science and Medicine* 44, no. 70: 1051–63.

Burtch, Brian. 1994. *Trials of Labour: The Re-emergence of Midwifery in Canada*. Montreal and Kingston: McGill-Queen's University Press.

Canadian Association of Midwives: http: //members.rogers.com/ canadianmidwives/canada/index.html

Canton, Marie. 2000. From Beginning to Birth, Centre Holds Monthly Gatherings for Expectant Mothers. *Northern News Service*, 2 August. http://www.nnsl.com/frames/newspapers/archive00–2/aug00/aug2_00birth.html

Canadian Women's Health Network. 1999. *Good News and Bad News for Aboriginal Midwives*. Volume 2. Summer. http: //www.cwhn.ca/network-reseau/2–3/inuit.html

Castellano, Marlene. 1982. Indian Participation in Health Policy Development. *The Canadian Journal of Native Studies* 1.

Chrystos. 1988. *Not Vanishing*. Vancouver: Press Gang Publishers.

Cohen, Mark. 1989. *Health and the Rise of Civilization*. New Haven: Yale University Press.

Cornacchia, Cheryl. 1999. Rebirth of Midwifery: Mohawk Women Reclaim their Art of Birthing – Using Modern and Ancient Wisdom. *Montreal Gazette*, November.

Couchie, Carol (Manitoba midwife). 2002. E-mail conversation. October.

Davis-Floyd, Robbie. 1992. *Birth as an American Rite of Passage*. Berkeley: University of California Press.

DeVries, Ray. 1996. *Making Midwives Legal*. Columbus: Ohio State University Press.

DeVries, R., C. Benoit, Edwin Van Teijlingen, and Sirpa Wrede, eds. 2001. *Birth by Design: Pregnancy, Maternity Care, and Midwifery in North America and Europe*. London: Routledge.

Dickason, O.P. 1992. *Canada's First Nations*. Toronto: McClelland & Stewart.

Dobyns, H.F. 1983. *Their Numbers Become Thinned: Native American Population Dynamics in Eastern North America*. Knoxville: University of Tennessee Press.

Donnison, Jean. 1977. *Midwives and Medical Men*. London: Heinemann.

Fiske, Jo-Anne. 1992. Carrier Women and the Politics of Mothering. In *British Columbia Reconsidered: Essays on Women,* edited by Gillian Creese and Veronica Strong-Boag. 198–216. Vancouver: Press Gang Publishers.

Gamble, Susan. 2000. Aboriginal Midwives First to Practise at Six Nations' Birthing Centre. Six Nations News Forum, Expositor Staff, Brantford. http://network54.com/Hide/Forum/message

Geertz, Clifford. 1983. *Local Knowledge*. New York: Basic Books.

George, J. 1999. Good and Bad News for Aboriginal Midwives. *Canadian Women's Health Network* (Summer): 10–11.

Greer, Darrell. 2000. Closer to Home – Birthing Centre Expansion to Benefit Moms Across Region. *Northern News Services*, 14 April. http://www.nnsl.com/frames/newspapers/archive00–1/apr00/apr14_00mid.html.

Halifax, Terry. 2000. The Business of Labour – Health Board Wants Legislation Before Midwives and Midwife Crisis – Caregiver Seeks a Birthing Centre South of 60. *Northern News Services*, 2 October. http: //www.nnsl.com/frames/newspapers/archive00–2/oct00/oct 2_00bir2.html

Hird, Carol, and Brian Burtch. 1997. Midwives and Safe Motherhood: International Perspectives. In *The New Midwifery: Reflections on Renaissance and Regulation*, edited by Farah Shroff, 115–45. Toronto: The Women's Press.

Iewirokwas Program (Pulling the Baby Out of the East). http://www.nativemidwifery.com/Home.html.

Inuit Women's Association of Canada. 1992. *Ikjurki (The Helper)*. Ottawa: The Inuit Women's Association of Canada.

James, Susan. 1997. Regulation: Changing the Face of Midwifery? In *The New Midwifery: Reflections on Renaissance and Regulation*, edited by Farah Shroff, 181–200. Toronto: The Women's Press.

Jeffries, T. 1992. Sechelt Women and Self-Government. In *British Columbia Reconsidered: Essays on Women,* edited by G. Creese and V. Strong-Boag, 90–5. Vancouver: Press Gang Publishers.

Jordan, Bridgette. 1992. Cosmopolitical Obstetrics: Some Insights from the Training of Traditional Midwives. *Social Science and Medicine* 28, no. 9: 925–44.

Kaufert, Patricia, and John O'Neil. 1993. Analysis of a Dialogue on Risk in Childbirth: Clinicians, Epidemiologists, and Inuit Women. In *Knowledge, Power, and Practice: The Anthropology of Medicine and Everyday Life*, edited by S. Lindenbaum and M. Lock, 32-54. Berkeley: University of California Press.

Kitzinger, Sheila, ed. 1988. *The Midwife Challenge*. London: Pandora Press.

Lepine, Freda (northern Manitoba Committee rep). June 2002. Conversation with authors.

Linehan, S. 1992. Giving Birth the "White Man's Way." *Health Sharing* 13, no. 2: 11-15.

Lowell, J. 1995. Rethinking Traditions: Women Taking Charge of Culture, Medicine and Each Other. *Herizons. Women's News, Feminist Views* 9, no. 1: 25-6.

Macaulay, A., T. Delormier, E.J. Cross, et al. 1998. Participatory Research with Native Community of Kahnawake Creates Innovative Code of Research Ethics. *Canadian Journal of Public Health* 89, no. 2 (March-April): 105–8.

Manitoba Midwifery Legislation: http: //www.gov.mb.ca/chc/statpub/free/index/html

Midwives Association of the NWT and Nunavut, 2002. midwives.nwt.nu@auranet.nt.ca; http://www.lex-nt.ca/

Morewood-Northrop, M. 1997. Community Birthing Project: Northwest Territories. In *The New Midwifery: Reflections on Renaissance and Regulation*, edited by Farah Shroff, 343–56. Toronto: The Women's Press.

National Aboriginal Health Organization: http://www.naho.ca

Newfoundland and Labrador Legislation: http://www.go.nf.ca/hoa/sr

New Brunswick Legislation: http://www.gnb.ca/justiceasriste/htm

Northwest Territories Legislation: http://www.lex-nt.ca/

Nova Scotia Legislation: http://www.gov.ns.ca/legc/sol.htm; http://www.gov.ns.ca/just/regulations/regs/index.htm

Nunavut Legislation: http://www.lex-na.ca/Nunavut Statutes current to 1 April 1999; http://www.nunavutcourtofjustice.ca/library/consolacts.htm

Oakley, Ann, and Suzanne Houd. 1990. *Helpers in Childbirth: Midwifery Today*. WHO: Hemisphere Publishing.

O'Neil, John. 1993. Aboriginal Health Policy for the Next Century. In *Royal Commission on Aboriginal Peoples. National Round Table on Health and Social Issues: Discussion Papers*. Ottawa: Royal Commission on Aboriginal Peoples.

O'Neil, John and Patricia Kaufert. 1990. The Politics of Obstetric Care: The Inuit Experience. In *Births and Power: Social Change and the Politics of Reproduction*, edited by W. Penn Handwerker. Boulder, CO: Westview Press.

O'Neil, John D., and Penny Gilbert. 1990. Childbirth in the Canadian North: Epidemiological, Clinical and Cultural Perspectives. Northern Health Research Unit, University of Manitoba.

Ontario Legislation: http://www.e-laws.gov.on.ca/home_E.asp?lang=en

Palmer, Martha (Manitoba Sub Committee on Aboriginal Midwifery). 2002 E-mail conversation. October.

Pauktuutit Inuit Women's Association: E-mail with Catherine Carry, October 2002.

Pauktuutit. Suvaguuq, Special Report on Traditional Midwifery. Vol. 10, no. 1. Pauktuutit Inuit Women's Association of Canada. Ottawa, 1995.

Ponting, J.R. 1998. Racism and Stereotyping of First Nations. In *Racism and Social Inequality in Canada*, edited by V. Satzemich, 269–98. Toronto: Thompson Educational Publishing.

Quebec Legislation: http://publicatinsdququebec.gouv.qc.ca/en/loisreglements/html/tel_mots-cles.dbml; http://www.lexum.umontreal.ca/ccq/en/index.html.

Rice, A. 1997. Becoming Regulated: The Re-emergence of Midwifery in British Columbia. In *The New Midwifery: Reflections on Renaissance and Regulation*, edited by Farah Shroff, 19-80. Toronto: The Women's Press.

Richardson, Luba Lyons. 2003. June. Personal communication.

Rothman, B.K. 1982. *In Labour: Women and Power in the Birthplace*. New York: Norton & Co.

– 2001. Spoiling the Pregnancy: Prenatal Diagnosis in the Netherlands. In *Birth by Design: The Social Shaping of Maternity care in Northern Europe and North America*, edited by R. DeVries, C. Benoit, E. Van Teijlingen, and S. Wrede. London: Routledge.

Royal Commission on Aboriginal Peoples. 1993. Aboriginal Health Policy for the Next Century. In *A Pathway to Healing*, 27–45. Ottawa: Communication Group.

– 1996. *Report of the Royal Commission on Aboriginal Peoples: Perspectives and Realities*. Volume 4, Minister of Supply and Services Canada, Ottawa 1996.

Rudmin, F. 1994. Cross-cultural Psycholinguistic Field Research: Verbs of Ownership and Possession. *Journal of Cross-Cultural Psychology* 25, no.1 (March): 118–32.

Saskatchewan Legislation: http://www.ucalgary.ca/library/law/legislat.htm#sask; http://www.qp.gov.sk.ca/; http:www.qp.gov.sk.ca/publications/index.cfm? fuseaction=home&c=1755&id=2 = References to Midwifery Practice

Schell, Lawrence, and Alice Tarbell. 1998. A Partnership Study of PCBs and the Health of Mohawk Youth: Lessons from Our Past and Guidelines for Our Future. *Canadian Journal of Public Health* (March-April): 833–40.

Shkilnyk, A. 1985. *A Poison Stronger Than Love: The Destruction of an Ojibwa Community.* New Haven: Yale University Press.

Six Nations Maternal and Child Care Centre, 2001: conversations with Ruby Miller, Maternal and Child Care Centre supervisor.

Smulders, B., and A. Limburg. 1988. Obstetrics and Midwifery in the Netherlands. In *The Midwife Challenge,* edited by Sheila Kitzinger, 235–49. London: Unwin Hyman.

Stonier, Jennifer. 2001. April. Personal communication.

Stout, Dion, M. Kipling, D. Gregory, and R. Stout. May 2001. *Aboriginal Women's Health Research Synthesis Project Final Report.* Prepared for Centres of Excellence for Women's Health, Women's Health Bureau.

Sullivan, Deborah A. and Rose Weitz. 1988. *Labor Pains: Modern Midwives and Home Birth.* New Haven: Yale University Press.

Thouez, J. 1992. The State of Health of the Cree and the Inuit of Northern Quebec. *Western Geographical Series* 27: 279–96.

Waldram, J., D. Herring, and K. Young. 1995. *Aboriginal Health in Canada.* Toronto: University of Toronto Press.

Wells, R., ed. 1994. *Native American Resurgence and Renewal.* Metuchen, NJ: The Scarecrow Press.

Wilson, Julie. 2001. April. Personal communication.

Yukon Legislation: http://www.lex-yk.ca/

I4

The Boundaries of Professional Belonging: How Race has Shaped the Re-emergence of Midwifery in Ontario[1]

Sheryl Nestel

PREFACE

In the summer of 1995, the interdisciplinary childbirth educator's training program that I had taught for several years – a collaboration between a suburban college and an urban hospital – received nearly triple its usual number of applications for the coming academic year. Even more unusual was that half of the students applying were women of colour, most of them trained midwives from Asia, Africa, Latin America, or the Caribbean. Childbirth education has been an overwhelmingly white avocation in Ontario (and elsewhere in North America) and the opportunity to develop a more diverse pool of childbirth educators was decidedly welcome in a city where "visible minority" people comprise more than half of the population. In the course of that academic year, these women and I jointly occupied a classroom where we shared a commitment to improving the experience of childbearing for women and those who support them. In a program where the political agenda was very explicit, and where the power dynamics of a racially mixed classroom were acknowledged (but remained predictably unequal), we struggled to understand the ways in which gender, race, class, sexuality, ethnicity, ability, and other dimensions of identity position both childbearing women *and* those who are involved in educational and health care programs directed at them (Nestel 1998).

Midwifery had been integrated into the Ontario health care system in 1994 and many of these women of colour had entered the childbirth educators training program as preparation for beginning the complex process of becoming registered as midwives through the newly formed College of Midwives of Ontario's Prior Learning Assessment program.

In the course of my association with this group of women, I was struck by the depth of their knowledge about childbearing, their commitment to humanized maternity care practices, and their clearly feminist positions on issues related to health care. And I was subsequently dismayed to see how with only one exception, they all retreated from their dreams to practice midwifery in Ontario. Through my relationships with these students, the contradiction between the presence in the province of hundreds if not thousands of immigrant midwives of colour and their virtual absence from the ranks of registered midwives in the province became more than a puzzling anomaly. Rather, I began to understand how this exclusion, indistinguishable from the many racist practices encountered by people of colour in Canada, constituted a personal injury to women whom I had come to know – a diminishment of the expertise and professional status that they had struggled to attain. In 1995, I began a doctoral research project to attempt to uncover the exceedingly tangled convergence of global and local politics that underlay this paradox.

In 1997 I gave my first public talk about racism in midwifery. While I had been prepared for the reactions of some in the audience who demanded to know why I was endangering the gains made for women by the midwifery movement, nothing had prepared me for what I was to hear the next day. A midwifery student with whom I was friendly called to ask whether "they were burning crosses" on my lawn. Needless to say, I was astonished by her question and I demanded to know to what she might be referring. She explained that the written version of the paper I had delivered on the previous day had been circulated in Ryerson University's Midwifery Education Programme that morning and that the responses of faculty had been furiously dismissive and, indeed, virulent. My work was seen as a gratuitous threat to midwifery's hard-won position in Ontario's medical care system. The imagery of racist and anti-Jewish violence that framed the student's question jarred me, but I don't believe that she chose her words carelessly. Images of burning crosses no doubt captured for her the intensity of what she had witnessed.

That this challenge to the progressive image of the midwifery movement in Ontario would engender a violent reaction should not come as a surprise. It is my guess that such a response reflects the deep resistance that white women have to acknowledging the limits of our own innocence and to viewing charges of racism as something more than the biased or hypersensitive imaginings of people of colour and anti-racist whites (Essed 1991, 272). As modern subjects, we understand ourselves to have coherent identities often constructed on a binary scale. We are either gay or straight, law-abiding or criminal, progressive or reactionary, etc. However, postmodern theories have been exceedingly useful in helping us to understand that our social identities and practices can be both multiple and contradictory – that women, for example, can be simultaneously oppressed by gender and privileged by race, class, sexuality, religion, or any other of a number of social positionings. Indeed, as Friedman argues, "Identity depends on a point of reference: as that point moves nomadically, so do the contours of identity, particularly as they relate to the structures of power" (1998, 22). When the point of reference for midwifery identity is patriarchal medicine, then indeed the midwifery movement in Ontario becomes intelligible as a liberatory movement poised to expand women's reproductive choices. However, this is but one story about the re-emergence of midwifery. When the point of reference for midwifery identity ceases to be patriarchal medicine and migrates to immigrant midwives of colour (Rattansi 1994; Nestel 1996/97), a story of domination rather than liberation emerges. This chapter foregrounds that story in the hope that those of us working for reproductive justice and other forms of social equity can begin to construct projects that, rather than effecting change along a solitary axis, might "multiply the sources of resistance in the many relations of domination that circulate through the social field" (Sawicki 1991, 45).

THE ISSUES OF RACE IN MIDWIFERY

The meagre representation of immigrant women of colour[2] among practising midwives in Ontario, as mentioned above, constitutes a frank paradox. The identities of these women as highly trained medical workers collide problematically with prevailing constructs of "immigrant women" or "visible minority women," which hold at their centre a woman victimized by her role as an unskilled domestic or industrial labourer or a dependent housewife restrained by patriarchal "cultural" norms (Smith 1994, 14). Received notions of "immigrant women"; the devaluing of non-European experience, credentials, and training; adherence to forms of feminist organizing that privilege the political skills and interests of white women; and acts of "everyday racism" (Essed 1991) have converged to create a predominantly white midwifery profession in a geographic space whose multiracial character is one of its most frequently invoked social signifiers (Abate 1998).

While "visible minority" people account for approximately 15 per cent of Ontario's total population (Statistics Canada 1999), in Toronto, the historical centre of midwifery activism, they account for more than one-third of residents in the Census Metropolitan Area (Chard and Renaud 1999, 20). However, the numbers of midwives expressing an interest in having their credentials recognized in the province has, since 1986, outstripped their proportion in the population at large, accounting for nearly half of those who, by 1994, had sought information from the College of Midwives and its predecessors about credentials assessment (TFIMO 1987, 331; CMO 1994a). Relatively few of these women, however, have succeeded in becoming registered as midwives.

The limited entry of immigrant midwives of colour into the midwifery profession in Ontario has also been an excruciatingly slow process. Prior to the graduation in September 1996 of the first class of the baccalaureate-granting Midwifery Education Programme only one out of the seventy-two registered midwives in Ontario was a woman of colour. The graduating class boasted two First Nations midwives and two additional women of colour, bringing the percentage of First Nations women and/or women of colour in midwifery ranks to approximately five per cent. By May 1998, there were 126 registered midwives, among whom were twelve women of colour and one First Nations woman, bringing the percentage of "visible minority" midwives to 10.3 per cent. More than seven years after the enactment of legislation designating midwifery as a legal, autonomous, and regulated health profession in Canada's most multicultural/multiracial province, First Nations women and women of colour continue to account for only about ten per cent of registered midwifery practitioners; midwifery and its various support structures remain dominated by white women.

As I will argue below, the overwhelming whiteness of the midwifery profession is linked to structural inequities related to race and to the historical conditions that have produced these, as well as to the midwifery profession's many complex and troubling interactions with groups popularly understood as "racially" different. This chapter represents an attempt to address the question posed by Ruth Frankenburg in her recent exploration of the social dimensions of white racial identity: "What are the social processes through which white women are created as social actors primed to reproduce racism within the feminist movement?" (1993, 5).

All too often in both academic knowledge production as well as movements of social change, racism and racially mediated discourses and structures are those elements that remain unnamed and unproblematized (Dei 1996, 66; Higginbotham 1992, 251; Barbee 1993, 348). Scholarship produced within critical anti-racism studies – and I include the work at hand within this category – seeks to re-centre concerns with racism in an attempt to understand "structural conditions that foster social discrimination" (Dei 1996, 46). According to anti-racist scholars, whiteness as a social identity yields a place of structural advantage to those who possess it (Harris 1993). Though a thorough discussion of the theoretical literature on racism is not possible here due to space limitations (see Nestel 1996/97 for a detailed description), it is important to note that the analysis at hand relies substantially on those approaches that foreground structural processes in the exclusion from social power and access to material resources of groups deemed racially different (Goldberg 1993; Anthias and Yuval-Davis 1992). Such approaches diverge from common understandings of racism as an expression of personal prejudice, arguing that "individuals do not have to actively express or practice racism to be its beneficiaries" (Shohat and Stam 1994, 19). In the words of Ebert, as a form of critique it is "not judgement but explanation; its concern is to explain how what we know, what we see, is related to what we do not see, to the historical limits of our knowledge and subjectivities and to the concealed material relations of power that produce them" (1996, 12).

METHODS

This chapter draws on material collected for a larger research project (Nestel 2000a), including extensive open-ended interviews with forty-six women collected between December 1997 and February 1999. The interviews lasted between forty-five minutes and four hours. They were transcribed and then coded using QSR NUD*IST computer software (Qualitative Solutions and Research, Non-numerical Unstructured Data Indexing Searching and Theorizing). Among those interviewed were seventeen immigrant midwives of colour, including both participants and non-participants in the College of Midwives' Prior Learning and Experience Assessment program, eight (practising and non-practising) white midwives, eight white midwifery students, five white members of official midwifery bodies, five women of colour and First Nations women who have been members of official midwifery bodies, and three midwifery students of colour. This study also relies on an extensive review of Ontario midwifery publications, documents, and records appearing between 1981 and 1995 (see Nestel 1996/97 for a more detailed description of the data).

PERSISTENT EXCLUSIONS:
MIDWIFERY'S RELATIONSHIP TO THE "OTHER"

There is evidence that non-European women have constituted a significant percentage of potential practitioners of midwifery in the province of Ontario both in the period prior to the introduction of legislation as well as in the period during which midwifery was integrated into the health care system. In a survey conducted in 1985 through the College of Nurses of Ontario, between 6,000 and 7,200 registered nurses and registered nursing assistants reported that they had formal midwifery training (Eberts 1987, 331). Approximately 35 per cent of these women reported that they completed their midwifery education in the West Indies, India, or the Philippines. Of the 621 women who reported an interest in practising midwifery upon legalization, 40 per cent had last practised in the West Indies, India, or the Philippines, indicating that immigrant women of colour probably constituted a significant percentage of such a group (Eberts 1987, 366).

It can be argued that estimates of the number of "racial minority" women in the ranks of trained midwives and among those interested in practising the profession are complicated by post-1985 trends in immigration. While immigration to Canada from Europe accounted for 77 per cent of immigrants in 1967, in 1987 only 22 per cent of immigrants were Europeans (Cumming et al. 1989, 12). In 1987, immigration from South and Central America (including the Caribbean) quadrupled from its 1967 rates (Cumming et al. 1989, 12). Nearly 40 per cent of Chinese immigrants, who comprise 26 per cent of adults in "visible minority" groups, arrived in the years between 1982 and 1991. The figures are similar for immigrants from the Philippines although they comprise only 7 per cent of the total "visible minority" group (Statistics Canada 1999). In addition, it is important to note that one-third of all Filipinos as well as one-third of all black women work as health care professionals (Boyd 1992, 303), suggesting that recent immigrant women from developing countries may be more likely to have training as health care workers, including midwifery training.

These figures indicate that the percentage of immigrant women of colour wishing to enter the midwifery profession may indeed be larger than that suggested in the 1987 report of the Task Force on the Implementation of Midwifery in Ontario (TFIMO). In fact, by May 1994, 46 per cent of the 900 requests for information about registration received by the College of Midwives of Ontario had come from women with midwifery training from the Philippines (25.1 per cent), Jamaica (3.4 per cent), Nigeria (3.4 per cent), Pakistan (2.9 per cent), India (2.4 per cent), Hong Kong (1.9 per cent), Ghana (1.4 per cent), China (1.4 per cent), Guyana (1 per cent), and Somalia (1 per cent) (CMO 1994a, 3). While the current exclusion of immigrant midwives of colour has very specific dimensions, its origins are discernible throughout the recent history of Ontario midwifery.

Ontario midwifery has occupied a predominantly white space since its inception. The Ontario Association of Midwives was founded in 1981 and included both local empirically trained midwives and midwives of European origin who received their training in formal midwifery programs outside of Canada. These midwives conducted home births and provided non-clinical support to women who chose or were compelled because of medical reasons to give birth in hospital (see also Sharpe, this volume).

Ruth Frankenberg (1993) has proposed that social geographies of race are constructed rather than naturally occurring. Social landscapes in which whiteness is the dominant racial identity in neighbourhoods, schools, and on the terrain of social and professional interaction are frequently constructed through deliberate choice. I would argue here that just such a landscape was cultivated in the early years of the Ontario midwifery movement and ultimately produced a movement dominated by white women. However, to construe such racial boundaries as impermeable would lead to a highly flawed analysis of racial dynamics in the Ontario midwifery movement. While interactions between immigrant midwives and white midwives were not particularly numerous and took place under circumstances characterized by their complexity, data from interviews with both white midwives and immigrant midwives who worked as labour and delivery nurses indicated that such encounters did occur. Indeed, middle-class white midwives met, interacted with, and formed a multiplicity of professional and personal relations with midwives of colour within the context of the hospital setting, where pre-legislation midwives served their clientele as labour support. Consequently, it can be argued that exclusionary policies and attitudes were enacted not from a racially bounded space of ignorance but from a position of knowledge, however limited, of the skills and aspirations of the women with whom white midwives came into contact in the pre-legislation period.

EXCLUSIONARY PRACTICES AND CREATION OF MIDWIFERY POLICY

Formed in 1985 and representing a merger of the organizations and interests of foreign-trained nurse-midwives (predominantly white and British) and local empirically trained midwives, the Association of Ontario Midwives (AOM) has been instrumental in the legalization of midwifery in the province (Bourgeault 1996, 56). While outreach to "foreign-trained midwives" (the term is never defined) is a stated goal in the AOM's early publications, this goal appears to have been consistently deferred. Reports of the "outreach committee" failed to appear in issue after issue of the AOM newsletter. By 1987, the committee was described as "currently inactive" (AOM 1987b, 12). While reactivation of the committee was recommended, its priority was to be "the needs and concerns of rural midwives" (12). A subsequent newsletter announced that the reactivated outreach committee was mandated to "define and address the concerns of rural midwives and minority group midwives ... particularly the Inuit issue ... [and] it was suggested that ads be put in ethnic newspapers." (AOM 1987c, 10). While First Nations midwifery was subsequently granted exemption from the constraints contained in the legislation, there is little indication that the issues of immigrant midwives of colour received similar serious consideration by the AOM or the state-appointed midwifery bodies on which its members served prominently.

The absence of women of colour from the social geography of midwifery has meant their exclusion from all the processes, both informal and formal, that have shaped professional practice. The impact of their absence was most clearly demonstrated in the composition of committees struck in the wake of a 1986 decision by Ontario Health Minister Murray Elston to integrate midwifery into the health care system. While the 1987 report of the TFIMO suggested that a short-term project be set up to "provide a means for the best qualified midwives, maternal child nurses, and others to integrate into the regulated profession of midwifery" (Eberts 1987, 153), two bodies in which midwifery activists featured prominently as appointees made decisions that would determine that many midwives of colour were structured out of practice.

In contrast to other policy-making bodies that preceded the establishment of the College of Midwives in 1994, the Curriculum Design Committee (CDC), struck in May 1989, and the body that implemented its recommendations, the Midwifery Integration Planning Project (MIPP), initiated in October 1990, featured no representation whatsoever of immigrant midwives of colour. Lack of representative voices was a persistent feature of midwifery bodies that made pivotal decisions in the period prior to legislation about who would be able to practise the profession once legalization occurred. The CDC's two most critical policy decisions in relation to immigrant midwives of colour were (1) to disqualify those who had not practised in Ontario from entering the vanguard corps of practising midwifery (Michener Institute, n.d.) and (2) to recommend that a baccalaureate degree be the appropriate academic qualification for midwives in Ontario (CDC 1990, 14).

The CDC recommendation that midwives with Ontario practice experience be given "first priority" to enter the profession (CDC 1990, 35) stood somewhat in contradiction to the recommendation of the TFIMO that while candidates were required to be resident in Ontario in the twelve months prior to a short-term midwifery integration project, practice in the province was not a prerequisite. The CDC recommendation was later codified in the admission criteria to the pre-registration program for midwifery held at Toronto's Michener Institute in the fifteen months prior to legalization and aimed at turning out a "carefully-selected, highly-competent and 'safe' cadre of midwives to act as ambassadors of the new midwifery and promoters of a professional image" for the new profession (Bourgeault 1996, 161). The criteria determined that while the candidates' experience must have been attained in the six years prior to application, thirty out of the sixty births required had to have been attended in Ontario.

While the requirement succeeded in keeping out and raising the ire of some apprentice, newly practising, and rural midwives, midwives of colour were the least likely to have had Ontario experience and therefore, despite other qualifications, the least likely to qualify for the Michener program and for immediate access to practice. Midwives of colour, as I have argued above, were less likely to be located within the monoracial social geography of the Ontario midwifery community. As a consequence, they were also less likely to establish apprenticeships that could link them to the social networks where midwifery was in demand and where clientele were likely to pay fees that could sustain a midwife in full-time practice. Some midwives of colour did, however, deliver babies within their communities, but social realities inevitably shaped the scope of their practice. One white midwife related in an interview how she had, in the early 1990s, struck a partnership with a midwife who had emigrated from a Latin American country. The fees that they were paid by their working-class Latin American immigrant clientele were well below the going rate of $600 and therefore both continued to work part-time – a situation that prevented them from accumulating the number of births necessary to be considered for the Michener program.

Other immigrant midwives of colour, while anxious to work in their profession, feared legal prosecution and deportation if they were to practise in the legal limbo that characterized the period prior to legalization.

While immigrant midwives of colour were unable to use their professional expertise in Ontario, practice experience acquired in the "Third World" enabled white Ontario midwives to qualify for registration in the province. Many members of the Association of Ontario Midwives travelled to locations outside of Canada where they were able to work as midwives despite their lack of institutional qualifications. Many did so in the years prior to legalization in order to acquire substantial experience within short periods of time. Immediately following the release of the TFIMO report, the Association of Ontario Midwives scrambled to find opportunities for supervised practice abroad so that its members could obtain the requisite number of births for participation in the pre-registration program that would produce the first group of practising midwives (AOM 1987a, 5). A significant number worked in independent midwifery clinics on the Texas/Mexico border, where Mexican nationals move illegally across the border to deliver their babies in U.S. territory (Ontario Association of Midwives 1981, 1; Barrington 1985, 69; AOM 1987c, 10). Still others found opportunities for practice in Jamaica (AOM 1988, 3), the Philippines (AOM 1988, 25), Brazil (AOM 1990, 24), Guatemala, or Haiti (Van Wagner 1991, 206). As I have argued elsewhere (Nestel 2000b), the fact that Ontario midwives produced themselves as professionals through knowledge of "Third World" women's bodies, while at the same time denying "Third World" women access to midwifery practice, raises troubling questions about the limits of global sisterhood.

A second policy decision, the adoption of baccalaureate preparation as the educational standard for midwifery practice, may indeed constitute an exclusionary measure in relation to immigrant midwives of colour. While "visible minority" women who have immigrated are more likely to be university trained than those born in Canada (15 per cent vs 10 per cent) (Statistics Canada 1995, 58), this statistic may not represent the educational attainments of nurses in this group, many of whom received their training in countries where, as in Canada, baccalaureate preparation for nursing is not the norm. While approximately 14 per cent of Canadian nurses have university degrees (Sedivy-Glasgow 1992, 28), some statistics indicate that less than one-half of one per cent of all foreign-trained nurses with formal midwifery education are university educated (Eberts 1987, 331). Baccalaureate equivalency has almost certainly constituted a significant roadblock on the major route to practice available for immigrant midwives of colour: the College of Midwives of Ontario's Prior Learning and Experience Assessment (PLEA) program.

"FOREIGN TRAINED" MIDWIVES AND THE PRIOR LEARNING AND EXPERIENCE ASSESSMENT PROGRAM

Initiated in 1994, what was then the Prior Learning Assessment program was designed to "assess the equivalency of applicants for registration with midwifery training and/or experience other than graduation from either the Pre-registration Program for Midwifery or the Ontario Midwifery Education Program" (CMO 1994b, 1). The second cycle of the program, which began in 1997 and added "Experience" to the assessment, required a number of steps including an orientation session; submission of a clinical experience portfolio; a two-part, profession-specific language exam required for all candidates *including* native speakers of English; the preparation of a baccalaureate portfolio; a three-stage, multifaceted assessment of midwifery knowledge including written, oral, and role play assessments; and a two-week course on midwifery in Ontario (CMO 1997). The cost of this process, while listed in the College of Midwives PLEA Orientation Booklet as CAD $3,015.00, can add up to much more when expenses for travel, documentation, study materials, childcare, booking time off work, etc. are figured in. Additional costs for either enrolling in requisite baccalaureate courses or paying a fee to sit a baccalaureate challenge exam can escalate costs to more than double the College's stated estimate. One immigrant midwife of colour estimated that her total costs for becoming registered in Ontario would come to over $10,000. In light of evidence cited above, that visible minority group members earn significant less than all whites in comparable occupational categories, it must be argued that the costs of professional registration contribute to racial stratification and exclusion in the case of midwifery.

Prior to the first cycle of the PLEA process, the CMO had received close to 1,000 inquiries about registration from trained midwives. While 337 women attended the 1995 PLA orientation, only 165 applications were received and eventually only 126 took the first language exam. Half that number (63) sat the second language exam, 56 submitted portfolios to the College, and 51 took the Multifaceted Assessment I exam. By March 1998, the PLEA program had produced only seventeen registrants (Nestel 1996/97). This represents a troubling rate of attrition over the four years of the program's existence. And yet the PLEA remains the only route of access to practice available to those trained midwives unwilling or unable to pursue a degree in the recently established university-based Midwifery Education Programme (see Kaufman and Soderstrom, this volume).[3] As discussed above, some statistics indicate that very few immigrant nurses trained as midwives possess baccalaureate degrees. These women will be required to upgrade their education to baccalaureate equivalency in addition to passing the controversial "profession-specific" language examination and rigorous clinical assessments cited above. The relative small number of PLEA graduates who are women of colour seems to indicate that the PLEA program is less easily negotiated by non-European midwives. One veteran Afro-Caribbean midwife, who served on a PLEA advisory committee and subsequently decided not to seek registration herself, has described the process as an "almost impossible effort."

ROUTINES OF RACISM

As Aida Hurtado and Abigail J. Stewart have observed, "people of Colour are experts about whiteness, which we have learned whites most emphatically are not" (1997, 308). Global injustices and institutional practices of racist exclusion frame the experience of immigrant midwives of colour in Ontario but they do not constitute the entire story. These macroprocesses are deeply enmeshed with, and indeed enacted through, racist microprocesses as well. Philomena Essed (1991) has explained the intersection of structural forces of racist exclusion and the routine recurrent practices of individual racism as "everyday racism."

One distinctive finding that has emerged from the interview material is that white midwifery aspirants seeking to enter the profession either through admission to the Midwifery Education Programme or the PLEA seem to possess the local knowledge that smoothes their entrance. For example, the Toronto Association of Aspiring Midwives (TAAM), a group of predominantly white women that has been meeting for several years to study clinical midwifery texts and discuss practice issues, boasts an acceptance rate to the MEP of well over fifty per cent of its members. Attached to various labour support organizations, midwifery practices, and other childbirth-related groups, TAAM members have been able to craft applications and prepare themselves for the interview process in ways that demonstrate an intimate knowledge of midwifery culture in the province. Study data have shown that those midwives of colour who have had close relationships with white midwives have been the most successful in entering practice in the province.

One such midwife attributes her success to her ongoing relationship with a white midwifery practice: "Having worked with the midwives here, I felt that there were certain practices that are different which they expect you to know – the things that are done here and that are done there."

This midwife, however, is a rare exception to the rule. Some women of colour who have attempted to gain local knowledge of midwifery through contact with practising midwives have encountered obstacles in the form of everyday racist practices. A woman who came close to finishing but ultimately dropped out of the PLEA program spoke about how, after seeking out a midwifery practice where she might learn about the local realities of practice, she was relegated to housekeeping work rather than treated as a colleague. Another woman described her efforts to find Ontario midwives who would allow foreign-trained midwives to familiarize themselves with Ontario practice. Regarded with suspicion by those she approached and relegated to a position of inferiority, she nonetheless frames her story to establish parity of status between Ontario midwives and those trained elsewhere: "I literally begged to see what they did. And it wasn't because I wanted to monitor them. It wasn't like that. It was to share the same love, the same experience. And they could have done the same."

Other immigrant midwives of colour have, in their interactions with midwifery institutions, encountered a racial "chilly climate" – behaviours, attitudes, and actions that conveyed to women of colour a sense of not belonging. A PLEA candidate described her strained attendance at meetings of the midwives' professional association, the Association of Ontario Midwives, an activity she felt was important to her future career in the profession: "I felt they portrayed this very elitist kind of attitude where 'we're very unique, nobody else is like us. Look at us, we've got it right.'"

For many PLEA participants, these routines of racism created routines of resistance. Reports of racist incidents were relayed from woman to woman and some interviewees reported that they and their colleagues began to regard the midwifery apparatus in Ontario as irretrievably racist. For some immigrant midwives of colour, rumours of racism caused them to reject participation in the process of becoming registered. One woman, a PLEA participant, commented: "Most of the people I talked to wouldn't even consider applying to do midwifery even thought they're midwifery trained."

SHAPING REPRESENTATION:
THE EQUITY COMMITTEE REPORTS

While I have argued that racist exclusions enacted in the establishment of the new profession of midwifery have occurred because of a variety of structural factors and everyday practices, I would like to posit here that forms of representation created by midwifery bodies and circulated in midwifery documents have been central in constructing subjectivities for immigrant midwives of colour that are antithetical to those that white midwives have created for themselves in their bid for professional closure and occupational power. As Stuart Hall has argued, representations have "a formative, not merely an expressive, place in the constitution of social and political life" (1992, 253) and as such must be examined for their material effects in the production of racist exclusions.

The first issue of *The Gazette*, published by the Ontario Interim Regulatory Council on Midwifery (IRCM) subsequent to its appointment by order-in-council in 1989, announced the formation of an Equity committee. The committee was to "ensure that the proposed College of Midwives is responsive to different groups who are interested in midwifery as a profession or as a service ... focusing on varied language and cultural groups, disadvantaged women and women in institutions" (IRCM 1990a, 4; see also Ford and Van Wagner, this volume).

The College of Midwives of Ontario and its various predecessors released, between 1990 and 1993, a series of Equity Committee reports.

Of these, a minority of pages are devoted to the issue of "immigrant and refugee women" (IRCM 1993; IRCM 1990b). Through their focus on victimization, the documents handily reproduce the discursive construct "immigrant women," which has come to signify "women of colour, women from Third World countries, women who do not speak English well and women who occupy lower positions in the occupational hierarchy" (Ng and Estable 1987, 29). While this construct, and its use by the midwifery movement, exemplifies the process by which racial identities are conferred upon groups and individuals, it is also paradigmatic in its demonstration of how "gender identity is inextricably linked to and even determined by racial identity" (Higginbotham 1992, 254).

The Equity Committee reports also reveal that significant control was exercised over how "equity" issues were to be defined in the public sphere. While the reports specify that the committee met with women who had practised midwifery in their countries of origin and were anxious to practise in Ontario, this issue was seen to be "in the jurisdiction of the Registration Committee" (IRCM 1993, 2) and not appropriate for inclusion in the reports. Removing the access to practice issue from the equity agenda and controlling how immigrant women's "difference" is understood have been important processes in the production of politically and culturally efficacious subjectivities for white midwifery activists in Ontario.

The equity issues that are subsequently ventriloquized in the reports speak primarily of linguistic and cultural barriers to adequate obstetrical care, of the negative obstetrical experiences of women who had undergone "female circumcision," and of the problems faced by political refugees in dealing with authority figures. While these are indeed of grave concern, showcasing them to the exclusion of other issues accomplished important cultural work for the struggling midwifery movement. Indeed, it produced immigrant and refugee women as a powerless and needy population and one that could be "saved" by the ministrations of Ontario midwives. Such an economy of meaning has no place for immigrant women of colour who are autonomous, competent, and sophisticated practitioners of midwifery.

As Ali Rattansi has pointed out, "identities, individual and collective, are conceptualized (in Derridean mode) as tending to be constructed in processes involving comparison, alterity, marginalization and opposition to other identities" (1994, 26). The identities of Ontario midwives have been carefully constructed in opposition to received notions about a number of other groups, including insensitive and patriarchal physicians, "primitive" historic and "Third World" midwives, and subservient nurses. Controlling the meanings of "difference" in relation to immigrant women has been critical in producing the subjectivity required for midwives to achieve occupational power and credibility in a hostile medical environment. It is, I would argue, a subjectivity in which whiteness plays a defining role.

RESISTING EXCLUSION AND MARGINALIZATION

"Marginality," as bell hooks has observed, "is ... more than a site of deprivation ... it is also a site of radical possibility, a space of resistance" (1992, 341). While it is beyond the scope of this paper, and likely well beyond my ken as a white researcher, to provide a thorough documentation and analysis of acts of resistance to racist exclusion in the re-emergence of midwifery in Ontario, some mention of those efforts that I am able to identify must be made. Indeed the few women of colour and First Nations women who have served on official midwifery bodies have used their positions to challenge exclusionary policies. Speaking at the inaugural meeting of the Interim Regulatory Council on Midwifery in 1989, Jesse Russell, a Métis woman from Thunder Bay, lost no time in inquiring how the Council would deal with traditional First Nations midwives (Ford 1992, 51).

Women of colour who participated in midwifery bodies saw their presence as critical to the achievement of equitable access to midwifery practice. When discussing her participation one women commented: "It made me feel that midwives from other countries have a chance. I was there not for me, but because we needed to give midwives from other countries a chance." Another woman talked about her efforts to argue that the midwifery principle of informed choice was meaningless unless resources were devoted to removing language barriers between midwives and clients.

CONCLUSION

I have argued here that the struggle for the legalization of midwifery and its subsequent implementation in Ontario represent racist processes inasmuch as they have enacted exclusions that impact systematically and dramatically on racialized[4] groups of women. Structural inequalities and symbolic processes in which racism plays a central role have not just gone unchallenged by the midwifery movement; they have, in fact, been essential to the formulation of politically efficacious strategies and midwifery subjectivities. Everyday practices of racism link with institutional policies in the marginalizing process. Positioned both symbiotically and hierarchically in the global and local economies, white midwives and midwives of colour can be seen to be embedded in systems of domination that are inextricably interlocked. Within these interlocking systems, race privilege can be deployed in order to mitigate gender subordination, giving white women a stake in the very system that oppresses them (Glenn 1992).

Systems of oppression capture everyone in their web, binding us to one another in ways that both constrain us and offer us a way out. The political potential of an inclusionary and anti-racist midwifery movement can only be imagined. By force of numbers alone, such a movement might have reconfigured maternity care in the province, unsettled prevailing representations of women of colour, and undermined racial segmentation in the medical labour force. Indeed, had power been shared, it might also have been gained. If there is even a glimmer of hope for devising feminist political projects that do not trample the rights of some women then we must inquire, consistently and repeatedly, after the differential impact of our organizing strategies on women in a variety of socially constructed locations. Such an inquiry can only happen in dialogue across difference, and such a dialogue must begin with an articulation of, and confrontation with, the ways that we are implicated in each other's subordination.

NOTES

1 An earlier version of this essay appeared in *Health and Canadian Society/ Santé et Société Canadienne* 4, no. 2: 315–41, (1996/97), Sheryl Nestel, " 'A New Profession to the White Population in Canada': Ontario Midwifery and the Politics of Race" and is reproduced here with their permission. I am grateful to Lesley Biggs, Ivy Lynn Bourgeault, George Sefa Dei, and Sherene Razack for their comments on the earlier version. This research was supported by a doctoral fellowship from the Social Sciences and Humanities Research Council of Canada.

2 The term "women of colour" is problematic but indispensable. While this phrase represents an act of self-definition and resistance to racist terminology by groups who have been subjected to racialized (see note 4 below) definitions and exclusions, it nonetheless fails to capture the multiple subject positions occupied by these women, eliding axes of difference along which women who share racialized status are positioned.

3 For a profile of cohorts, see Stewart and Pong, 1998.

4 The term "racialized" is used here to signal that race is a historically and socially constructed category of differentiation and not in any way a "natural" one. "Racialization" then can be seen as a process through which racial significance comes to be conferred upon a wide range of human attributes.

REFERENCES

Abate, George. 1998. Visible Minorities Will be Majority by 2000. *Globe and Mail*, 18 June, A6.

Anthias, Floya, and Nira Yuval-Davis. 1992. *Racialized Boundaries: Race, Nation, Gender, Colour and Class and the Anti-Racist Struggle*. London and New York: Routledge.

Association of Ontario Midwives (AOM). 1987A. *AOM Newsletter* 3, no. 2.

– 1987b. *AOM Newsletter* 3, no. 3.

– 1987c. *AOM Newsletter* 3, no. 4.

– 1988. *AOM Newsletter* 4, no. 1.

– 1990. *AOM Newsletter* 6, no 1.

Barrington, Eleanor. 1985. *Midwifery is Catching*. Toronto: New Canada Publishers.

Barbee, Evelyn. 1993. Racism and U.S. Nursing. *Medical Anthropology Quarterly* 7, no. 4: 346-62.

Bourgeault, Ivy Lynn. 1996. Delivering Midwifery: An Examination of the Incorporation of Midwifery in Ontario. Ph.D. dissertation, Graduate Department of Community Health, University of Toronto.

Boyd, Monica. 1992. Gender, Visible Minority, and Immigrant Earnings Inequality: Reassessing an Employment Equity Premise. In *Deconstructing a Nation: Immigration, Multiculturalism and Racism in 90s Canada*, edited by Vic Satzewich. Halifax: Fernwood.

Chard, Jennifer, and Viviane Renaud. 1999. Visible Minorities in Toronto, Vancouver and Montreal. *Canadian Social Trends*. Autumn: 20–5.

College of Midwives of Ontario (CMO). 1994a. *Language and Prior Learning Assessment for Midwifery Project Phase III, Multifaceted Intensive Assessment*. Application for Access to Professions and Trades Demonstration Project Fund Part B: Project Information, May. Toronto, Ontario.

– 1994b. *Policies on Prior Learning Assessment*. PLA Orientation Session #1. October, 1994. Ontario Institute for Studies in Education. Photocopy.

– 1997. *Prior Learning and Experience Assessment 1997/98 Orientation Booklet*. Toronto: College of Midwives of Ontario.

Cumming, Peter A., Enid L.D. Lee, Dimitrios G. Oreopoulous. 1989. Access! Task Force on Access to Professions and Trades in Ontario. Ontario Ministry of Citizenship.

Curriculum Design Committee (CDC). 1990. *Report of the Curriculum Design Committee on the Development of Midwifery Education in Ontario*.

Dei, George Sefa. 1996. *Anti-Racism Education Theory and Practice*. Halifax: Ferwood.

Ebert, Teresa L. 1996. *Ludic feminism and after: Postmodernism, Desire, and Labor in Late Capitalism*. Ann Arbor: University of Michigan Press.

Eberts, Mary (Chair). 1987. Report of the Task Force on the Implementation of Midwifery in Ontario. Ontario Ministry of Health.

Essed, Philomena. 1991. *Understanding Everyday Racism: An Interdisciplinary Theory*. Newbury Park, NJ: Sage.

Ford, Anne Rochon. 1992. The Importance of an Equity Approach in Consumer Perspectives on Midwifery. In *Shaping Midwifery – Report of the National Invitational Workshop on Midwifery Research and Evaluation*. McMaster University, Hamilton, Ontario, 13–15 November.

Frankenberg, Ruth. 1993. *White Women, Race Matters: The Social Construction of Whiteness*. Minneapolis: University of Minnesota Press.

Friedman, Susan Stanford. 1998. *Mappings: Feminism and the Cultural Geographies of Encounter*. Princeton: Princeton University Press.

Glenn, Evelyn Nakano. 1992. From Servitude to Service Work: Historical Continuities in the Racial Division of Paid Reproductive Labour. *Signs* 18, no. 1: 1–43.

Goldberg, David Theo. 1993. *Racist Culture*. Oxford, UK and Cambridge, Mass: Blackwell.

Hall, Stuart. 1992. New Ethnicities. In *"Race," Culture and Difference*, edited by James Donald and Ali Rattansi, 252–59. London: Sage.

Harris, Cheryl. 1993. Whiteness as Property. *Harvard Law Review* 106, no.1707: 1709–91.

Higginbotham, Evelyn Brooks. 1992. African American Women's History and the Metalanguage of Race. *Signs* 17, no. 2: 251–79.

hooks, bell. 1992. Marginality as a Site of Resistance. In *Out There: Marginalization and Contemporary Cultures*, edited by R. Ferguson, M. Gever, TT. Minh-ha, and C. West. Cambridge, Mass. and London, England: MIT Press.

Hurtado, Aida, and Abigail J. Stewart. 1997. Through the Looking Glass: Implications of Studying Whiteness for Feminist Methods. In *Off White: Readings on Race, Power and Society*, edited by Michelle Fine, Lois Weis, Linda C. Powell, and L. Mun Wong. New York and London: Routledge.

Interim Regulatory Council on Midwifery (IRCM). 1990a. *The Gazette*. Vol. 1, no. 1.

– 1990b. "Report on the Visit to Ottawa."

– 1993. *Midwifery and Immigrant and Refugee Women: Report of the Equity Committee of the Interim Regulatory Council on Midwifery*.

Michener Institute. No date. *The Michener Institute Hospital Information Package – Pre-registration Program for Midwifery*.

Midwifery Students, Ryerson Polytechnic University. 1997. *Equity Checklist for Interviewers*. Photocopy.

Nestel, Sheryl. 1996/97. "A New Profession to the White Population in Canada": Ontario Midwifery and the Politics of Race. *Health and Canadian Society/Santé et Société Canadiene* 4, no. 2: 315–41. text

– 1998. Atalanta's Daughters: Tales of Identity, Reflexivity and Accountability in Feminist Knowledge Production. *trans/forms* 3 / 4: 167–85.

– 2000a. Obstructed Labour: Race and Gender in the Re-emergence of Midwifery in Ontario. Ph.D. dissertation, Department of Sociology and Equity

Studies in Education, Ontario Institute for Studies in Education, University of Toronto.

– 2000b. Delivering Subjects: Race, Space and the Emergence of Legalized Midwifery in Ontario. *Canadian Journal of Law and Society* 15, no. 2: 187–215.

Ng, Roxana, and Alma Estable. 1987. Immigrant Women in the Labour Force: An Overview of Present Knowledge and Research Gaps. *Resources for Feminist Research* 16, no. 1: 29–33.

Ontario Association of Midwives. 1981. *Issue: Newsletter of the Ontario Association of Midwives* 1, no.1.

Rattansi, Ali. 1994. Western Racisms, Ethnicities, and Identities in a 'Postmodern' Frame. In *Racism, Modernity, and Identity on the Western Front*, edited by Ali Rattansi and Sallie Westwood, 15–86. Cambridge: Polity Press.

Sawicki, Jana. 1991. *Disciplining Foucault*. New York: Routledge.

Sedivy-Glasgow, Marie. 1992. Nursing in Canada. *Canadian Social Trends* (Spring).

Shohat, Ella, and Robert Stam. 1994. *Unthinking Eurocentrism: Multiculturalism and the Media*. New York: Routledge.

Smith, Yvonne Bobb. 1994. The Social Construction of Immigrant Women Identity. Unpublished paper, Department of Adult Education, Ontario Institute for Studies in Education, University of Toronto.

Statistics Canada. 1999. Statistics Canada 1996 Census Nation Tables. http://www.statcan.ca/english/Pgdb/People/Population/demo40b/jt

Stewart, Diane, and Raymond Pong. 1998. *A profile of the 1997 cohort of applicants to the Midwifery Education Program and a comparison of the 1993, 1994, 1995, 1996, and 1997 cohorts of applicants.* Centre for Rural and Northern Health Research, Laurentian University and Lakehead University. Working paper w98-5, March.

Van Wagner, Vicki. 1991. With Woman: Community Midwifery in Ontario. Unpublished paper, Faculty of Environmental Studies, York University, Ontario.

Missing Pieces and New Developments: Challenges and Opportunities

Ivy Lynn Bourgeault and Cecilia Benoit

In the introduction to this volume we described how our collection of chapters represents a snapshot in the continuing dialogue about the so-called "new midwifery" in Canada. Several important issues have been addressed in the preceding pages, including the historical roots of what we argue are not one but a variety of emerging models of midwifery care in different parts of the country. The volume also traces the international antecedents of these emerging models, the pivotal role played by legislators and other stakeholders, and the impact of subsequent legislation in the different provinces discussed. Other chapters have focused much-needed attention on the politics of public funding for midwifery services, lingering interprofessional tensions between midwives and physicians and midwives and nurses, the inevitable dilemmas that result from formal educational models that attempt to train midwives for practice, as well as the advantages and disadvantages of organizing midwives' work so that continuity of client care is front and centre. The research presented has enabled us to move beyond earlier, more inwardly focused analyses of midwifery to a more critical reflection of the profession and its place within the occupational division of labour and within the larger Canadian society. In doing so, we are joined by others who are also focusing on the key challenges and opportunities facing the midwifery profession in the new century, as well as equity issues and different models of practice and education (Biggs et al. 1996/97, Burtch 1994; DeVries et al. 2001; Bourgeault 2002; MacDonald and Bourgeault 2000).

Despite the breadth of topics covered herein, our volume nevertheless falls short, not least of all due to limitations of geographic coverage and areas of study. For example, there is scant research reported on midwifery developments in the north or in Atlantic Canada. By contrast, there is a heavy focus on midwifery developments in Ontario, largely because it is here that midwifery is furthest along in the integration process. There is also a greater concentration of scholars – both within the profession and within the social sciences – conducting research on issues concerning the emerging models of midwifery and midwifery integration. As this group of scholars branches out and as new scholars surface in the other provinces and territories where midwifery develops, we look forward to more comparative analyses that show that there is not necessarily one or even a few styles of midwifery integration but perhaps several provincial, regional, and territorial variations.

In terms of areas of study, several important topics have not been addressed due to length restrictions and time constraints. One such issue is that of the critical role played by organized consumer groups in the politicization and eventual integration of midwifery in pockets across the country. As was the case in other jurisdictions, certain consumer groups were integral in getting the issue of midwifery on the government's agenda in the first instance and they were critical players in the evolution of the midwifery model of practice (see Bourgeault, Declercq, and Sandall 2001). Organized consumer groups also played a large role in sustaining midwifery through the challenges of the integration process. Hopefully this topic will be explored more fully in subsequent research and writings.

Another issue that we did not address as fully as we would have liked is the impact of the models of practice on midwifery practitioners and students. In a comparative piece on nursing and midwifery in Canada, Sweden, and the Czech republic, Benoit and Heitlinger (1998) describe how various models of practice shape the "caring dilemma" that these female health professions face. British midwife and social science scholar Jane Sandall (1997) has focused on the similar "continuity of care" project undertaken by particular groups of midwives in the UK and what impact this may have on the larger midwifery profession in terms of recruitment, retention, and burnout. This dialogue has surfaced both at provincial midwifery meetings as well as at the national midwifery research conference held in Vancouver in 2001. We anticipate that future research will focus more critically on the midwifery models of practice described in this volume, compare them with others models that are just getting underway in other parts of the country (e.g., Manitoba) or are already in place in other countries, and reflect on the variety of modes of implementation of these models.

More challenges or potential opportunities are arising for the profession from the looming human resources crisis in the maternity care division of labour. As more and more physicians abandon the practice of obstetrics across the country, what are the implications for Canadian midwives, their core values and emerging models of practice? Added to these changes is the altering landscape of health care in Canada with rapidly increasing health care reforms including regionalization; devolution of authority; mergers and closures of hospitals, particularly those with low volume maternity services in predominantly rural and remote areas (Benoit et al. 2002); and the response to these changes with broad sweeping reviews such as the Romanow Commission. How the profession responds to these contemporary concerns will be critical to its existence and evolution.

The scholarship of the emerging models of midwifery across Canada will continue. We look forward to the future of this dialogue between midwives, social scientists and interested others with the development of a new journal – the *Canadian Journal of Midwifery Research and Practice*. In addition to accepting submissions related to the profession and practice of midwifery, we are pleased to note that the editors highlight the importance of articles related to midwifery from a social science perspective. Indeed, we believe that we are on the cusp of a new and what is sure to be fruitful future for midwifery scholarship in our country, which until a mere decade ago viewed midwifery as an artifact of the past. If nothing else, *Reconceiving Midwifery* has shown readers that midwifery is in fact alive and well in this country, and there is promise of further growth in the years to come.

REFERENCES

Benoit, Cecilia, Dena Carroll, and Alison Millar. 2002. But Is It Good For Women's Health? Regionalizing Maternity Care Services in British Columbia, Canada. *Canadian Review of Anthropology and Sociology* 39, no. 4.

Benoit, Cecilia, and Alena Heitlinger. 1998. Women's Health Caring Work in Comparative Perspective: Canada, Sweden & Czechoslovakia/Czech Republic as Case Examples. *Social Science and Medicine* 47, no. 8: 1101–11.

Biggs, C. Lesley, Brian Burtch, and Farah Shroff. 1996/97. Special Issue of *Health and Canadian Society/Santé et Société Canadienne* on Midwifery.

Bourgeault, Ivy L. 2002. The Evolution of the Social Science of Midwifery and Its Canadian Contributions. *Canadian Journal of Midwifery Research and Practice* (Winter) no. 1(2): 4-8.

Bourgeault, Ivy L., Eugene Declercq and Jane Sandall. 2001. Changing Birth: Consumers, Politics and Policy. In *Birth by Design: the Social and Cultural*

Aspects of Maternity Care in Europe and North America, edited by Raymond Devries, Cecilia Benoit, Edwin R. Van Teijlingen, and Sirpa Wrede. Routledge: New York.

Burtch, Brian. 1994. *Trials of Labour.* Montreal and Kingston: McGill-Queen's University Press.

DeVries, Raymond, Cecilia Benoit, Edwin R. Van Teijlingen, and Sirpa Wrede, eds. 2001. *Birth by Design: The Social and Cultural Aspects of Maternity Care in Europe and North America.* Routledge: London.

MacDonald, Margaret, and Ivy L. Bourgeault. 2000. The Politics of Representation: Doing and Writing "Interested" Research on Midwifery. *Resources for Feminist Research.*

Sandall, Jane. 1997. Midwives' Burnout and Continuity of Care. *British Journal of Midwifery* 5, no. 2: 106-11.

Contributors

CECILIA BENOIT, Ph.D. is a professor in the Department of Sociology at the University of Victoria, British Columbia, Canada and grant facilitator for the Office of Vice-President, Research. Cecilia has published journal articles and book chapters on midwifery in Canada and a number of other high-income countries, comparative health and welfare systems, and midwives' caring work in cross-national perspective. She is author of *Midwives in Passage* (1991) and *Women, Work and Social Rights* (2000), co-author of *Society: The Basics, First and Second Canadian Editions* (1999, 2002) and co-editor of *Professional Identities in Transition* (1999) and *Birth By Design* (2001). She serves on the executive of one of the five national Centres of Women's Health, NNEWH (located at York University). Some of her most recent research projects have involved collaboration with Dena Carroll and focused on narratives of Aboriginal midwifery in British Columbia (1995), non-urban women's access to maternity care (2002), and the health concerns of Aboriginal women in Vancouver's Downtown Eastside (forthcoming, 2003). Other projects have involved investigation of the working conditions, health status, and exiting experiences of sex workers. The latter study has been written up into a report, "Dispelling Myths and Understanding Realities: Working Conditions, Health Status, and Exiting Experiences of Sex Workers." Cecilia is co-principal investigator of "Risky Business: Experiences of Youth in the Sex Trade," one of the six target projects funded under the Canadian Institutes for Health Research (CIHR) program, Healthy Youth in A Healthy Society. She is also principal investigator on a second CIHR-funded longitudinal study, "Marginalized Populations' Work, Health and Access to Services."

IVY LYNN BOURGEAULT, Ph.D. (bourgea@mcmaster.ca), is an assistant professor in Health Studies and Sociology at McMaster University, Canada. She is a recent recipient of a Canada Research Chair in Comparative Health Labour Policy and has held a New Investigator Award with the Canadian Institutes for Health Research for a five-year study of the impact of gender and location on human resources decision making in Canada and the United States. Ivy has published extensively in national and international journals not only on midwifery in Canada and the United States but also on alternative medicine, patient consumerism, and the relations between health professions and the state. Recent co-authored books include *Medicine, Nursing and the State* (1999) and *Heal Thyself* (2000), both with Garamond Press. Ivy was active within the midwifery and alternative childbirth movement for several years, including a position on the board of directors of the Toronto Birth Centre committee. Her Ph.D. is from the Department of Community Health (Medical Sociology Program) from the University of Toronto, and her thesis was entitled "Delivering Midwifery: An Examination of the Process and Outcome of the Integration of Midwifery in Ontario."

ROBBIE DAVIS-FLOYD, Ph.D., is a cultural anthropologist specializing in medical, ritual, and gender studies and the anthropology of reproduction. She lectures at childbirth, midwifery, and obstetrical conferences around the world. She is author of over seventy articles and of *Birth as an American Rite of Passage* (1992), co-author of *From Doctor to Healer: The Transformative Journey* (1998) and *The Anatomy of Ritual* (forthcoming), and co-editor of eight collections, including *Childbirth and Authoritative Knowledge: Cross-Cultural Perspectives* (1997), *Cyborg Babies: From Techno-Sex to Techno-Tots* (1998), *Daughters of Time: The Shifting Identities of Contemporary Midwives* (a special triple issue of *Medical Anthropology* 20:2-3/4, 2001), and *Mainstreaming Midwives: The Politics of Change* (forthcoming). Her research on global trends and transformations in health care, childbirth, obstetrics, and midwifery is ongoing. Her present projects address change in Mexican and Brazilian midwifery and obstetrics. For the academic year 2002–03, she is serving as Mather Visiting Professor in the anthropology department at Case Western Reserve University in Cleveland, Ohio. She serves permanently as senior research fellow, Department of Anthropology, University of Texas Austin.

ABOUT THE CONTRIBUTING AUTHORS

LESLEY BIGGS received her Ph.D. from the University of Toronto, 1989, Department of Behavioural Science, Faculty of Medicine. She is the former head of the Department of Women's and Gender Studies, University of Saskatchewan. Her research interests include sociology of health care professions, particularly alternative healers such as mid-wives and chiropractors. In addition, she is currently developing re-search in the gendered body. She was chair of the Midwifery Advisory Committee to the government of Saskatchewan, which recommended that midwifery be legalized in the province.

DENA CARROLL is a member of the Chippewa of Nawash First Nation Band, located in Cape Croker, Ontario. She currently works as a con-sultant on Aboriginal health issues in British Columbia and some other jurisdictions and is a community member and member of the RNT Committee of the National Network on Environment and Women's Health (NNEWH), one of the five national Centres of Women's Health. She was formerly with the Aboriginal Health Policy Branch in B.C.'s Ministry of Health, where she was primarily responsible for the minis-try's consultation on the aboriginal midwifery legislation issue in that province. Dena has partnered with Cecilia Benoit to co-author a num-ber of articles including narratives of Aboriginal midwifery in British Columbia (1995), non-urban women's access to maternity care (2002), and health concerns of Aboriginal women in Vancouver's Downtown Eastside (forthcoming, 2003).

ELAINE CARTY is professor and director of the University of British Columbia Midwifery program and professor in the UBC School of Nursing. She received her master's degree and midwifery certificate from Yale University. She has been an activist for the legalization of midwifery in Canada for twenty-five years and was one of the founding members of the midwifery service at Children's and Women's Hospital. The issues facing women with disabilities/chronic illness during preg-nancy, birth, and the postnatal period are also a focus of her research.

ANNE ROCHON FORD is a freelance writer and consultant on women's health issues in Toronto. She has worked extensively in this area for the past twenty years, with a particular focus on reproductive health, over-prescription of pharmaceuticals, midwifery, breast cancer, and women's health policy. She has served on several committees related to the inte-gration of midwifery in Ontario and was a founding member of DES

Action, the Ontario Breast Cancer Support and Resource Centre, the Canadian Women's Health Network, and the Toronto Women's Health Network. She is currently the coordinator of Women and Health Protection, a national working group focused on strengthening Canada's health protection laws for the enhancement of women's health.

SUSAN JAMES is the director of the Midwifery Education Programme/ Programme de Formation des Sages-Femmes at Laurentian University, Sudbury, Ontario. She practised midwifery in Edmonton, Alberta for eight years. She began her career as a case room nurse in 1973 and worked in all areas of hospital maternity care, taught prenatal classes, and taught undergraduate nursing at the University of Toronto before moving to Alberta to study midwifery. In addition, she was politically active in the process of regulation and implementation of midwifery in Alberta, acted as the coordinator of the Canadian Confederation of Midwives, and provided midwifery assessment consultation to the College of Midwives, in Ontario and British Columbia. Her doctoral work was a phenomenological study of relations between women and their midwives. Her current research is in the area of relational ethics, focusing on relations among health care providers and on interdisciplinary health issues in northern, rural, and remote Canada.

PATRICIA KAUFERT is a British-trained social scientist who did her Ph.D at the Centre of West African Studies, University of Birmingham. After coming to Canada in 1977, she was retro-fitted as a health researcher, courtesy of a postdoctoral fellowship and a National Health Research Scholar Award from Health Canada. Her areas of specialty in women's health include midwifery, menopause, and mammography. She is a professor in the Department of Community Health Sciences at the University of Manitoba.

KARYN KAUFMAN, RM DrPH, is a professor in the Faculty of Health Sciences at McMaster University and director of the Ontario Midwifery Education Programme offered through the consortium of Laurentian, McMaster, and Ryerson Universities. She also is appointed to the graduate faculty at McMaster, and the University of Toronto and a member of master's and doctoral thesis committees for students pursuing interests in maternity care. She is a practising midwife in Hamilton, Ontario and member of the board of the Association of Ontario Midwives.

JUDE KORNELSEN, Ph.D., has been studying midwifery and home birth in British Columbia since 1992, with a particular interest in exploring differences between home birthing and hospital birthing women's relationships to technology. Currently she is a visiting social scientist at the University of British Columbia's School of Nursing and part of the Midwifery Research Group at the British Columbia Centre of Excellence for Women's Health. Through the centre she has conducted research into the consequences – both intended and unintended – of introducing midwives into the health care system. Current research includes a study of perinatal and community health nurses' attitudes towards midwifery, a study of the experiences of those who applied to register with the college of midwives in B.C., a study of midwives' experiences post-registration, and a study of physicians' attitudes toward midwifery.

MARGARET MACDONALD, Ph.D., is a medical anthropologist specializing in gender and health with particular interests in women's reproductive health. She has conducted ethnographic research in both Canadian and international settings. Her work encompasses an interest in cultural representations of the body, health, and illness, as well as the social organization and ideology of health practitioners themselves. Her work on midwifery in Canada focuses on a series of interrelated tensions around the fundamental tenets of midwifery philosophy, knowledge, and practice: the meaning of tradition, natural birth, and home birth, and the place of medical technology within midwifery. She has a paper in the December 2001 issue of *Medical Anthropology* entitled "Postmodern Negotiations with Medical Technology: The Role of Midwifery Clients in the New Midwifery in Canada." She is also engaged in a new study on the impact of international maternal and infant health policy and programs on traditional birth attendants and birthing women in Africa. She is with the Department of Anthropology at York University.

DENISE MARION is a British-trained midwife who has worked in northern communities as an outpost nurse. Her thesis for her M.Sc. in Community Health and Epidemiology at Dalhousie University was "Women Who Choose Midwifery Care in Nova Scotia: A Retrospective Survey and Selected Interviews." She lives in the Ottawa area and is a recent Primary Health Care Nurse Practitioner graduate.

SHERYL NESTEL currently teaches in the Department of Sociology and Equity Studies of the Ontario Institute for Studies in Education of the University of Toronto. She has published several articles in the area of race and reproduction and is working on a book about the role of race in the re-emergence of midwifery in Ontario. She is a former childbirth educator and childbirth reform activist.

KRISTINE ROBINSON is a registered midwife and currently chair of the College of Midwives of Manitoba. She runs a clinic for pregnant teenagers. Her M.Sc. research was on midwifery in New South Wales, Australia.

MARY SHARPE is a registered midwife in Ontario. Over the last thirty years, Mary has worked as a teacher, childbirth educator, lactation consultant, and midwife. She began attending home births in 1976 and since 1979 has been practising as a midwife in Ontario. In addition to her current midwifery practice, she is working toward a doctoral degree in Adult Education and Community Development at the Ontario Institute for Studies in Education at the University of Toronto, where she is exploring woman/midwife relationships. She is a faculty member in the Ontario Midwifery Education Programme at Ryerson University in Toronto. She has served as a midwifery assessor for the Alberta government and the British Columbia College of Midwives. Mary has six children and at the time of publication has had the privilege of being the midwife for five of her six grandchildren.

BOBBI SODERSTROM is an associate professor at Ryerson University in the Midwifery Education Programme. For the first seven years, she was the coordinator of clinical placements, a job that includes providing in-service for clinical preceptors. Bobbi has been in practice as a midwife since 1984 in Ottawa. Besides her midwifery training, she has a Bachelor of Science in Nursing and a Masters of Library Science. She is also credentialed as an International Board Certified Lactation Consultant. Research interests include clinical education, preceptor education, and professional liability. Bobbi was instrumental in developing the first professional liability insurance program for Canadian midwives.

HÉLÈNE VADEBONCOEUR holds a master's degree in Community Health from the Université de Montréal and is pursuing a doctorate on obstetrical practices in Applied Social Sciences at the same institution. Her master's thesis was on the legalization of midwifery in Quebec, from which she has published several articles in both French and English. She is the author of a book on VBAC, the only book on the subject in French, published in 1989 called *Une autre césarienne? Non merci*. Between 1990 and 1995, she worked for several government health institutions, (including the Unité de coordination des projets-pilotes de pratique sage-femme of the Quebec Ministry of Health and Social Services, regarding the application of the law authorizing the experimentation of midwifery. Her main research interests include childbirth issues, violence against women, and women's health.

VICKI VAN WAGNER has been a practising midwife since 1980. She is a faculty member in the Ontario Midwifery Education Programme at Ryerson University in Toronto. As part of the movement to gain recognition for midwifery in Canada, she has served on several midwifery policy-making bodies including the Association of Ontario Midwives, the Interim Regulatory Council on Midwifery, and the College of Midwives. She is currently working on her Ph.D. at York University, focusing on the history and politics of evidence-based practice. Other research interests include midwifery care and education in remote communities, reproductive technologies, and the creation of family in the queer community. Vicki practises part of the year in Toronto, Ontario and part of the year in Inukjuak, a remote Inuit community in Nunavik, northern Quebec.

Index

AUTHORS